Inside National Health Reform

CALIFORNIA/MILBANK BOOKS ON HEALTH AND THE PUBLIC

ılth Reform

JOHN E. McDONOUGH

University of California Press

BERKELEY   LOS ANGELES   LONDON

Milbank Memorial Fund

NEW YORK

University of California Press, one of the most distinguished university presses in the United States, enriches lives around the world by
advancing scholarship in the humanities, social sciences, and natural
sciences. Its activities are supported by the UC Press Foundation and
by philanthropic contributions from individuals and institutions. For
more information, visit www.ucpress.edu.

The Milbank Memorial Fund is an endowed operating foundation that
engages in nonpartisan analysis, study, research, and communication
on significant issues in health policy. In the Fund's own publications,
in reports, films, or books it publishes with other organizations, and in
articles it commissions for publication by other organizations, the Fund
endeavors to maintain the highest standards for accuracy and fairness.
Statements by individual authors, however, do not necessarily reflect
opinions or factual determinations of the Fund. For more information,
visit www.milbank.org.

University of California Press
Berkeley and Los Angeles, California

University of California Press, Ltd.
London, England

Library of Congress Cataloging-in-Publication Data

McDonough, John E. (John Edward)
    Inside national health reform / John E. McDonough.
        p. ; cm.   (California/Milbank books on health and the public ; 22)
    Includes bibliographical references and index.
    ISBN 978-0-520-27019-0 (cloth : alk. paper)
        1. Health care reform—United States.   I. Milbank Memorial Fund.
II. Title.   III. Series: California/Milbank books on health and the
public ; 22)
    [DNLM: 1. Health Care Reform—United States.   2. Federal
Government—United States.   3. Health Care Costs—United
States.   4. National Health Programs—United States.   5. Politics—
United States WA 540 AA1]
    RA393.M244   2011
    362.1'0425—dc22   2011003834

Manufactured in the United States of America

20 19 18 17 16 15 14 13 12 11
10 9 8 7 6 5 4 3 2 1

This book is printed on Cascades Enviro 100, a 100% post consumer
waste, recycled, de-inked fiber. FSC recycled certified and processed
chlorine free. It is acid free, Ecologo certified, and manufactured by
BioGas energy.

To the memory and legacy of
Senator Edward Moore Kennedy,
whose life and example have inspired millions
to achieve health care justice

Contents

Illustrations follow page 100

Tables

Foreword

CARMEN HOOKER ODOM, *President, Milbank Memorial Fund*

SAMUEL L. MILBANK, *Chairman, Milbank Memorial Fund*

The Milbank Memorial Fund is an endowed operating foundation that works to improve health by helping decision makers in the public and private sectors acquire and use the best available evidence to inform policy for health care and population health. The Fund has engaged in nonpartisan analysis, study, research, and communication since its inception in 1905.

Inside National Health Reform by John E. McDonough is the twenty-second book of the series of California/Milbank Books on Health and the Public. The publishing partnership between the Fund and the University of California Press encourages the synthesis and communication of findings from research and experience that could contribute to more effective health policy.

On March 23, 2010, President Obama signed the Affordable Care Act (ACA), following seventy-five years of efforts by U.S. Presidents and Congresses to establish a national health insurance framework. Experienced as a state legislator, legislative advisor, professor of public health and social policy, and consumer health advocate, McDonough writes about the twenty-two-month process that led to the passage of the ACA and provides readers with a comprehensive analysis of the law itself in *Inside National Health Reform*, his second book in the California/Milbank series.

As Senior Advisor on National Health Reform for the U.S. Senate Committee on Health, Education, Labor and Pensions, McDonough was deeply involved in the legislative process leading to the passage of the ACA. In the first section of his book he provides readers with an overview of prior health reform efforts over the years and then an insider's account of the complex and challenging road leading to this landmark law, detailing the thousands of hours of meetings, debates, negotiations, compromises, and sacrifices made by Democrats and Republicans alike as well as the many outside stakeholders involved. In the second section, McDonough explains in detail the ten titles comprising the ACA that affect almost every aspect of the U.S. health care system, and anticipates the challenges in implementing the ACA and how it will be revisited and revised repeatedly in the years to come.

A confessed Democrat, McDonough has successfully represented both sides of the legislative aisle in writing his book, having written extensive notes throughout the process, conducted more than 125 interviews with both congressional and administration staffers, and pored through the copious literature on the health reform process and the complex U.S. health care system itself.

Those interested in learning in depth about the history behind and contents of the ACA and about the U.S. lawmaking process will be well rewarded in reading *Inside National Health Reform*.

Preface

The Affordable Care Act (ACA), signed into law by President Barack Obama in March 2010, is a landmark law in the history of health and social welfare policy in the United States, on the same level as the Social Security Act of 1935 and the Medicare and Medicaid Act of 1965. This is true whether one regards the law as monumentally good or monumentally bad. Few federal laws in U.S. history approach it in terms of scope, breadth, and ambition.

Unlike its 1935 and 1965 peers, the ACA is also monumentally complex and challenging to comprehend. The law's ten titles address nearly every aspect of the U.S. health care system, sometimes clarifying, improving, and simplifying, and other times adding further layers of complexity. The ACA's complexity reflects that of the American health care system, a diverse, decentralized, and poorly understood behemoth. No system in any other advanced nation is so fractured and difficult to understand, whether in financing or the delivery of medical services. The system's sizable and ever-growing intricacy is the reason that comprehensive legislative reform of the system is challenging to explain and to understand.

I wrote this book to help Americans better understand what the ACA really is, what it contains, what it seeks to accomplish, how it is structured, how its financing works, and how so many of its diverse elements came to be. In the wake of the law's signing and the congressional elections of November 2010, many Americans want to revisit the actions of the Obama administration and the Democratic majorities in the U.S. Senate and House that passed the law. Some want to repeal it in toto while others want various provisions altered or eliminated. Others hope to see the law implemented as enacted in whole or in major part or even expanded beyond its current scope. Still more find themselves perplexed and uncertain what to believe and how to regard the law. All perspectives can benefit from a deeper and more nuanced explanation of the ACA's essential architecture, features, purposes, and background. Indeed, understanding the ACA is also a helpful path to better understand the U.S. health care system.

This book seeks to provide that better understanding by approaching the law as it was written, as a federal statute. (For the most part, this book does not describe the ACA's implementation process, which evolves nearly every day.) Just as a book is composed of chapters, so a federal law is made up of titles, each with a distinct purpose, structure, content, theme, and rhythm. While much statutory language is plain and understandable, some is nearly incomprehensible to laypersons and experts alike. Some parts are clear in purpose and execution, while other parts leave wide space for interpretation in rulemaking and implementation. Some provisions are fully funded within the structure of the law itself, while others are left to the uncertainties of the federal appropriations process. Some provisions have already taken effect in 2010 and 2011, but major portions will wait until 2014 or even 2018. Many elements are vital to achieving the intended policy outcomes, while others were inserted only to gain votes needed for passage. They are all part of the process and the final product.

In the early days of the ACA legislative process in 2008 and 2009, a common and bipartisan refrain was "We all agree that doing nothing is not an option." In U.S. health policy circles, this assertion was warmly greeted as a welcome repudiation of Altman's Law, coined by Stuart Altman, of the Heller School at Brandeis University. It goes like this:

> Almost every American and advocacy group supports some form of
> Universal Health Insurance. But if it's not their preferred version,
> their second best alternative is to maintain the status quo.[1]

By approving the ACA, by the barest possible margins, the Obama administration and the Democratic majorities in the Senate and House rejected the status quo and set the U.S. health care system on a path to reform and improvement. Since its signing, one part of American society has begun energetic efforts on many fronts to use the law to implement health system reform while another large portion is now engaged in strenuous efforts to repeal or substantially weaken the law. As we take a second look at what was produced in the congressional process, I hope this account of the Affordable Care Act will help Americans to draw informed insights and conclusions.

Acknowledgments

It takes a village to create a book such as this. I am deeply indebted to all those who helped in so many ways to make this book a reality.

The Milbank Memorial Fund and the University of California Press were essential partners in every stage of this book's development. Sincere thanks to the Fund's president, Carmen Hooker Odom, its chairman, Samuel Milbank, and its president emeritus, Daniel Fox, as well as to Kathleen Andersen, Heidi Bresnahan, Gail Cambridge, and Tara Strome. Special thanks to Janet Reed Blake, Hannah Love, David Peattie, Marilyn Schwartz, Karen Seriguchi, Gerald van Raavensway, and Lynne Withey from the Press for their invaluable support. I am honored to have this book as my second in the distinguished California/Milbank Books on Health and the Public.

This book would not have been written without major support from Hunter College in New York City and its new Roosevelt Public Policy Institute, where I worked for most of 2010 as the first Joan H. Tisch distinguished fellow in public health; there I found the space and time to write because of this wonderful community's generosity and commitment to public policy and public health. Special thanks to Hunter president Jennifer Raab and the Tisch Family—especially Joan, Laurie, and Jonathan. Also at Hunter, sincere appreciation to Judith Friedlander, Christine Gebbie, Jacqueline Mondros, Ellen Murray, Ken Olden, Sindy Pierre-Noel, Fay Rosenfeld, Darrell Wheeler, and all the participants in my faculty seminar on the Affordable Care Act.

I express deep gratitude to all those colleagues and friends who read and commented on earlier drafts of the entire or select portions of the manuscript, including a good number of current congressional and administration staff who cannot be named—thank you for your trust and support. Those who can be named include Shawn Bishop, David Bowen, John Colmers, Allan Coukell, Karen Davenport, Karen Davis, Neleen Eisinger, Christie Ferguson, Liz Fowler, Daniel Fox, Connie Garner, Gerry Goodrich, Ed Howard, Joe Hutter, Andy Hyman, Chris Jennings, Jon Kingsdale, Nick Littlefield, Howard Markel, Taryn Morrissey, Len Nichols, Jonathan Oberlander, Peter Orszag, Kavita Patel, Ron Pollack, Rob Restuccia, John Rother, and Deborah Trautman. None of these good people are responsible for errors or misjudgments in this book—they are all my responsibility. Special thanks to the more than 125 persons who consented to be interviewed, mostly on a confidential basis, for this effort.

And thanks to my family—Devlin, Jax, and Amy—who inspire me on a daily basis. Words cannot express my appreciation and love for my wife, Janice Furlong.

Abbreviations

ACA	Affordable Care Act (PPACA as modified by HCERA)
ACO	Accountable Care Organization
ACT!	Affordable Care Today
ADL	Activities of Daily Living
AHA	American Hospital Association
AHIP	America's Health Insurance Plans
AHRQ	U.S. Agency for Healthcare Research and Quality
AMA	American Medical Association
ARRA	American Recovery and Reinvestment Act of 2009
BBA	Balanced Budget Act of 1997
BRT	The Business Roundtable
CBO	Congressional Budget Office
CBPP	Center on Budget and Policy Priorities
CER	Comparative Effectiveness Research
CHA	Catholic Health Association
CHIO	Community Health Insurance Option
CHIP	Children's Health Insurance Program
CHIPRA	Children's Health Insurance Program Reauthorization Act of 2010
CLASS	Community Living Assistance Services and Supports
CMS	U.S. Centers for Medicare and Medicaid Services
CPI	consumer price index
DHHS	U.S. Department of Health and Human Services
DME	Durable Medical Equipment

DSH	Disproportionate Share Hospital Payments
ERISA	Employee Retirement and Income Security Act of 1974
FAH	Federation of American Hospitals
FDA	Food and Drug Administration
FMAP	Federal Medical Assistance Percentage
FPL	federal poverty level
FQHC	Federally Qualified Health Centers
HCAN	Health Care for America Now
HCBS	Home and Community Based Services
HCERA	Health Care and Education Reconciliation Act of 2010
HELP	U.S. Senate Committee on Health, Education, Labor and Pensions
HIAA	Health Insurance Association of America
HIPAA	Health Insurance Portability and Accountability Act of 1996
HIT	health information technology
IHS	U.S. Indian Health Service
IOM	Institute of Medicine
IPAB	Independent Payment Advisory Board
JCT	Joint Committee on Taxation
MA	Medicare Advantage
MedPAC	Medicare Payment Advisory Commission
MMA	Medicare Prescription Drug Improvement and Modernization Act
NFIB	National Federation of Independent Business
NGA	National Governors Association
NHSC	National Health Service Corps
NIH	National Institutes of Health
PCORI	Patient Centered Outcomes Research Institute
PhRMA	Pharmaceutical Research and Manufacturers of America
PPACA	Patient Protection and Affordable Care Act
SCHIP	State Children's Health Insurance Program
SEIU	Service Employees International Union
SGR	sustainable growth rate
USPSTF	U.S. Preventive Services Task Force

Introduction—A Meeting in Minnesota

I joined about forty persons in a nondescript conference room somewhere near Saint Paul, Minnesota, in late April 2008. Most were veterans of the 1993–94 national health reform campaign conducted during the first two years of President Bill Clinton's administration; a smattering of folks such as me, who would be involved in the next round, were also in attendance. That effort began with fanfare and high hopes in January 1993 when the president named first lady Hillary Rodham Clinton to lead a five-hundred-person task force to develop comprehensive health reform legislation. It ended in utter failure in the fall of 1994, when neither the House nor the Senate could agree on even a slender package of incremental reforms. The failure was one of many contributing factors in the loss of Democratic control of the Senate and House of Representatives in the November 1994 midterm elections.[1]

By late April 2008, Senator John McCain had already clinched the Republican presidential nomination more than a month earlier, and Democratic senators Barack Obama and Hillary Clinton were still more than a month from bringing closure to their state-by-state trench warfare for the Democratic nomination. There were still traces of snow on the ground to match the chilly, wet Minnesota weather.

Sitting around a hollow-squared table were Republicans and Democrats, most of whom had been staffers on key House and Senate committees, aides to key senators and House members, Clinton administration officials, and an assortment of others who had watched the catastrophe unfold from perches inside or outside the government. They had come at the invitation of former Minnesota senator Dave Durenberger, a Republican moderate who left the Senate in 1994; he was the only member of his caucus with seats on both Senate committees that had been key to health reform's fate

(Senate Finance and Senate Labor and Human Resources, later changed to Health, Education, Labor and Pensions, or HELP). Also corralling us was Len Nichols, a health economist with a sweet Arkansas drawl who was a former Clinton administration budget official using his perch at the New America Foundation to help advance the next round of national health reform any and every way he could.

Nearly everyone around the table believed an effort to achieve comprehensive health reform would happen if the Democrats won the White House in November. No one thought Democrats would win sixty or more seats in the U.S. Senate, which would enable them to proceed without Republican support. All three leading Democratic candidates (Obama, Clinton, and former senator John Edwards) had produced similar reform plans. McCain also produced a reform plan, which differed sharply from Democratic designs.

Many of these veterans had painful memories going back further than 1993–94. In July 1988, in a bipartisan celebration, President Ronald Reagan signed into law the Medicare Catastrophic Coverage Act, the largest expansion of Medicare benefits since their inception in 1965. The new law sought to fill gaping holes in Medicare, including coverage of outpatient prescription drugs, and it had been approved with overwhelming bipartisan support. Less than eighteen months later, facing a rebellion from senior citizens angry about their newly required contributions to pay for the program, President George H. W. Bush signed into law a complete repeal of the 1988 act.

Agreement that a reform effort would be mounted did not imply confidence that reform would succeed. Many, especially the Republicans in the room, expected a repeat of prior defeats. If reform somehow passed, some even predicted a repeat of the 1988–89 repeal experience with Medicare Catastrophic. Attendees had gobs of interesting comments and advice:

Conference organizer Nichols observed: "The single greatest impediment is the belief that it can't be done."

David Nexon, who in 1993 was a key health staffer for Senator Edward M. Kennedy's Labor and Human Resources Committee and who in 2008 was working at AdvaMed, the trade association for the medical-device industry, warned: "It can never happen unless everyone moves fast and takes advantage of momentum. Get it done early and with a real sense of urgency."

David Broder, the *Washington Post* columnist and coauthor of *The System*, the definitive account of the Clinton health reform fiasco, recalled:

"Newt Gingrich, in a brilliant way, as he saw Democrats make health care a defining issue, realized if he could create defeat, the disillusionment would benefit Republicans in the 1994 elections."

Nick Littlefield, the former staff director in 1993 for Senator Kennedy's committee and now a lawyer representing pharmaceutical and biotechnology clients, noted: "Everyone sees things differently; everyone sees things through their own experiences. We can't get this done unless we talk with each other."

Chip Kahn, who in 1993 was a key executive at the Health Insurance Association of America, a leading opponent of the Clinton plan, and by 2008 was the chief of the Federation of American Hospitals, a national association of for-profit hospitals, observed: "I'll join any coalition, but they are long on principles and not good at solutions. Everyone protects their little corner. And we're not always honest with each other. This is a 50-50 nation. And most reform proposals represent different worldviews."

In 1993, Christine Ferguson was the key health aide for Senator John Chafee (R-RI), the leading Republican Senate moderate whose alternative plan featured a mandate on individuals to purchase health insurance. Though rejected at that time by Democrats, it bears striking resemblance to the 2010 health reform law approved by Democrats with zero Republican votes. She noted: "Our key problem is that we have not defined our goals. What are we trying to achieve? Some say we want high-quality care that is accessible and affordable. Now others say it's more about cost containment."

John Rother, in both reform epochs a senior leader at AARP, the massive senior citizens' lobby, reflected on the 1989 failure to sustain the Medicare Catastrophic Coverage Act: "We could not overcome the barrier of explaining it to the American public. It was an insiders' game until the momentum gathered for repeal, and by then it was too late."

Congressman Jim Cooper (D-TN), the only elected official in the room, was the leading House Democrat who opposed the Clinton plan: "I feel like a cicada—I come out every fifteen years and hope it feels good. A lot has happened over the past fifteen years. Congress has dumbed down—so much so that I have to explain to members the difference between Medicare and Medicaid. I want change to happen. Quick or not, I want it to be inevitable. The last time got a whole lot of nothing. The Wyden-Bennett bill has the best chance right now. It's controversial stuff, but if there is a bipartisan center, it's this bill."

In the end, Durenberger and Nichols took the comments and cooked up "ten commandments" for presidential leadership on health care reform:

- Exercise political will. Presidential leadership is critical.
- Communicate to the public. The vision, principles, and goals of health reform must be understood.
- Choose the right advisors and surrogates. They should be those who have your trust and the trust of the public.
- Empower the Congress. Delegate to Congress the details of legislation.
- Manage partisanship. Focus on messages and policies that bring people together.
- Calibrate the timing. Use all deliberate speed in moving the issue to Congress to begin work.
- Manage stakeholders. Keep them in the circle (at the table) but not at the center.
- Involve the states. Recognize the steps that the states have taken while acknowledging their limitations.
- Determine the scope. Decide whether it is better to go after a "big bang" bill linking coverage, cost, and quality or a "baby bang" bill that may be easier to pass.
- Negotiate procedural roadblocks. Congressional leaders have to agree on a process before legislative work begins.

I noticed a different theme in sidebar conversations. Republicans would comment with bitterness: "Those Democrats *never* talked with us, even with the moderates. There was a deal to be made, and they blew it because they wouldn't talk with us and wouldn't listen." Democrats were equally sharp: "These Republicans never wanted a deal. Every time we approached them on their terms, they changed the terms of the deal." Fourteen years later, the wounds were still open and hurting, the disagreements gaping, and a sense of common vision nowhere to be found. I left Saint Paul more disquieted than reassured.

· · ·

Barack Obama was the eighth U.S. president to undertake a serious effort to achieve some form of comprehensive national health reform, following Franklin Roosevelt, Harry Truman, John Kennedy, Lyndon Johnson,

Richard Nixon, Jimmy Carter, and Bill Clinton. Of those, only Lyndon Johnson succeeded, with the enactment of legislation in 1965 creating Medicare and Medicaid. That landmark was the conclusion of a thirteen-year effort to create national health insurance for senior citizens, and its passage proved to be the start, only the opening chapter, in an ongoing process to expand, modernize, stabilize, finance, and reorganize the U.S. health care system.

Similarly, President Obama's signing of the Affordable Care Act (ACA) in March 2010 ended seventy-five years of efforts by U.S. presidents and Congresses to establish a national health insurance framework. As with Medicare and Medicaid, enactment of the new law is only chapter 1, with much more to follow. There will be controversy, threats, financial stress, modifications, deletions, improvements, and limits in many directions. Many Americans' lives will be saved and improved, and more than a few burdened. There will be surprises aplenty, welcome and distressing. At the heart of it will be the perpetual effort to shape and reshape a health care system to meet the values and expectations of a diverse and divided public. The ACA is a landmark law, on a par with the Social Security Act of 1935 and the Medicare and Medicaid law in 1965. Whether one likes or hates it, it is helpful to understand it.

I wrote this book to help the American public understand what happened, how it happened, and why it happened in the twenty-two months between the start of the congressional health reform process in June 2008 and the signing of the health reform laws in late March 2010—not the implementation process, which is fast-moving and constantly changing. I want to help people understand not just the issue, the need, the controversies, and the cause but also the Affordable Care Act itself, as a law, as a federal statute. Most Americans I meet can name one or several aspects of the law, though few have an appreciation for the scope, complexity, and ambition of the whole. When I explain the ACA to individuals or groups, I begin by outlining and explaining the law's ten titles to give a sense of the statute's architecture and purpose. I usually find interest and appreciation for the opportunity to understand it better—what it is, what it does, why it does it, and how it came to be. There is a lot in the ACA, and a lot that is surprising. The premise of this book is that the statute matters and demands understanding.

A note on labeling: I refer to the final health reform law as the Affordable Care Act (ACA), though even this requires explanation. On December 24, 2009, and March 21, 2010, respectively, the U.S. Senate and the House of Representatives enacted the Patient Protection and Affordable Care Act

(PPACA), which President Obama signed on March 23; on March 26, the Senate and House approved the Health Care and Education Reconciliation Act (HCERA), making numerous significant changes to PPACA, which the president signed on March 30. In this book, the term *ACA* refers to the final health reform law as amended by the Reconciliation Act, and *PPACA* refers to the original legislation and statute, unamended by the HCERA.

I bring an assortment of experiences to the task of writing this book. Between June 2008 and January 2010, I served on the staff of the U.S. Senate Committee on Health, Education, Labor and Pensions (HELP), one of two Senate committees with principal health policy jurisdiction. My job title was senior advisor on national health reform, and I was a small part of an enormous team of mostly anonymous Senate, House, and administration staffers who worked long hours to develop, refine, and push reform legislation through the challenging Capitol Hill process. I joined the HELP Committee at the request of Massachusetts senator Edward M. Kennedy, who chaired the committee, to help him on the major legislative priority of his career and life. After his death in August 2009, I worked for Iowa senator Tom Harkin, who succeeded him as chair.

Prior to working in Washington DC, I was the executive director of Health Care For All, a Massachusetts consumer health advocacy organization. In that role, I participated in the conception, birth, infancy, and toddlerhood of the Massachusetts health reform program, which became law in 2006 with the support of the Republican governor, Mitt Romney; the Republican president, George W. Bush; and massive Democratic majorities in the state Senate and House of Representatives. More than any of us imagined at the time, Massachusetts reform became an essential template for federal reform. Before that, I worked for five years as an associate professor at Brandeis University's Heller School, and prior to that I served for thirteen years as a member of the Massachusetts House of Representatives, representing an inner-city Boston district. During my time in the State House, I became deeply engaged in health policy and bolstered my interest by earning a master's degree in public administration from the John F. Kennedy School of Government at Harvard University and a doctorate in public health from the School of Public Health at the University of Michigan.

I came to Washington DC a veteran of state health reform. Specifically, I was involved in three major Massachusetts reform drives: in 1988, when Michael Dukakis was governor (the law was passed, never fully implemented, and ultimately repealed); in 1996, when I cochaired the state legislature's Health Care Committee; and in the 2006 Romney effort. From a distance, I watched and supported the ill-fated effort in 1993–94. I took to Washington two assumptions about process: First, every major health reform campaign takes much more time and political capital than anyone imagines possible—far beyond most people's patience. Second, being in any major health reform effort, state or national, feels like barreling down a mountain on a creaky bus on a dirt road with no guard rails, the possibility of crashing always at hand. On both counts, the 2008–10 process did not disappoint.

I bring to the task of writing this book the experience of having seen the ACA develop and evolve from inside Capitol Hill, plus the experience of watching many other reform campaigns win and lose, especially in Massachusetts. This book is not intended as a definitive narrative history of the ACA; rather, I seek to explain the law and to provide a context for understanding how it came to be. Informed readers will notice gaps in many juicy episodes of the health reform process; that is because I tell the legislative process story principally to inform the main part of this book, the chapters on each of the ACA's ten titles. This book is not meant to be the story of the U.S. health justice movement, which has worked for decades across the nation to address the inequities in our health care system. Also, some will find the process within the House of Representatives not as extensively described as in the Senate. To this, I plead guilty, first, because I observed the Senate more closely on a daily basis, and second, because—unfairly but true—the basis of the ACA is much more the version that was developed in the Senate as PPACA.

The book is organized into two main sections:

The first section, Preludes and Process, sets the context for reform and describes the legislative process leading to the law's signing in March 2010. Chapter 1 provides an overview of prior health reform efforts and key U.S. health policy developments since the demise of the Clinton effort. Chapter 2 describes the seminal 2006 Massachusetts reform and discusses two roads not taken in 2009–10. Chapter 3 describes health reform efforts in 2007 and 2008—outside Capitol Hill—including activities in the presidential campaigns of Barack Obama, Hillary Clinton, John Edwards, and John McCain, plus efforts by outside groups to lay the foundation for reform. Chapter 4 describes the legislative process leading to reform between June 2008 and March 2010, with emphasis on the procedural elements most important to understanding the final statute.

The second section, Policies, includes ten chapters, one for each of the ten titles of the ACA. Each chapter includes descriptions of key sections plus information to understand the structure, development, and significance of key elements within each title. The ten titles are:

I.   Quality, Affordable Health Care for All Americans (coverage)

II.   The Role of Public Programs (Medicaid and the Children's Health Insurance Program)

III. Improving the Quality and Efficiency of Health Care (Medicare and more)

IV.   Prevention of Chronic Disease and Improving Public Health

V.   Health Care Workforce

VI.   Transparency and Program Integrity

VII. Improving Access to Innovative Medical Therapies (biopharmaceutical similars)

VIII. Community Living Assistance Services and Supports (CLASS Act)

IX.   Revenue Provisions

X.   Strengthening Quality, Affordable Health Care for All Americans (the "Manager's Amendment"), plus the Health Care and Education Reconciliation ("sidecar") Act.

Part II is the spine of this book. The ACA can best be understood by taking a deep dive into its structure and content, and that requires exploring each of the ten titles. The law touches nearly every aspect of the U.S. health care system—so exploring the law means exploring the U.S. system circa 2010. Some readers will find the detailed view to be revealing and engaging, while others may find section descriptions challenging. I hope all readers will emerge with a deeper appreciation of the actual stuff of the law itself.

The final chapter includes conclusions and observations on the process and substance of U.S. health reform in 2010.

Three sets of sources inform this book. First, during my time in the Senate, I kept extensive notes and materials accumulated along the way, as well as a journal. Second, in writing this book, I conducted more than 125 interviews with congressional and administration staffers, plus participants from key stakeholder organizations. Finally, I relied on public documents, as well as journalistic and other accounts from cited sources. All congressional and administration staff comments were provided on a "background" basis (that is, anonymously). In cases where I rely on staff accounts of key events and activities, I used the information only when verified by at least one other source.

A word about author bias—I can't deny it. I was baptized a Democrat and moved to Washington DC to help Senator Kennedy achieve his lifetime mission of universal health care, and I worked with Democratic members and staffers to help him achieve that ambition. I have strived to present positive, negative, and neutral information important to understanding and making judgments about the ACA. More than anything else, I hope this book will help readers achieve a good understanding of this remarkable law. And because this is not a mystery novel, I lay out my conclusions here with details in the last chapter. The first five conclusions glance back at the legislative process and substance of the ACA; the second five look to the future. These are the looking-backward conclusions:

- The ACA is a landmark law and a landmark in U.S. health and social welfare policy. The statute is replete with numerous smaller and significant landmarks. It is an achievement in the realm of health policy—and it is also an achievement in social policy and in distributive justice—leveling the huge imbalance between classes in our society.

- The ACA was an accomplishment of individuals and also of a national movement, the health justice movement. Though this book focuses on the work of individuals and organizations based in Washington DC, the ACA could not have happened without vigorous, longstanding, and passionate efforts by hundreds of thousands of Americans—including many movement participants who reject the ACA as insufficient. In the process, the ACA became, and continues to be, the flashpoint between two incompatible movements, the health justice and the tea party movements.

- Bipartisanship was seriously and sincerely pursued by a few leaders from both parties and was not possible. The differences were too stark, the political bases too alienated from each other, and the stakes too high for a deal that could have satisfied enough of the partisans on both sides.

- Compromises, negotiations, trades, and deals were necessary, not scandalous. They are the principal form of currency in Washington DC and indeed in every democratic legislative assembly on the planet. It is how legislative business gets done.

- The 2008–10 health reform debate was a debate about values. It was also about money, politics, media, culture, and more, but most of all, it was and will continue to be about values.

These conclusions look forward:

- Like Social Security, Medicare, and Medicaid, the ACA will be revisited and revised repeatedly for years to come. Congress will revisit the law in 2011 and 2012 and would have done so regardless of the 2010 midterm election results, in which Republicans won control of the U.S. House of Representatives.

- The affordability of health insurance, and the affordability of health insurance policies for new exchange enrollees, will be two key challenges—over the short, medium, and long term—and especially long term. (Exchange plans are discussed in chapter 5.) To achieve deficit-reduction targets for the second decade of the law, between 2020 and 2029, changes were made to affordability provisions that will make health insurance policies unaffordable for many of those in need of subsidies. Fixing these subsidies to ease the harm will lower the currently favorable deficit projections for the second decade of the law.

- The ACA's fiscal future is as uncertain as its affordability guarantees—and it is tied to the nation's economic outlook. This uncertainty swings in both directions: in other words, there is a real possibility that the ACA will perform better than expected. For example, had the Clintons' reform achieved passage in 1994, implementation would have benefited from two huge and unpredicted phenomena: first, record low medical inflation in the mid- to late 1990s, and second, the immense economic boom of the late 1990s. Also, the track record over thirty years shows that major health reforms tend to perform better than predicted by the Congressional Budget Office.

- The ACA has the potential to do more to meet the health needs of America's racial and ethnic minorities, and more to reduce racial and ethnic health disparities, than any other law in living memory. Among the many ways the ACA can be described is as a landmark civil rights law: "the civil rights act of the 21st century," in the words of Representative James Clyburn (D-SC).

- The implementation of this law is already proving to be among the most challenging implementations of a federal law in many decades. Stay tuned.

. . .

A word about congressional staff—the men and women who work on Capitol Hill or in states and districts on behalf of members. So much gets written about the senators and representatives and the Congress itself. Not much gets said about the thousand employees of Congress outside Washington DC or the twenty-nine thousand who inhabit the Capitol and the six legislative office buildings, three for the Senate (Russell, Dirksen, Hart) and three for the House (Rayburn, Longworth, Cannon), connected by a web of subway lines, subterranean passages and an array of cultures, norms, and everyday practices.[2] A key part of a staffer's job is to be as anonymous as possible to the news media. So it was revealing for me, however briefly, to become a part of the congressional staff and to see their work up close.

In any occupational category, including congressional staff, workers populate a bell curve: there are the fantastics, the horribles, and the great middle. I left Washington DC deeply impressed with the commitment, talent, skill, and character of the many men and women who make their way to Capitol Hill to work in one of the most challenging legislative and political environments anywhere. This is a bipartisan observation—I have seen staff from both parties work incredibly long hours, seven days a week, constantly on call, sacrificing sleep and time with loved ones, to help achieve their bosses' goals and objectives because they believe in their bosses and those goals, in their political party, in their own skill and professionalism, and in the U.S governmental process, especially the legislative variety. Some work directly for members as aides or policy experts; some work for committees, on either the majority or the minority side; some work for the nonpartisan offices such as the legislative counsel or the Congressional Budget Office; some work in support capacities literally to make the trains run on time or feed other staff. Whether they are there for three months or three years or thirty years, it is an honorable place and calling to make part or all of a career.

At the risk of neglecting many, here are the names of some key staffers with whom I worked and watched and who played invaluable roles in making the ACA happen: Cybele Bjorklund, David Bowen, Stephen Cha, Mark Childress, Tony Clapsis, Brian Cohen, Debbie Curtis, Bill Dauster, Chris

Dawe, David Dorsey, Jack Ebeler, Neleen Eisinger, Jim Esquea, Caroline Fichtenberg, Yvette Fontenot, Liz Fowler, Connie Garner, Andrew Garrett, Ches Garrison, Carolyn Gluck, Tim Gronniger, Andrea Harris, Ruth Katz, Cathy Koch, Tom Kraus, Jenelle Krishnamoorthy, Sarah Kuehl, Jacqueline Lampert, Kate Leone, Caya Lewis, Tamar Magarik Haro, Craig Martinez, Bill McConagha, Taryn Morrissey, Liz Murray, Michael Myers, Mary Naylor, Karen Nelson, Kavita Patel, Wendell Primus, Purva Rawal, Terry Roney, Stacey Sachs, Andy Schneider, David Schwartz, Naomi Seiler, Jeremy Sharp, Dan Smith, Topher Spiro, Russ Sullivan, Jeff Teitz, Michele Varnhagen, Kelley Whitener, Tim Westmoreland, and Portia Wu.

.   .   .

Finally, a word about Senator Edward M. Kennedy. From 1969, when he first called for universal health insurance in a speech at Boston City Hospital, he was the nation's leading, longest-lasting, and most determined advocate for national health reform. At times, he pushed as far to the left as possible, and at other points he defined the vital center, the political sweet spot where real change happens, to save and improve the lives of millions. His instincts and gut, more than anyone else's, helped to shape and define the agenda of the health justice movement for more than forty years. The staggering scope of his interests and passions, combined with his indelible ties to America's history, always helped to elevate the moral urgency and immediacy of the cause.

After Senator Kennedy's passing, his HELP Committee staff director, Michael Myers, defined the senator's most compelling gift. Everyone has heard the countercultural expression "The personal is political," he observed. Senator Kennedy proved the opposite, that "the political is personal." The senator never forgot or neglected the indispensable importance of personal relationships to political progress. The strong and personal bonds of affection he fashioned with partisans on all sides opened innumerable windows of opportunity for progressive change, small, medium, and large.

The senator played a role in the 2008–10 health reform process far different from what anyone had imagined it would be, most of all him. As the debate moved from generalities to specifics, this time he avoided the details he had always mastered better than any of his colleagues and stayed focused on the overall mission and the vital few strategic choices, such as implanting funding for health reform in President Obama's first budget proposal to Congress and leaving the door open for use of the budget reconciliation process. Just as Woody Allen observed that 90 percent of life is just showing up, so Senator Kennedy—even in the course of his fatal illness—always showed up when it mattered: in the Senate chamber in July 2008 for a crucial Medicare vote, at the Democratic National Convention in August 2008, at the first bipartisan meeting of senators on health reform in November 2008, at key confirmation hearings in early 2009, at the March 2009 White House Health Reform Summit, and so many more. When he could not show up anymore, his widow, Vicki Reggie Kennedy, always showed up in his stead to carry his torch. He always spread the same message: This is the moment. This time we will prevail.

There were many heroes in health reform between 2008 and 2010, inside and outside government, people who took enormous personal risks to achieve what they thought was right. They all walked in Senator Kennedy's footsteps and share the achievement with him. I am honored to dedicate this book to his memory and his legacy.

PART I

Preludes and Process

．　　．　　．　　．　　．

About thirty years ago, former U.S. surgeon general Julius Richmond and the health researcher Milton Kotelchuck wanted to answer a question: How does public health knowledge get translated into public health policy, action, legislation, and law? More broadly, how does knowledge get translated into public policy? The answer, they concluded, involves three ingredients: the knowledge base, social strategy, and political will.[1] The *knowledge base* is the science-based evidence necessary to make judgments and decisions. The *social strategy* is a plan of action by which knowledge can be translated into policy. *Political will* is society's desire and commitment to develop and fund programs to implement the strategy. All three in sufficient measure set the stage for a positive policy outcome—a deficiency in any one will more often result in failure.

The process leading to signing of the Affordable Care Act in March 2010 is a compelling example of this model's relevance. In this first part, I use the Richmond-Kotelchuck model as an organizing framework to describe the process leading to the ACA's signing.

Chapter 1 reviews the knowledge base, the policy case for comprehensive national health reform developed over many years. Chapter 2 describes the development of a key building block of the social strategy, the health reform law enacted in Massachusetts in 2006, and considers two potential social strategies not taken. Chapter 3 explores the development of political will in its early stages, the prelude to the legislative process played out in the 2008 presidential campaign and in preparations by key system stakeholders. Chapter 4 presents political will in action—the extraordinary commitment of President Barack Obama, House Speaker Nancy Pelosi, Senate Majority Leader Harry Reid, and other key Senate and House leaders to win the ACA's passage.

While all three ingredients are indispensable for success, large-scale reforms more often fall short in political will than in the other two ingredients. The legislative process between 2008 and 2010 leading to the ACA's passage was ultimately all about the third ingredient, political will.

1. The Knowledge Base—
Why National Health Reform?

In national politics South Dakota is a reliable red state, a backer of Republican candidates in every presidential election since 1968—even rejecting its homegrown Democratic candidate, George S. McGovern, in 1972. Reflecting this orientation, of the fifty-one Democratic U.S. senators in the 110th Congress (2007–08), South Dakota senator Tim Johnson was ranked the thirty-ninth most liberal.[1] The state's "red" designation does not diminish the hurt that many residents experience from having inadequate or no health insurance. As the national health reform campaign heated up in the spring of 2009, Senator Johnson—himself the victim of a congenital brain illness—asked his constituents to write him describing problems they experienced getting insurance and medical care for themselves and their families. He circulated these messages to his Senate colleagues in May. A few of those stories, edited slightly for clarity and grammar, are shared below.

> I am a 58-year-old teacher at Roslyn School in northeast South Dakota. Our school is closing in June of 2010, which means I will be losing my job and my health insurance. I am a type 1 diabetic, and I had heart bypass surgery in 2005. My husband is also a teacher at Roslyn, so we will both be losing insurance. I am exploring other options and have been told that I cannot stay on our group policy or transfer to another policy after our jobs cease because of my medical condition. What am I to do after 39 years of teaching to acquire adequate health coverage?

> We currently have health insurance. We pay approximately $8,000 a year and have a $10,000 deductible per person. We average another

---

A note about terminology: *Health reform* is a blanket term used by health policy professionals to encompass the reform of any policy or delivery system relating to the nation's health system. Health care reform is a part of health reform.

$6,000 out of pocket for medical expenses, since we have had no major health issues. When we were shopping for insurance over four years ago, my husband and I were refused coverage by Blue Cross/Blue Shield, and our two boys were offered coverage, but not for anything they had previously been treated for. . . . I would be very grateful if there was another option for those of us that do not have health insurance through an employer.

My wife had lung cancer in 1990, and for that reason we cannot get health insurance of any kind. Now she has lung cancer. As of April 24, 2009, we have no insurance. I am not a rich man. We are taking tests now. I expect the cost of all these tests and the treatment will wipe us out. I have gone door to door for Obama to get some kind of insurance, but it will be coming too late. I own my business, but I think it will take everything I have. Do I worry about my wife? Yes, I do. I don't know how I will ever be able to pay for all this.

I am a small business owner for over 30 years. I lost my health insurance several years ago. Could not afford the premiums any longer. I ended up in the hospital from food poisoning and again later for heart problems. Now my finances are a big mess and I am filing for bankruptcy. I am 55 years old and it's going to be very difficult to start over again, but what else can I do? . . . How can a small business operator like me survive?

I am 31 years old, married, and have four children and one stepchild ranging from 2 to 13 years old. My husband works on the family farm. . . . We can't afford health insurance because it costs too much. I have medical problems that I can't afford, so I don't go to the doctor. . . . I was healthy up 'til 2003 when I had my second to last children, and from there I have had problems. I have Raynaud's disease, had pre cancer two times, my gallbladder does not function right, and my teeth are unreal and painful. . . . It's not fair that I fear I won't live to see my children grow into adults and their children because I can't afford medical.

Government getting involved in health care will DESTROY the excellent health care we now have!!

WHEN DID U.S. LEADERS BEGIN PUSHING FOR HEALTH CARE REFORM?

Fixing medical care and health insurance in the United States has been a public policy concern for about a century. Often credited as the first national political leader to focus on this issue, Theodore (Teddy) Roosevelt called for some form of national health coverage in 1912, when he was the unsuccessful presidential candidate of the Bull Moose Party, though he had made no reform effort in his earlier years as president. His cousin Franklin Delano Roosevelt was the first chief executive to attempt establishing national health insurance during his White House tenure. FDR tried several times to instigate a national discussion; he considered including health insurance in legislation that became the Social Security Act of 1935 but retreated when opposition from the American Medical Association threatened to unhinge the entire effort. In 1943 he directed aides to begin working on national health insurance legislation, but he died in 1945 before any bill was introduced. FDR's efforts showed for the first time how difficult achieving reform would be, how powerful interests could thwart the process, and how critical presidential leadership was. "The only person who can explain this medical thing is myself," FDR told his treasury secretary, Henry Morgenthau, in 1943.[2]

Harry S. Truman adopted FDR's plan as his own and urged Congress in repeated messages to enact it into law, the first time in late 1945. In many respects the Truman-FDR plan was the most ambitious ever promoted by a U.S. president—proposing what many would recognize today as a Canadian-style single-payer public health insurance scheme well before Canada had such a plan of its own. Yet the legislation filed in Congress by his allies was purposefully vague, in part to avoid the jurisdiction of the Senate Finance Committee, which sponsors believed would never give the bill a legitimate hearing. Further, his lackluster efforts to promote the cause left his supporters disheartened and his opponents triumphant, demonstrating the indispensability of presidential leadership in thwarting the inevitable and potent backlash from powerful interests. Toward the end of his tenure as president, he quietly authorized his aides to work on less ambitious legislation to provide health insurance coverage for the elderly—the start of a thirteen-year legislative process.[3]

In 1961, John F. Kennedy took up the cause of health insurance for senior citizens with vigor. Though he did not realize success before his November 1963 assassination, he laid the groundwork for his successor. It was Lyndon Baines Johnson, boosted by new and strong Democratic majorities in the Senate and House, who in 1965 achieved the passage of Medicare and Medicaid, the nation's most ambitious health insurance advance until 2010, opening new chapters in U.S. health policy history that continue unfolding to this day. LBJ's lessons for his successors were many: move legislation early and quickly, leave the details and credit to Congress, see the president's role as summoning the nation's political will, and don't let budget writers hold you back. These strategies gave the nation its first momentous health reform law—even though it was restricted to elderly persons and some disabled and poor individuals. At the time, many believed the 1965 law was only a prelude to a full Medicare for All system, which would arrive sooner rather than later.[4]

Richard M. Nixon embraced the goal of universal health insurance with a twist. Rather than advance publicly sponsored coverage à la Medicare, he proposed private coverage for most Americans, strengthened by federal mandates: most employers would be required to cover their workers, and individual workers would be required to enroll. His plans were waylaid by the Watergate scandal, which ended Nixon's presidency in 1974 as well as another chance at reform.[5] In his other legislative efforts, including approval of a 1973 law to promote the development of health maintenance organizations (the first form of "managed care"), Nixon was the first president to attempt meaningful reform in the delivery of health care services in order to hold down the rising costs of health insurance and medical care—a preoccupation that attracted the attention of every succeeding chief executive, committed to universal coverage or not.[6]

Jimmy Carter advanced a national health reform plan that resembled Nixon's formulation, offering catastrophic coverage with an employer mandate and a new federal "HealthCare" program to replace Medicare and Medicaid for all elderly, disabled, and low-income individuals; it was tied to a package of reforms to constrain physician and hospital costs and was intended to be phased in over time. The cost control part of the plan was introduced in June 1979, halfway through the third year of Carter's difficult term in office, showing that his passion for coverage was eclipsed by his determination for cost control. His signature legislation to contain hospital costs passed the Senate and was defeated in the House. Carter's experience demonstrated the risk of waiting to move on an issue as volatile as health reform, and the difficulty in sustaining a reform agenda.[7]

Universal coverage reemerged as a compelling political issue in 1993, when Bill Clinton staked his young presidency on achieving national health reform, placing Hillary Rodham Clinton in charge of the cause and a five-hundred-person White House task force. That effort, begun with high hopes and optimism, foundered in Congress, and the backlash from the failed effort along with a lackluster economy and other political setbacks in the early Clinton administration helped Republicans reclaim control of the Senate and House of Representatives in the November 1994 midterm elections. This failure taught Democrats lessons galore, among them: the president should not micromanage the congressional process, and the effort should not threaten the coverage of Americans who want to keep what they have. Some wondered if comprehensive health reform was just too much to achieve.[8] The 1993–94 failure weighed on the minds of political veterans who reengaged in 2008–09, inside and outside of government, and helped create both motivation and a determination to get it right.

No more presidential efforts were made to achieve comprehensive national health reform until the inauguration of Barack Obama in January 2009.

THE EVOLUTION OF UNIVERSAL COVERAGE AS AN ISSUE

But what drove eight of the thirteen presidents since 1933 to work for national health reform and, specifically, for some form of universal health insurance coverage? In the beginning, back in the late nineteenth and early twentieth centuries, national health reform was about income security, replacing income that had been lost as a result of illness or disability—that was it. Germany started a form of national insurance coverage in 1883 under Chancellor Otto von Bismarck, other nations followed, and the push slowly spread to the United States. In 1912 Teddy Roosevelt advanced the idea in his failed presidential campaign, though anti-German sentiment of the time was one of many factors stalling the notion. In the 1930s, there was policy logic in tying health insurance to Social Security in FDR's New Deal reforms—health and disability coverage together—but the merger could not achieve political logic. With the lack of government action, private health insurance began to emerge in the 1920s and 1930s, first in Texas and California, and then across the nation. It started mostly as nonprofit and hospital- or physician-controlled and spread as a private, for-profit commercial enterprise only after World War II, chiefly as an employee benefit offered by employers. During the World War II wage- and price-control regime, buying health insurance for workers was discovered as a way that employers could circumvent federal wage controls in the competition for scarce labor, and it was advanced by a crucial Internal Revenue Service ruling that money paid by employers for health insurance premiums was not taxable as wages. In 1954, President Dwight D. Eisenhower signed legislation enshrining that practice and interpretation into federal law—a fateful move that became a central part of the reform conversation in 2009–10.[9]

While many developed nations devised health systems reliant on varied forms of public coverage, the United States endorsed and promoted a system of private health insurance, mostly through employers, for those who could afford it. Beginning in 1965 with the creation of Medicare and Medicaid, the federal government and states began a long process to fill in the holes by providing public or publicly sponsored private coverage to select groups. Medicare and Medicaid were expanded incrementally to cover politically attractive and needy populations; the Children's Health Insurance Program was created in 1997 to extend coverage to many uninsured children and their parents. Various state governments stepped in with their own coverage expansions and innovations, with and without federal support.

· In spite of the expansions, the number of Americans without any health insurance has grown nearly every year since data were first collected. During the Clinton health reform efforts, about 37 million Americans lacked coverage. By the time the Obama effort got under way, the number had risen to approximately 47 million, a number that reached 50.7 million by 2010 with the impact of the economic downturn.[10] Official estimates looking ahead to 2019 projected that, without reform, the number would rise to between 54 and 61 million.[11]

Though the uninsured are a diverse population, some trends in their numbers are clear. People without insurance tend to be poorer and younger adults, racially and ethnically diverse (just over half non-Caucasian), employed in businesses with fewer than fifty workers, less educated, and more likely to live in Sunbelt states than their insured counterparts. And being uninsured has health consequences. During the past decade, the Institute of Medicine has released a series of reports to document the relationship between a lack of insurance and poor health.[12] In 2009, the IOM updated its findings to inform the congressional health reform process:

> A robust body of well-designed, high-quality research provides
> compelling findings about the harms of being uninsured and the
> benefits of gaining health insurance for both children and adults.
> Despite the availability of some safety net services, there is a chasm
> between the health care needs of people *without* health insurance and
> access to effective health care services. This gap results in needless
> illness, suffering, and even death.[13]

The IOM, in its earlier reports, had estimated that approximately eighteen thousand Americans die every year due to a lack of health insurance. In 2009, another group of researchers, using more recent data, concluded that the number of deaths due to a lack of health insurance was closer to forty-five thousand.[14]

During the decade prior to the 2009–10 reform effort, awareness had grown of access problems that affected not only the uninsured but also the "underinsured": those whose health insurance policies contained limitations, loopholes, and cost-sharing requirements that placed them at financial jeopardy in the event of serious illness or injury. Cost sharing takes various forms, including co-payments at the point of service, deductibles that require a set patient payment before insurance payments begin, or co-insurance requiring patients to pay a set percentage of all medical bills. Studies show as many as twenty-five million underinsured adult Americans in 2007, up fully 60 percent since 2003.[15] Recent research has attempted to quantify the proportion of Americans facing bankruptcy whose financial problems were related to medical costs and has determined that the majority of those undergoing bankruptcy proceedings had burdensome medical debts, and that a majority also had health insurance policies leaving them exposed to serious financial harm.[16]

COST AND QUALITY EMERGE AS HEALTH CARE CONCERNS

Concerns about the cost of medical care can be traced back to the early twentieth century. Prominently, the Committee on the Cost of Medical Care, sponsored by seven leading national foundations (and, initially, the American Medical Association), was formed in 1926 and produced twenty-six research reports in its five years of existence. Its reports calling for voluntary health insurance available to all Americans as well as reform of the health care delivery system were blasted as dangerously radical by the AMA, and the group disbanded in 1932.[17] President Truman's speeches in favor of national health insurance focused on the financial consequences and economic catastrophes faced by families confronted with major illness.[18]

It was not until the creation of Medicare and Medicaid in 1965 that rising health care costs became a prominent concern for the federal and state governments, assuming a prominence that has only grown in each succeeding decade. These two new programs accelerated medical inflation on the government's dime. Ever since, federal and state governments have constantly sought ways to reduce medical-related spending or at least to reduce its relentless rate of growth. From the late 1960s into the 1980s, the most common tools were regulatory; beginning in the late 1970s and then more actively in the 1980s and 1990s, federal and state governments sought to use market forces and competition to tame spending.

The market approach has met with mixed success at best. International comparisons of health spending have always shown the United States to be among the most expensive nations in the share of its gross domestic product devoted to medical care, but until about 1980, it was bunched among the leading nations. Only in the 1980s did the United States break from the pack and become a health-spending outlier.[19] In the 1990s, health spending as a percentage of GDP leveled off for a brief number of years as managed care reached critical mass; then, in the 2000s, excess spending again broke loose. Market boosters claim the United States has yet to try serious competitive reform in health services—what's clear is that the market orientation to date has yet to show results that can tame the relentless rate of growth of health spending.

Quality is a different, though related, story. For the last half of the twentieth century, Americans believed they enjoyed the highest-quality medical care in the world. Every U.S. hospital had a "quality assurance" office to make sure things stayed that way. Yet inside the medical professions, many frontline practitioners were dubious of the assurance, witnessing poor care on a daily basis. In the 1970s and 1980s, U.S. manufacturers had begun to address a growing industrial crisis by applying lessons from the burgeoning industrial sector of Japan, which had been taught innovative approaches to improving quality by Americans such as W. Edwards Deming. Deming had been shunned in the late 1940s by American corporations that felt no need to pay attention to the quality of their products in the Pax Americana following World War II. When American corporate leaders began traveling to Japan in the 1970s to investigate the Asian success story, they were often referred to Deming.[20]

A small number of medical practitioners, particularly a Boston pediatrician named Donald Berwick (named by President Obama in 2010 to head the federal Centers for Medicare and Medicaid Services), began in the 1980s to explore the applicability of industrial quality-improvement principles to medical care.[21] Berwick founded the Institute for Healthcare Improvement in Boston to train physicians, nurses, and other medical professionals in the use of industrial quality-improvement tools to improve the delivery of medical services. With remarkable speed, the underlying paradigm in U.S. medical care shifted from "quality assurance" to "quality improvement," with a new core assumption: no matter how good or how bad you believe the quality of your organization or medical practice to be, every day you have multiple opportunities to improve its quality at all levels.[22]

The other paradigm-busting principle of the new movement proposed that improving quality saves money and resources—good quality can cost less than bad quality—by getting work done right the first time and eliminating rework. In 1994, Harvard surgeon Lucian Leape published an article called "Error in Medicine," drawing the broad medical community's attention for the first time to the enormous human and economic burden of errors and injuries in medicine.[23] In 1999 the Institute of Medicine published a report, *To Err Is Human,* estimating that between forty-four thousand and ninety-eight thousand Americans die each year in U.S. hospitals due to preventable medical errors.[24] For the first time, systemic poor quality in U.S. medical care became a national concern.

Since 1990, as the quality-improvement paradigm has deepened and spread, a belief has taken root in many influential circles that waste and inefficiency in the U.S. health care system is exacting an enormous financial toll. Physician leaders and others assert that as much as one-third of all U.S. medical spending—estimated at $2.7 trillion in 2010—is spent on unnecessary and inefficient care as well as administrative waste.[25] As this conviction took hold, so did the belief that an effective strategy to eliminate waste and inefficiency could be the source of enough savings to pay for universal coverage for all Americans as well as the gateway toward a more affordable, efficient, and sustainable system.

Health care policy has long been divided into three domains: access, quality, and cost. Every policy initiative involves at least one, often two, and frequently all three. Usually, a health policy initiative results in a positive impact on one or two of these domains, with a negative impact on one or two, thus requiring tradeoffs when making a policy change. Rarely, one can win a health policy trifecta by positively influencing all three. An example is public funding for childhood vaccinations, which enhances access to health care services, improves the quality of life, and reduces the costs of illness.

In the heady days leading to the 2009–10 national health reform campaign, health system and political leaders became convinced that a health reform campaign focused on expanding coverage for all Americans, combined with systemic reform addressing quality, could be such a trifecta. Improving quality and controlling costs were seen as symbiotic, not at odds. Done right, they could open the political pathway to universal coverage for all Americans and improve the quality and efficiency of the system. It was an intoxicating blend, and it caught the imagination of key political leaders, including Senate Finance Committee chair Max Baucus (D-MT):

> Ensuring access to meaningful health coverage is a fundamental goal of health care reform, but there are also other vital priorities we must pursue. Among them is the critical need to improve the value of care provided in our health care system. We must take steps to ensure patients receive higher quality care, and do so in a way that reduces costs over the long run. In short, the U.S. must get better value for the substantial dollars spent on health care.[26]

WHAT HAPPENED TO FEDERAL REFORM AFTER THE
1993–94 CLINTON HEALTH REFORM FAILURE?

The cause of national health reform did not perish with the demise of
the Clinton effort in 1994. In fact, the period 1995 to 2008 saw a series
of successes and failures on incremental and not-so-incremental reforms
advanced by each political party. Advances and defeats both had consequences for the health reform drive between 2008 and 2010.

In January 1995, Republicans took control of the U.S. Senate for the first
time since 1987 and the House of Representatives for the first time since
1955. The new Speaker of the House, Newt Gingrich (R-GA), did not include
health care among the priorities in his caucus's "Contract with America,"
though it quickly appeared on his legislative agenda. Proposals were made
to reduce the federal budget deficit and to finance tax cuts by instituting
far-reaching changes in Medicare and Medicaid, including "block granting"—or handing over—the latter program to states with a fixed budget.
The Clinton administration's refusal to agree to those proposals ignited two
federal government shutdowns in late 1995 and early 1996, each ending in a
Republican retreat. In that era, deficit reduction required bipartisan support
to advance.

In 1996, President Clinton signed into law the Health Insurance Portability and Accountability Act (HIPAA) to provide portability and continu-
ity of coverage in the private, employer-based health insurance market
for workers and their families when they lost their jobs, thus establishing
nationwide "guaranteed issue" in the group market for eligible workers—a
guarantee that they could obtain health insurance. The law also addressed
privacy, administrative simplification, and other reforms. In the wake of
the dual defeats of the Clinton health plan in 1994 and Republican proposals to change Medicare and Medicaid in 1995, HIPAA's passage showed
that Congress had not lost interest in health reform or the ability to work
on it in a bipartisan manner. Its success was due to joint leadership by
Senators Nancy Kassebaum (R-KS) and Edward M. Kennedy (D-MA)—
a welcome achievement in a harshly partisan environment. From the
Kassebaum-Kennedy accomplishment, hopes rose for more health policy
breakthroughs, incremental or otherwise.

In July 1997, in an agreement between the Republican-controlled Congress and President Clinton, Congress approved the Balanced Budget Act
to balance the federal budget by 2002, relying heavily on cuts and savings in Medicare payments to hospitals, physicians, home health agencies,
nursing homes, and other providers; these were not done to "reform" the

programs, but simply to finance deficit reductions and tax cuts. Among its smaller provisions, the BBA established a new Medicare physician-payment formula called the sustainable growth rate (SGR), under which physicians face across-the-board payment cuts if the cost of their aggregate level of services to Medicare enrollees exceed the law's targets. The BBA also reformed the program by which private health insurers participated in Medicare, tightening the program and giving it a new name, Medicare + Choice.

The health industry learned an important lesson in the years between 1993 and 1997. The Clinton reform failure did not take health care off the table. In fact, lowering public payments to hospitals, physicians, and other providers assumed a higher profile after the Clinton reform collapse, and the changes were all negative for the health sector—deep reimbursement cuts as growing numbers of uninsured patients came through their doors. At least the Clinton plan provided major coverage expansions and new revenues to accompany the harsher medicine. This lesson was not forgotten as key industry players, especially hospitals, considered their prospects and options for 2009.

The Balanced Budget Act also established the Children's Health Insurance Program (CHIP), which provides federal matching funds to states that expand coverage to lower-income children and their parents, the largest expansion of taxpayer-financed health insurance since Medicare and Medicaid's creation in 1965. The drive to create CHIP began with Kennedy, who teamed up with Senator Orrin Hatch (R-UT) in February 1997. The unlikely duo maintained momentum for their cause in an environment otherwise focused exclusively on budget and tax cutting. Like the larger BBA of which CHIP was a small part, this was a bipartisan win—and one achieved over the objections of senior Republican leaders. CHIP also was a source of Hatch's enduring belief in 2009 that together he and Kennedy could formulate a bipartisan comprehensive health reform bill; Kennedy did nothing to disabuse Hatch of that hope. CHIP's initial authorization expired in 2007, and the reauthorization process in 2007 and 2008 was contentious, as President George W. Bush vetoed several bills he deemed too expansive; although the Senate overrode the veto, the House could not win over enough Republicans to achieve enactment. CHIP reauthorization was part of the Democrats' unfinished agenda when President Obama took office in January 2009.

Following the Clinton plan's demise in 1994, the nation unexpectedly experienced a period of record low inflation in medical spending, spurred significantly by the practices of managed-care companies, including aggressive for-profit health maintenance organizations, to cut costs and erect care barriers between patients and providers. Across the nation, an anti-managed-care backlash erupted, fueled by angry consumers and even angrier physicians. A bipartisan backlash led to the enactment of patients' bills of rights in more than thirty-five states in the last half of the 1990s and triggered a drive for a national patients' bill of rights in Congress. The federal effort stalled over whether patients should be empowered to sue their health insurance providers in state courts, and about six years of work in Congress went without an enactment. The Clinton administration extended patients' rights protections via executive order to enrollees in Medicare, Medicaid, and federal workers' health plans—and many insurers voluntarily softened their practices at the urging of employer clients. The issue did not die. Title I in the Affordable Care Act includes most provisions that were part of the patients' bill of rights agenda (though not the right to sue), and these sections were among the most touted by Democrats in their efforts to promote the new law.

In the 2000 presidential campaign, both the Republican candidate, Texas governor George W. Bush, and the Democratic candidate, Vice President Al Gore, committed themselves to passing an outpatient prescription-drug benefit for Medicare enrollees. Bush made good on his pledge, succeeding in December 2003 with a minority of Democrats to pass the Medicare Prescription Drug Improvement and Modernization Act (MMA). The prescription plan—called Part D—relied on private health plans and the market to provide drugs to seniors; the law also delivered hefty payment increases to private insurance plans that provided comprehensive coverage to seniors in the portion of Medicare called Part C, also known as Medicare Advantage (and formerly known as Medicare + Choice). Part D implementation was rocky, as many confused seniors faced a blizzard of new private drug-plan choices where easy comparisons were hard to make. Democrats, who preferred a public delivery model such as exists in Medicare Parts A (hospital services) and B (physician services), promised to change the law when they took power. By the time of the 2008 presidential election, the disruption had subsided and Part D became a nonissue in the general election campaign between Senators John McCain and Barack Obama. There was one aspect of Part D especially helpful to the 2009 health reform effort: If the MMA had not passed, any viable health reform proposal would have had to include a prescription drug benefit for seniors, which would have ballooned the total cost of the reform law. MMA took a costly and contentious issue off the Democrats' to-do list, an issue that would likely have prevented any agreement between Democrats and the pharmaceutical industry.

A lingering issue in this period involved Medicare's physician payments and the sustainable growth rate. In the 1997 Balanced Budget Act, Congress set maximum aggregate limits for physician payments, with automatic cuts if those limits were exceeded. The expected ten-year savings, about $12 billion, were small relative to the other BBA savings, though they grew over time. In 2002, payment cuts were mandated and took effect. Since then, to prevent across-the-board cuts to Medicare's physician payments, Congress has stepped in periodically with short-term fixes, the costs of which have grown dramatically over time as Congress has been unable to agree on a longer-term solution. Looking ahead to 2009, Democrats were convinced they could include a permanent SGR fix in their reform legislation and thus guarantee support from a large portion of the nation's physician community for health reform.

HIPAA, CHIP, patient rights, SGR, Medicare—all these incremental federal changes and issues debated between 1994 and 2008 demonstrated the endurance and inevitability of health policy as an ongoing concern, and each in its own peculiar way helped set the stage for the dramatic process yet to come.

One other significant change involved the federal government's roller-coaster-like fiscal outlook. The 1993–94 Clinton health reform process played out in the context of a sizable and controversial federal budget deficit, dramatized to great effect by the 1992 and 1996 third-party presidential candidate Ross Perot. In the late 1990s, the rapidly growing national economy—combined with the major budget cuts included in the 1997 BBA and other laws—changed the nation's fiscal outlook dramatically. In 1998, the federal government experienced its first budget surplus in thirty years, $70 billion, and the Congressional Budget Office projected growing surpluses year by year, reaching $380 billion in 2009.[27] In the early years of the new century, President George W. Bush and the Republican-controlled Congress approved two rounds of major tax cuts in 2001 and 2003, the Medicare prescription drug program, and two wars in Afghanistan and Iraq—none of which were paid for with revenue increases, savings, or spending cuts. As a result, the nation quickly reentered an environment of chronic federal budget deficits. In early 2007, new Democratic majorities in the House and Senate reinstituted so-called pay-go rules requiring all new federal spending to be financed by revenues or savings. The severe national economic crisis of 2008 and accompanying deep recession—combined with measures to stabilize and stimulate the economy—significantly worsened the nation's economic balance sheet, influencing the actions of all participants in the health reform process.

THE CONGRESSIONAL BUDGET OFFICE

When considering the major difference between passing laws in, say, 1935 or 1965 versus 2010, many knowledgeable sources cite three letters, C-B-O. When it comes to the federal budget, few voices are as consequential as that of the Congressional Budget Office, established in 1974 and as essential as breathing in the work of the U.S. Congress, though ignored or unknown by the vast majority of Americans. In January 1994, the CBO determined in its official review of the Clinton health plan that all health insurance premiums collected by proposed state health "alliances" should be considered federal revenues, meaning that the Clinton proposal, if implemented, would have vastly increased the size and scope of the federal budget. While Congress can ignore the CBO's conclusions, that opinion forced congressional committees to begin seeking alternative reform structures, precipitating the final collapse of the plan in September 1994.[28] CBO opinions matter.

The CBO is located on the fourth floor of the bland Ford Office Building near the base of Capitol Hill, and consists of 250 employees, mostly economists and public policy experts whose job is to advise the Senate and House of Representatives on the federal cost and other consequences of pending legislation. When Congress commits itself to passing legislation that will not worsen the federal budget deficit—to which both chambers concurred regarding national health reform—the CBO is the agreed-upon scorekeeper, even as senators and representatives criticize its opinions. The CBO issues studies, reports, briefs, letters, presentations, testimony, and most importantly, federal cost estimates on pending legislation. It does not take positions on pending bills, though it offers informal advice on how it would score potential policy options—advice often used by congressional staff in designing legislation to achieve an acceptable score. Staffers complain about the amount of time required to court the CBO staff. The CBO's professionals are known to work long hours to meet the demanding agendas of Congress, and congressional leaders often complain of their slowness. Senator Richard Durbin (D-IL), for example, jokes: "That's what it's going to say on my tombstone: 'He was waiting for CBO.'"[29]

The CBO director is named by the House Speaker and Senate president (recommended by the Budget Committee chairs in both chambers) to a four-year term. In 2007, Peter Orszag took the position and immediately highlighted health reform as a key opportunity to address federal budget problems, producing an unusual two-volume set of health-reform-related budget options for the new administration and Congress.[30] In 2009, Orszag left the CBO to become President Obama's first director of the Office of Management and Budget, and Douglas Elmendorf was appointed to fill the remainder of his term.

ELUSIVE PUBLIC OPINION

One area that did not show marked change between 1994 and 2009 was public opinion. The differences among Americans regarding the future of the U.S. health care system remained deep and fundamental. In 2008, the Harvard School of Public Health and Harris Interactive conducted a public opinion survey on American attitudes about the U.S. health care system. One question asked whether the U.S. has the best health care system in the world. Nearly seven in ten Republicans (68 percent) believed the American system is the best, while only three in ten Democrats (32 percent) and four in ten Independents (40 percent) felt that way.[31] These differences are reflected in attitudes about specific aspects of the system. In an earlier 2008 national survey, 58 percent of Republicans said they were "satis-fied" with the quality of health care in this country, but only 20 percent of Democrats offered the same opinion. While 94 percent of Democrats thought it a "very serious" problem that many Americans do not have health insurance, only 55 percent of Republicans felt the same way.[32]

In presidential election surveys since 1988, health care has been one of the six most important issues for voters, though only in 1992 was it one of the top two; in 2008 it ranked third.[33] Yet the overall level of support to address health care masks striking differences among citizens and between the parties on the preferred nature of reform, with Democrats placing a higher priority on health reform than Republicans, favoring a more expansive role for government in addressing the problem, and expressing a greater willingness to consider new taxes to pay for it.

One other factor must be recognized, the decades-long decline in public trust in government, at its lowest level in half a century in 2010:

> Just 22% of Americans say they trust the government to do what is right "just about always" (3%) or "most of the time" (19%). The current level of skepticism was matched previously only in the periods from 1992 to 1995 (reaching as low as 17% in the summer of 1994), and 1978 to 1980 (bottoming out at 25% in 1980). When the National Election Study first asked this question in 1958, 73% of Americans trusted the government to do what is right just about always or most of the time.[34]

Mollyann Brodie, of the Kaiser Family Foundation, has noted that "public support cannot pass health reform, while strong public opposition can kill it."[35] The history of attempts to achieve national health reform shows a familiar pattern: early support weakens as details become available and opposition groups hone their anti-reform messages. Many hoped that 2009 would be different.

2. Social Strategy— Massachusetts Avenue

In October 2008, one month before the presidential election, the staff of the U.S. Senate Committee on Health, Education, Labor and Pensions (HELP) was already preparing for a legislative effort to enact national health reform in the new Congress set to convene in January 2009. The committee chair, Senator Edward M. Kennedy (D-MA), had directed us to bring together key system "stakeholders" to see whether they could find consensus on a path to reform.

We assembled about twenty and gave them the moniker "the Workhorse Group," intending to work them hard to reach consensus. They sat around tables in the HELP Committee's spacious hearing room on the fourth floor of the Dirksen Senate Office Building, named after the late Illinois Senator Everett Dirksen, the Republican minority leader in the 1960s and a key player in passage of that decade's civil rights laws; his memory is often invoked in discussions of the Senate's history of bipartisanship. At the table were representatives of consumer, disease advocacy, business, insurance, physician, hospital, labor, pharmaceutical, and other organizations. Some chiefs were there: Chip Kahn of the Federation of American Hospitals, the trade group of for-profit hospitals; Karen Ignagni, president of America's Health Insurance Plans; Ron Pollock, executive director of Families USA, a leading consumer advocacy group. Others were represented by staffers or lobbyists.

We decided to focus the first meeting on coverage for all Americans. We conceptualized three avenues we could travel in search of consensus:

- The first we called *Constitution Avenue*, meaning a radical, systemic shift away from the current system, in which most Americans get insurance through their jobs. It could be achieved with a government-run Canadian-style "single payer" system replacing private insurance with public coverage, sometimes called "Medicare for All." Or it could be done through the private sector, through the Healthy Americans Act, the scheme devised by Senator Ron Wyden (D-OR), which replaced employer coverage and Medicaid with an individual choice of private plans. Either way, employer-based coverage was eliminated.

- The second we called *Independence Avenue*, meaning an incremental "go slow" approach to minimize conflict. The federal government could support state high-risk pools to cover those with preexisting conditions, subsidize uninsured lower-income folks, expand Medicaid a bit, and implement limited insurance-market reforms. Though it did not come close to universal or even a major expansion, and though it would disappoint and anger many on the Democratic and progressive side because it would fall far short of their expectations, it might get done quickly as a bipartisan measure.

- The third we called *Massachusetts Avenue*, meaning reform based on the key elements of the near-universal coverage law enacted in Massachusetts in 2006. Those elements include deep and systemic health insurance market reform, a mandate on individuals to purchase insurance, subsidies to make insurance affordable, and an insurance "exchange" to connect people easily with coverage.

After ninety minutes of talking, we wanted them to choose. We would not let them leave without getting a sense of their preferences.

"How many want to go down Constitution Avenue?" I asked. Zero hands were raised.

"OK, how many want to take Independence Avenue?" Zero hands.

"All right, how many want to travel down Massachusetts Avenue?" Of the twenty or so in the room, fifteen hands went up. Impressive, I thought.

I noticed the five unraised hands all belonged to business representatives: those from the Business Roundtable, the National Federation of Independent Businesses, the U.S. Chamber of Commerce, the American Benefits Council, and the National Retail Federation.

"What's up?" I asked.

"Couldn't we have a Wisconsin Avenue?" asked Paul Dennett from the American Benefits Council, a large corporate-benefits coalition.

"Sure," I said. "Wisconsin, Pennsylvania, Rhode Island, whatever. You five folks get together, work out what your Wisconsin Avenue looks like, bring it back. Let's compare it with Massachusetts Avenue, and if that's where people want to go, that's what we'll do."

They came back the following week but had no alternative avenue to propose. They said they just wanted us to know two things. First, if by "Massachusetts Avenue" we meant fifty different coverage plans, state by state, they would not participate in our process because they wanted national uniformity and not a state-based patchwork. Second, if we planned to alter a federal law known as the Employee Retirement Income Security Act (ERISA) of 1974, which sets the federal legal framework for employer-provided health insurance, especially a prohibition on states' ability to tell employers what to do regarding worker health benefits, they were out the door. We told them neither concern was high on our list, and they chose to stay and participate.

The broad support to travel on Massachusetts Avenue was not a huge surprise. By October 2008, this approach had become the accepted direction among nearly all major Democratic officeholders who wanted health reform to be a top priority in 2009, including the three major Democratic presidential candidates: New York senator Hillary Clinton, former North Carolina senator John Edwards, and Democratic nominee Barack Obama (though candidate Obama had opposed an individual mandate). Still, it was revealing. Before the election, before the congressional process was actively engaged, a 2006 Massachusetts law had already become the essential template for national reform. How did this happen?

MASSACHUSETTS HEALTH REFORM EXPLAINED

Boston's historic Faneuil Hall was the site at which Republican governor Mitt Romney chose to sign into law the health reform legislation that the state Senate and House of Representatives had just overwhelmingly approved. The date was April 12, 2006. The hall's stage is prominent, yet Romney's team built an even higher stage on top of it for the speeches and the signing—better for the abundant national media on hand. Senator Edward M. Kennedy, the Democratic lion of the U.S. Senate, was there to celebrate his and Romney's partnership, which had secured the federal financing essential to make the law possible. The Democratic leaders of the state House and Senate, Sal DiMasi and Bob Travaglini, respectively, joined him onstage. Feeling outnumbered by Democrats, Romney gave a speaking role to a representative from the Heritage Foundation, the conservative Washington DC think tank that had provided some key policy ideas embedded in the new law. Romney's people handed out beige buttons with the phrase *Making History in Healthcare*. On the back in tiny print were the words *Made in Mexico*. A three-person fife-and-drum corps, dressed in tricorn hats and breeches, marched and played down the center aisle to open the ceremony.

"This isn't 100 percent of what anyone in this room wanted," Romney said. "But the differences between us are small."[1] Kennedy joked that when he and Romney agreed on a legislative matter, "that means at least one of us hasn't read the bill."

The differences may have been small within the left-leaning universe of Massachusetts policy making, yet the law's passage drew a firestorm of double-barreled criticism across the nation from the political right and left. The *Wall Street Journal* editorial page positioned itself as the law's most persistent conservative critic, backed up by like-minded think tanks and policy voices. On the left, advocates for a single-payer system regularly attacked the law in columns, articles, and speeches. Leaders on both ends of the political spectrum instantly recognized Massachusetts reform as a harbinger of national policy developments to come—it made sense to hit back early, often, and hard.

When the Massachusetts reform process began in 2003, the newly inaugurated governor may have had his eye on national consequences, but most did not. Many were surprised to see Romney express any interest in expanding coverage. In his 2002 gubernatorial campaign, he showed no interest at all. Yet in his first months as chief executive, he created an in-house task force to develop a plan to cover the state's five to six hundred thousand uninsured residents. Whether his interest was triggered by national ambitions, policy concerns, his wife's battle with multiple sclerosis, or something else, we never knew.

Others got the same idea around the same time. The Blue Cross and Blue Shield of Massachusetts Foundation launched its own "Roadmap to Coverage" process in 2003, hiring the Washington DC–based Urban Institute to scope out policy options for universal coverage and beginning a series of "policy summits" at the John F. Kennedy Library in Boston to bring attention to the issue and to provide a stage for political leaders to address the issue. Also in 2003, my organization, Health Care For All, launched a broad advocacy coalition named Affordable Care Today (ACT!) to write universal coverage legislation for introduction in the new legislative session in 2005 and to craft a parallel statewide ballot initiative for the November 2006 state elections if reform had not been achieved by then.[2]

Another force shaped the process. Since 1997, Massachusetts had run its Medicaid program (called MassHealth) under special terms negotiated through a so-called Section 1115 waiver with the federal government. These waivers are time limited, generally for two to five years, and require negotiations with the U.S. Department of Health and Human Services (DHHS) for renewal. The Massachusetts waiver, first negotiated during President Bill Clinton's administration, permitted the state to enroll more residents in Medicaid than were allowed in other states and provided a special pot of money to assist key safety net hospitals (chiefly Boston Medical Center and the Cambridge Health Alliance) in meeting their obligations.

When Massachusetts officials began negotiations in 2004 with the administration of President George W. Bush for a third waiver, DHHS officials assured them it would be renewed, with one proviso. The special pot of extra money known as "special payments to disproportionate share hospitals" (amounting to about $350 million per year) would not be continued under a new waiver, set to start on July 1, 2005. In Massachusetts, $350 million is a lot of money, and the news set off alarm bells. Governor Romney reached out and formed a partnership with Senator Kennedy to scheme how to keep the extra federal dollars coming. At that moment, the state's mundane desire to retain federal dollars merged with the policy goal of universal coverage to create a new policy imperative. Romney and Kennedy proposed that Massachusetts keep receiving the extra payments, and in return the state would shift the use of those dollars away from safety-net hospitals and use them instead as subsidies to help lower-income individuals and families purchase health insurance. And they would tie this structure to establishing the first mandate in the nation's history for individuals to purchase health insurance coverage. Let us do this, they implored the Bush administration, and you can take credit for universal coverage in one state at no new cost.

In late January 2005, on his last day as U.S. Secretary of Health and Human Services, so late in the day that the music from his goodbye party could be heard in the distance, former Wisconsin governor Tommy Thompson signed a new three-year Section 1115 waiver for Massachusetts—under the condition that the state legislature enact a law to implement the proposed system and that the system be up and running no later than July 1, 2006. If the timetable was not met, the state would lose all three years of supplemental payments, $350 million times three, $1.05 billion.

Massachusetts put a financial gun to its head that made passage of universal coverage legislation a policy, political, and financial necessity and the Bush administration provided the bullets. Still, the road to legislative enactment was contentious, with policy differences dividing the governor, the Senate, and the House. Romney proposed an individual mandate for all residents to purchase health insurance and the creation of an "insurance exchange" (suggested by Heritage). The ACT! coalition appreciated the governor's commitment to universal coverage and opposed his skinny, stripped-down benefits package, preferring a mandate on employers to cover their workers, not one on individuals. The Senate was cautious, favoring neither mandate, opting for incremental expansions and small insurance-market reforms. The House, the last to show its hand, surprised everyone by embracing both individual and employer responsibility, along with a robust expansion resembling the ACT! proposals.

An arduous conference process dragged on for months, deadlocked over employer responsibility. On a Sunday morning in late January 2006, a frustrated Romney visited the private residences of Speaker DiMasi and President Travaglini, leaving handwritten letters asking them to hurry up and finish. In March, business leaders brokered an agreement between the two legislative leaders—a smallish fine (compared with the cost of health insurance) of $295 per year on most employers for each worker without health insurance. All remaining issues—including three years of state funding for Boston Medical Center and Cambridge Health Alliance to hold them harmless—were wrapped up in weeks, paving the way for the April signing ceremony at Faneuil Hall.

Though there were fights aplenty on the path to enactment, Romney's observation that "the differences between us are small" was on the money. Applauding at the bill signing were Democrats and Republicans, business organizations, consumer and disease advocacy groups, health insurers, and medical groups such as the Massachusetts Hospital Association and the Massachusetts Medical Society. Of the major constituencies, only organized labor was split. The Service Employees International Union supported the new law, while the state and national AFL-CIO blasted the law for its lack of a tough employer mandate and the inclusion of an individual mandate. Shortly after the signing, all the major constituencies joined in a statewide campaign, including paid TV advertising, to educate the public about the new law.

The new law became known as Chapter 58, the fifty-eighth bill signed in 2006. It was not designed as comprehensive health reform; it was crafted to respond to the threat and opportunity provided by the Bush administration's determination to withdraw more than $1 billion that the state had assumed would continue to flow into its health care system. In some ways, Chapter 58 expanded on approaches taken by other state health reform efforts; in other ways, it broke new ground. At its core, it combined three policy elements, like the legs on the three-legged stool.

The first leg was systemic reform of health insurance markets for individuals and small employers, the most troubled parts of the nation's insurance system. Massachusetts had already implemented reforms in these markets in 1991 and 1996, eliminating exclusions for preexisting conditions and requiring insurers to take all qualified applicants, a practice called *guaranteed issue*. Chapter 58 established a new marketplace for individuals and employers called the Massachusetts Health Insurance Connector Authority. (Romney called it the Exchange, and the legislature chose *Connector* to deny him naming rights.)

The second leg was a mandate on all residents to purchase a minimum level of health insurance or face a state income tax fine as high as half the cost of coverage. Guaranteed issue without an individual mandate tempts some individuals to delay purchasing insurance until they know they will incur a medical expense. The resulting "adverse selection" drives up insurance premiums for those with coverage to unsustainable levels, leading many to drop coverage in a continuous "death spiral." This concern was not hypothetical—Massachusetts had instituted guaranteed issue in its individual market in 1996 without a mandate and watched premiums double. Other states saw similar results; some, such as Maine, New Jersey, New York, and Vermont, held on to the reforms and higher premiums; others, including Kentucky, New Hampshire, and Washington, repealed guaranteed issue within a few years of passage.

The third leg was subsidies to make coverage affordable for those subject to the mandate who otherwise could not afford insurance. Affordability involves the cost of premiums along with cost sharing in the form of co-payments, deductibles, and co-insurance. Controlling the cost of premiums without addressing cost sharing can leave low- and moderate-income families with insurance exposed to bankruptcy-inducing costs. Indeed, research shows that most of those who face bankruptcy due to "medical debt" had health insurance that included excessive cost sharing.

The three legs of the stool—insurance-market reforms, an individual mandate, and subsidies—are inseparable. Take one or two away, and there is no chair on which to sit. While the individual mandate can assume various forms, some mechanism to avert adverse selection is essential. The private sector coverage portions of Title I of the ACA embrace this triad. While the ACA and Chapter 58 differ in many ways, the coverage idea in both is the same.

Still, differences abound, and a key one is timing. While the ACA

includes some reforms that take effect in 2010 and 2011, the core features—drawn from Chapter 58—do not take effect until 2014, nearly four
years after enactment. Consider, in contrast, the pace of Massachusetts
implementation following the law's signing in April 2006:

June 2006—The Connector is established.

July 2006—Expansions and coverage restorations in the state Medicaid
program become effective, adding fifty thousand newly enrolled persons.

October 2006—Enrollment opens in Commonwealth Care, new subsidized coverage for uninsured persons with incomes up to three times
the federal poverty level (that is, up to $32,490 for an individual in 2010).

July 2007—Individual and small-group health insurance markets merge.

July 2007—The individual mandate takes effect; penalties for individuals without coverage become effective December 31, 2007.

Over two years, the numbers of persons covered by the various aspects
of Chapter 58 mounted, leveling off at about 425,000 in 2008. By 2009,
coverage of non-elderly adults had reached 95 percent, up from 88 percent
in 2006 before reform implementation, by far the best performance in any
state in the nation.[3]

A common criticism of Chapter 58 is its failure to stop rising health costs
and insurance premiums. Chapter 58 included provisions to address rising
costs that have proven insufficient, and by 2011, the state was continuing
to grapple with additional measures. Still, there is a tendency to criticize
laws for failing to accomplish objectives they were never designed to meet.
Chapter 58 was designed to expand coverage to about a half million uninsured and to avoid the loss of at-risk federal money. Those objectives were
accomplished. In the wake of reform, the state has also undertaken one of
the most ambitious efforts by any state to reform its system to control costs.

Others complain that the law triggered a physician shortage, especially
in primary care. Before Chapter 58, some geographic regions experienced
physician shortages and many persist, as they would have without Chapter
58. Massachusetts reform has triggered a sustained effort to address workforce needs. There is irony in this: Massachusetts has the highest rate of
physicians per capita of any state, including one of the highest rates of
primary care physicians (129 per 100,000 persons versus 90 for the nation
as a whole).[4] News stories describing workforce challenges would lead one
to believe Massachusetts is the only state facing these pressures. One
response to this depiction comes from the state's physician community;

surveyed in 2009, 70 percent said they supported the law while 13 percent indicated opposition, and only 7 percent said the law should be repealed.[5]

After passage, Chapter 58 became the nation's early Rorschach test on national health reform. The political right attacked it as a bloated government scheme that would drive up costs and lessen liberty. The political left, especially single-payer advocates, portrayed it as the last gasp of the political establishment to thwart their preferred solution. Especially challenged by the backlash was one of its principal promoters, Mitt Romney, who voluntarily vacated his position as governor in 2007. Because so many Republicans and conservatives had embraced an individual mandate prior to the ACA process, Romney miscalculated that such a mandate would appeal to the national Republican base, and he has been compelled repeatedly to defend the Massachusetts law, which bears striking resemblance to the coverage provisions in Title I of the ACA. Romney can rightly assert that the ACA includes an additional nine titles (plus a reconciliation bill); moreover, the ACA tilts toward federal control and uniformity. Yet his need to reconcile the law he proudly signed with the federal law he needs to delegitimize is primarily evidence of transformed sentiment among Republicans and conservatives. A Republican individual mandate plan generated in 1993–94 as an alternative to Clinton health reform has become the most vilified example of Democratic excess in 2009–10.

In the end are the individuals whose lives have been helped and saved by Massachusetts reform. Among them is Ibby Caputo, who in 2007 at age twenty-six was given a diagnosis of acute myelogenous leukemia and a prognosis of six weeks to live without treatment. Shortly before her diagnosis, Caputo had moved from out of state to Cape Cod to intern at a radio station and work at a coffee shop. She had no medical insurance when she got her diagnosis, and she qualified right away for coverage under Chapter 58. Now, $913,425.15 in bills later, she is alive and well and working as a staff writer at the *Washington Post*, where she wrote an account of her experience.[6]

CALIFORNIA TRIES AND STUMBLES

After the passage of Chapter 58 and the resultant national attention, policy makers in numerous states were encouraged to look at ways to expand coverage.[7] Some did, and many others chose to wait to see what the federal government might have in store. California made the most aggressive effort to fashion its own health reform plan—resembling the Massachusetts plan—though instead offered the nation a cautionary tale on the hard road to reform. In 2007, California's Republican governor, Arnold Schwarzenegger, teamed up with the Democratic state assembly speaker, Fabian Núñez, to advance a plan that imposed an individual mandate on Californians to obtain health insurance; created a new state purchasing pool to help individuals and businesses buy insurance; imposed guaranteed issue on the individual health insurance market; created subsidies to lower the cost of insurance for income-eligible persons and expanded the state's Medicaid and CHIP programs; and imposed a "pay or play" requirement on employers to cover their workers or pay a tax to the state.

While the plan won approval in the state assembly in late 2007, it faltered and died in the Democratic-controlled state Senate in early 2008. Unlike Massachusetts, where most major stakeholder interests supported reform, in California nearly every key constituency—including consumers, business, insurers, labor unions, and the health industry—split apart over the plan. A promising and ambitious plan, an intense political brawl, and nothing accomplished after a huge effort—which was the harbinger for national reform, Massachusetts or California?[8]

ROADS NOT TAKEN

Massachusetts Avenue is a good locale to explore two choices on "Constitution Avenue" that were not taken in the 2009–10 process: first, the option to establish a Canadian-style single-payer public financing system to replace private health insurance and second, a private sector variant of that approach, the Wyden-Bennett Healthy Americans Act.

Single Payer

Early in my time in the Senate, single-payer proponents—led by organizers from the California Nurses Association—visited to seek Senator Kennedy's support for single payer as the path to national reform. We asked them how many senators they knew supported their preference. "We haven't done a head count," they said, and they never provided one. Senator Kennedy's health team had done one—the Medicare for All legislation he sponsored earlier in the decade had garnered zero cosponsors.

A year later in the fall of 2009, as Senator Bernie Sanders (I-VT) prepared to offer an amendment on the Senate floor to substitute a single-payer alternative for the Senate health reform bill, I sat down with one of his aides. "How many votes are you sure of?" I asked. We counted: Sanders, Sherrod Brown (D-OH), Roland Burris (D-IL), Jeff Merkley (D-OR)—we guessed these without confirmation. Senator Tom Harkin (D-IA) was a single-payer supporter, but as Kennedy's successor as HELP Committee chair, his vote was uncertain. Perhaps Carl Levin (D-MI) or Russ Feingold (D-WI)? Beyond that, all maybes. It would be a minor miracle, we agreed, if yea votes for the amendment broke into double digits. "Let's say it ends up nine for and ninety-one against—what does that prove?" I asked. "Bernie wants a vote," he said.

In early December, Sanders got his chance to force a Senate roll-call vote on single payer. Majority Leader Harry Reid had assured him that his amendment would reach the floor, and he kept his word. Sanders did not count on physician-senator Tom Coburn (R-OK) exercising his right to demand that the full text of his amendment be read on the Senate floor—a move that would devour fifteen hours of increasingly scarce floor time. After the Senate clerk had spent several hours reading his amendment, Sanders threw in the towel and withdrew. Thus ended the moment for single payer on the Senate floor.

Sanders soon joined forces with Senator Ron Wyden in seeking to create a waiver enabling states to establish comprehensive alternatives to the ACA's coverage programs as long as those programs covered as many as and cost no more than the new law—a provision that Sanders hoped could be used by Vermont and other states to establish their own single-payer plans. Pushback from the CBO that the provision would be difficult to score led Senate staffers to write the waiver so that no state could obtain one prior to 2017, which is how PPACA's section 1332 of Title I was structured. Sanders and Wyden pushed during the January 2010 House-Senate merger process to allow two states to obtain waivers in each of the years 2014, 2015, and 2016—something the CBO said would not add further costs. The senators, though, got stiff pushback from House leaders, especially Energy and Commerce chair Henry Waxman (D-CA). Any possibility of further changes expired on January 19, when the results of the special Massachusetts Senate election halted the House-Senate bill merger process.

In the U.S. House of Representatives, single-payer supporters numbered about 80 in the 435 member chamber, and they were determined to put the chamber on record. Representatives John Conyers (D-MI) and Dennis Kucinich (D-OH) were the lead sponsors of House single-payer legislation. Kucinich had promoted single payer in his long-shot run for the 2008 Democratic presidential nomination. Annoyed at the unwillingness of the media to discuss single payer, he used the opportunity during a Democratic presidential debate in late 2007 to pose a question to himself instead of asking a fellow candidate a question. "Is it true," he asked himself, "that you are the only candidate who supports a universal single-payer not-for-profit health care system?" His answer was yes.[9] When the moment came for a single-payer roll-call vote during the House health reform debate in early November 2009, supporters demurred (as House Speaker Nancy Pelosi had urged), fearing the potential impact of such a debate on the tenuous margin needed to pass the House health bill and deciding that a lopsided defeat might do more harm than good. Representative Anthony Weiner (D-NY) withdrew his amendment the day before the final vote, announcing:

> I have decided not to offer a single-payer amendment to the health reform bill. Given how fluid the negotiations are on the final push to get comprehensive health care reform that covers millions of Americans and contains costs through a public option, I became concerned that my amendment might undermine that important goal.[10]

Replacing private health insurance with public health insurance has been the gold standard for many Americans since Harry Truman tried it in the 1940s. Progressives want to push private insurance out of the picture and lower the system's administrative costs. Conservatives dislike the elimination of private health insurance choices as well as the power it would give to the federal government. Medicare—Parts A and B—signed into law in 1965 is a version of Truman's vision, though only for the elderly and some disabled persons. Since then, reform efforts have focused on establishing some form of a public-private hybrid.

Numerous states have considered single-payer proposals within their borders since the 1980s, though no such legislation has been signed into law. In two states, voters had the opportunity to adopt a single-payer system through proposed ballot initiatives, and in both cases, the proposals were trounced. In California in 1994, less than two months after the final defeat of the Clinton initiative, voters rejected the idea 73 to 27 percent; in Oregon in 2002, voters dismissed the proposal 78 to 22 percent.

The single-payer choice presented a dilemma for Senator Kennedy. He had promoted single payer consistently in the 1970s and in his final decade was the lead Senate sponsor of Medicare for All legislation. But Kennedy believed there was no way such legislation could get to President Obama's desk. He was determined not to miss this opportunity in 2009 to achieve national reform and so—in spite of his personal preference—backed the Massachusetts Avenue approach.

A similar dynamic played out in the Democratic presidential campaign. One key lesson many Democrats took from the 1993–94 Clinton reform failure was not to threaten the coverage that about 80 percent of Americans had and that the large majority did not want to lose. As they formulated their health reform planks, lead contenders John Edwards, Hillary Clinton, and Barack Obama all made the same guarantee: if you like the coverage you have, you can keep it. The single-payer candidate, Kucinich, failed to achieve significant support despite being the only candidate agreeing with the Americans who supported that option—who made up a sizable proportion of Democrats. So while single payer was preferred by many Democrats, it also was not a deciding issue.

In the legislative process, single-payer advocates pressed their case through the efforts of the California Nurses Association, Physicians for a National Health Program, and the Healthcare-Now coalition. The Senate HELP Committee and House committees, on several occasions, gave single-payer advocates a seat at the hearing table; the Senate Finance Committee did not, leading to an act of civil disobedience and eight arrests at a May 2009 Finance hearing when the single-payer voice was excluded from a panel of interest groups.[11] Single-payer advocates, passionately as they believed in their cause, were unable to convince even sympathetic lawmakers that there was a way to get a Medicare for All bill to the president's desk.

Despite the passage of the ACA, the single-payer option will not disappear from the political landscape.

Healthy Americans Act

Single payer was not the only game-changing plan on Constitution Avenue. Senator Ron Wyden, the Oregon Democrat, crafted his own ambitious plan in 2007 after three years crisscrossing the nation hearing stories from Americans about their frustrations with the health system. He discovered a pattern:

> We held a large number of Town Hall meetings in the early part of the new century to talk about health reform. One person would stand up to say, "We want single payer," and a lot of people clap. Then another stands up and says, "We don't want all that government," and a different bunch of people clap. Then both sides look sullen at each other because there hasn't been progress. Then someone would stand up and say, "We want what you people in Congress have," and the entire room would erupt in applause, people on both sides.[12]

From that insight, Wyden constructed the Healthy Americans Act. In its original version, every adult and business contributed—based on ability to pay—to a federal fund that paid private insurance companies for each person they enrolled. Like the Massachusetts Connector, state "Health Help" agencies would enroll uninsured individuals in private coverage, except Wyden's agencies were a one-stop source for everyone to enroll in the plan of his or her choice (except Medicare enrollees, who would keep their current coverage). Medicaid was eliminated, and its enrollees were covered along with everyone else. Wyden's original plan eliminated all employer coverage; his amended version allowed businesses the option to continue covering their workers, though in a way that weakened his plan's savings and the stability of its structure.

As mainstream Democrats embraced the mantra "If you like what you have, you can keep it," Wyden advanced a radical, privately based plan that would have become the new, dominant market for nearly all U.S. health insurance. Two aspects made Wyden's plan especially noteworthy. First, he persuaded the Congressional Budget Office, Congress's nonpartisan budget scorekeeper, to do a preliminary fiscal analysis, released in May 2008, concluding that Wyden's plan covered nearly all Americans, would be budget neutral by 2014, and would decrease the federal deficit in years thereafter. Wyden's plan achieved this eye-catching benchmark because, in addition to taxing nearly all individuals and businesses, his plan proposed eliminating the current federal tax deduction for employer-provided health insurance—the largest, fastest-growing federal tax expenditure, costing $188 billion in 2004[13]—and replacing it with a smaller, slower-growing individual deduction.[14]

Second, in 2007 and 2008 Wyden persuaded eight Senate Republicans to cosponsor his legislation, including New Hampshire's Judd Gregg, Iowa's Charles Grassley, Tennessee's Lamar Alexander, South Carolina's Lindsay Graham, and his lead cosponsor, Utah's Robert Bennett. This was an early encouraging sign that bipartisanship, even for ambitious reform, was achievable. Those paying close attention noticed that several Republican endorsers accompanied their cosponsorship with objections to various provisions such as the employer mandate—Alexander and Gregg both stated they would not vote for the bill as written.[15] Also expressing reservations were several Democratic cosponsors, including Debbie Stabenow (D-MI), who opposed eliminating Medicaid, a feature that made the package especially attractive to Republicans.

In the midst of Wyden's early advances came setbacks. The ranking Republican on Senate Finance, Grassley, who cosponsored the 2007 bill, refused to do so in 2008, not wanting to undermine his relationship with Finance chair Max Baucus. Baucus never warmed to Wyden's proposal, concerned that Wyden would repeat the Clintons' fatal mistake by proposing to change coverage for all Americans, including those satisfied with their current plans, most significantly by eliminating entirely the exclusion of employer health insurance premiums from income taxes (section 106 of the Internal Revenue Code). The Washington DC stakeholder community echoed Baucus's concerns. Though some individual business leaders supported the plan, as did labor's Andy Stern, the president of the Service Employees International Union, most business and labor leaders gave the plan a firm, public thumbs down. The liberal Center for Budget and Policy Priorities drew up a report highlighting the plan's weaknesses and flaws, especially the way it would erode the affordability of insurance subsidies over time.[16]

As momentum gathered for the Massachusetts Avenue approach, Wyden and his bill were marginalized. He had one ace in his sleeve—his seat on the Senate Finance Committee. From that perch, he promoted his plan at every Finance reform hearing, in a way that alienated some fellow Democrats. He openly hoped that if the prevailing approach faltered, his would be the backup plan, writing a *Washington Post* op-ed to that point in August 2009 just as the emerging tea party movement made its mark opposing reform in town hall meetings across the nation.[17] As that possibility faded in late 2009, Wyden proposed amending the Senate bill to allow anyone with employer-sponsored coverage to claim from an employer the dollar value of the insurance and use it to purchase coverage through an exchange. Again, Wyden faced vocal and determined opposition from business and labor—two forces rarely on the same side. Finally, in December, needing Wyden's vote to get to the needed sixty votes in the Senate, Baucus and Wyden agreed to cosponsor an opt-out option for a sliver of workers—those for whom the cost of purchasing employer coverage would be between 8 and 9.5 percent of the family income. It was a narrow victory, but a victory nonetheless.

"I take pride in being part of a bipartisan group that has been on the right side of history," Wyden reflects.[18] Still, his chief partner, Utah Republican Bob Bennett, lost his reelection bid in 2010 to a tea-party-associated rival who used Bennett's association with Wyden against him—a signal of what might have occurred more broadly had Wyden's bill gained traction. Wyden had a different view of the reform opportunity in 2009–10 than did his colleagues and most stakeholders. His ideas may return to see another day.

Early on, the strategy for national health reform, version 2009–10, was set. It was Massachusetts Avenue.

3. Political Will I—Prelude to a Health Reform Campaign

The scene: a Democratic presidential primary debate in Las Vegas, Nevada, on November 15, 2007, less than two months before the pivotal Iowa caucuses. After a shaky showing in the prior debate, Senator Hillary Rodham Clinton was urged by aides to challenge Senator Barack Obama on inadequacies in his health reform proposal, which was projected to cover fewer uninsured Americans than her plan because of the lack of an individual mandate to purchase health insurance. Here is the key exchange moderated by CNN's Wolf Blitzer:

SENATOR CLINTON: Well, I hear what Senator Obama is saying, and he talks a lot about stepping up and taking responsibility and taking strong positions. But when it came time to step up and decide whether or not he would support universal health care coverage, he chose not to do that. His plan would leave fifteen million Americans out. That's about the population of Nevada, Iowa, South Carolina, and New Hampshire. I have a universal health care plan that covers everyone. I've been fighting this battle against the special interests for more than fifteen years, and I am proud to fight this battle. You know, we can have different politics, but let's not forget here that the people who we're against are not going to be giving up without a fight. The Republicans are not going to vacate the White House voluntarily. . . . [cheers, applause]

MR. BLITZER: All right. Senator Obama.

SENATOR OBAMA: Well, let's talk about health care right now because the fact of the matter is that I do provide universal health care. The only difference between Senator Clinton's health care plan and mine is that she thinks the problem for people without health care is that nobody has mandated—forced—them to get health care. That's not what I'm seeing around Nevada. What I see are people who would love to have health care. They—they desperately want it. But the problem is they can't afford it, which is why we have put forward legislation [*cheers, applause*]—we've put forward a plan that makes sure that it is affordable to get health care that is as good as the health care that I have as a member of Congress. [*applause*]

MR. BLITZER: All right. . . .

SENATOR CLINTON: Wolf, I—Wolf, I cannot let that go unanswered. You know, the most important thing here is to level with the American people. Senator Obama's health care plan does not cover everyone. He starts with children, which is admirable—I helped to create the Children's Health Insurance Program back in 1997. I'm totally committed—[*applause*]—

SENATOR OBAMA: That's not true, Wolf.

SENATOR CLINTON: —to making sure every single child is covered. He does not mandate the kind of coverage that I do. And I provide a health care tax credit under my American Health Choices Plan so that every American will be able to afford the health care. I open up the congressional plan. But there is a big difference between Senator Obama and me. He starts from the premise of not reaching universal health care. . . .

SENATOR OBAMA: —states that she wants—she states that she wants to mandate health care coverage, but she's not garnishing people's wages to make sure that they have it. . . . She is not—she is not enforcing this mandate. And I don't think that the problem with the American people is that they are not being forced to get health care. . . . The problem is, they can't afford it. And that is why my plan provides the mechanism to make sure that they can. [*applause*][1]

National health reform was a front-and-center issue in Democratic primaries and in the general election, to an extent rarely seen in the history of presidential elections. In the Democratic primaries, the defining issue became whether to include an individual mandate as part of reform, and in the general election whether to tax employer-provided health insurance. More than settling those issues, the challenge for reformers was to create an expectation that reform had to happen. Most of the time, generating political will does not happen spontaneously—it is developed and nurtured over time to take advantage of political opportunity when it arises. In this chapter, we will explore the presidential campaign and, before that, the activities between 2005 and 2008 of stakeholders who wanted to make sure that health reform mattered.

GATHERING MOMENTUM

While the Democratic primary campaigns provided heat and electricity to health reform, interest groups, key stakeholders, and influential individuals committed to achieving what was missed in 1993–94 had been working hard on reform well before Americans focused on the 2008 presidential sweepstakes. Their work was critical in generating the energy exhibited in the Democratic campaigns. While many were familiar progressive groups, the early action also involved nontraditional and surprising reformers—both groups and individuals. Consider six—the American Medical Association, the Federation of American Hospitals, the trade group for the medical-device industry known as AdvaMed, the Business Roundtable, the Pharmaceutical Research and Manufacturers of America, and America's Health Insurance Plans.

No organization has been more associated with opposition to national health reform than the AMA, the nation's largest, most influential physician organization. The AMA's opposition to the health reform designs of Presidents Roosevelt, Truman, and Johnson were potent and, with the exception of LBJ's plan, effective. In 1993–94 the AMA was conflicted and ineffective as insurers, business groups, and drug companies spearheaded the effort to kill Clinton-care. At the same time, a shrinking AMA membership and the growing memberships of a dizzying array of other physician organizations have made its work more difficult. Looking ahead to 2009, the AMA approached the prospect of national health reform differently. At the organization's 2005 strategic planning meeting, support for covering the uninsured and for participating in broader health reform had already emerged as top priorities. Leading up to the 2008 presidential elections, the AMA spent $16 million to invest in TV, newspaper, and subway ads, and more to promote health reform as a 2008 election issue. It had eight reform priorities, the top of the list including a fix to the flawed Medicare physician-payment system, medical-liability reform, and universal coverage. This time, unlike all the others, the AMA wanted reform and wanted to be a leader in helping to make it happen.[2]

Few individuals were more identified with opposition to the Clinton plan than Chip Kahn. As a leader of the Health Insurance Association of America (HIAA) in 1993, he dreamed up a TV advertising series featuring "Harry and Louise," a fictional middle-American couple worrying about the effects of the Clinton plan on their own coverage. "There's got to be a better way," they sighed, to devastating effect.[3] In 2001, after stints on Capitol Hill as a top health policy aide to House Republicans and time as president of the HIAA, Kahn was hired as the chief of the Federation of American Hospitals, the national trade organization of for-profit hospitals—not a liberal or social-justice-oriented association. At a 2006 federation meeting in Florida, he was summoned by his staffers into a raucous session:

> Staff told me I had better get in the room fast because everyone is angry. My members told me they were sick and tired of incremental health reform measures. They wanted universal coverage NOW. I said we won't get it. They told me they wanted the Federation to stand for this right away. They felt the path we were on was unsustainable with the levels of uncompensated care and the expectation that hospitals would take care of everyone, plus this byzantine financing scheme.[4]

His member revolt led Chip in early 2008 to formulate a proposal for a "Health Care Passport"—a pathway to universal coverage within the existing private health insurance structure. "My people said we're not interested in incremental anymore, and they put me in a different place."

AdvaMed, the national trade organization for the burgeoning medical-device industry, was another atypical party. Formed in 1974 as the Health Industry Manufacturers Association, it took its current name in 2000 to create a higher profile. As part of an effort to create a stronger federal presence, in 2005 it hired David Nexon as senior executive vice president. For twenty years before that, as Senator Edward M. Kennedy's senior health policy chief, Nexon was called the "dean of health policy in the U.S. Senate." In mid-2008, AdvaMed released its own universal coverage plan including Massachusetts-like insurance subsidies and an individual mandate. Nexon's fingerprints were visible all over it. While making clear it wanted to be a player, AdvaMed offered no suggestions for how to pay for the plan.

The Business Roundtable is just one of countless business voices in Washington DC. Yet as a voice for America's largest corporations, with $6 trillion in annual revenue and twelve million employees, it displays a more moderate disposition than harder-edged competitors such as the U.S. Chamber of Commerce and the National Federation of Independent Business (NFIB). Because all its members provide employee health coverage, it wanted to create greater efficiency and value for the medical services it purchased and to stop footing the bill for the uninsured. In September 2008, Business Roundtable president John Castellani released a four-part health plan calling for greater consumer value, a reorganized private health insurance market, an individual mandate, and subsidies for the lower-income uninsured. As for the other business groups, NFIB leader Todd

Stottlemyer publicly supported health reform, an eye-popping and short-lived turnaround from the organization's prior role as the business community's leading galvanizer against the Clinton plan. In 1993–94, the U.S. Chamber initially supported Clinton-care and its employer mandate, until NFIB browbeat it into opposition. This time, the Chamber started out hostile and browbeat NFIB into opposition. NFIB's new pro-reform stance was short-lived, as Stottlemyer left in early 2009, and the group soon returned to its prior anti-reform position. But in the early days of 2007 and '08, Stottlemyer and NFIB had teamed up with the Business Roundtable, AARP, and the Service Employees International Union (SEIU) to form the Divided We Fail coalition to promote a positive reform agenda throughout 2008.

The pharmaceutical industry was among the most vociferous and effective opponents of the 1993–94 Clinton health reform plan, investing tens of millions in opposition advertising. Working with the Bush administration and Republican congressional leaders, the industry and its trade organization, the Pharmaceutical Research and Manufacturers of America (PhRMA), won a major victory in 2003 with passage of the Medicare Modernization Act (MMA), which created a Medicare outpatient prescription-drug benefit relying on the private market without government cost controls. PhRMA's president, Billy Tauzin, had been a Republican congressman and the House Energy and Commerce Committee chair who brokered the MMA deal and then left Congress to head the drug trade group. While the MMA was a Republican victory, the industry had allies aplenty among Democrats who took control of the Senate in 2007. Among them was Senator Max Baucus (D-MT), chair of the Senate Finance Committee and one of the few leading Democrats to vote for the MMA. Also friendly was Senator Kennedy, whose Health, Education, Labor and Pensions (HELP) Committee had jurisdiction over the Food and Drug Administration and whose home state of Massachusetts was a base for many drug and life sciences firms. In 2008, Kennedy began meeting with industry leaders, particularly Pfizer's new president and CEO Jeff Kindler, to avoid a repeat of 1993–94. Well before an industry deal on health reform was reached with Baucus and the White House in July 2009, Pfizer began TV and other advertising to promote reform, signaling its intention to play a different role this time.

The health insurance industry—with its principal trade organization, America's Health Insurance Plans (AHIP)—was perhaps the most surprising player. And its president, Karen Ignagni, was a surprising leader. The daughter of a Rhode Island firefighter, she had been a staffer for U.S. Senator Claiborne Pell (D-RI) and was an AFL-CIO health policy director during the Clinton health reform process. Looking ahead to 2009, she was the face and voice of the U.S. health insurance industry and determined to steer a different course:

> In March 2006, my Board began an important strategic conversation—what position would we take after the 2008 election? We discussed the Clinton era and what happened. Back then, they decided not to advance proposals, and so our only choice was to say yea or nay. We did not want to do that again and wanted this time to play a leadership role. In November 2006, we became one of the first national organizations to adopt the principle that all Americans should be covered.[5]

AHIP began releasing proposals: in March 2007, on improving health care quality; in December 2007, on how states could achieve guaranteed issue; in May 2008, on cost containment; in November 2008, on how to achieve guaranteed issue federally; and in March 2009 on how to eliminate insurance rating based on health status and gender. To many, AHIP's proposals did not go far enough, though it was clearly an industry whose position was evolving—so it was not surprising when President Obama turned to Ignagni for a comment at the White House health reform summit on March 5, 2009. She told him, "We hear the American people about what's not working. We've taken that seriously. You have our commitment to play, to contribute, and to help pass health care reform this year."[6]

Business, insurers, manufacturers, medical organizations were all calling for comprehensive reform, all issuing principles and priorities, all stating that doing nothing to fix health care was unacceptable. An era of health reform good feeling had broken out and lasted well into 2009. Seasoned observers knew it would not last once actual legislation appeared, though many wondered if this time things just might be different.

Of critical importance in sustaining the focus and good feelings were key national health foundations, many of whom had been preparing for a new reform opportunity for years. The Robert Wood Johnson Foundation, led by Risa Lavizzo-Mourey, supported early efforts to connect congressional staff from both parties with researchers and promoted initiatives to build a robust community voice in the legislative process; the foundation also financed efforts to achieve multistakeholder and bipartisan consensus, including the Health Reform Dialogue and the Bipartisan Policy Center (both described shortly); it played an essential role in developing a robust health prevention part of the reform agenda. The Kaiser Family Foundation, run by former New Jersey Human Services commissioner Drew Altman, provided key polling data throughout the process, and became a key go-to organization for fast access to critical data and information; the Kaiser Foundation's Diane Rowland, one of the nation's leading experts on

Medicaid, was keenly involved in that part; its private insurance expert, Gary Claxton, consulted extensively with every congressional staffer involved in the private-insurance-market portions of the ACA. The upstart Atlantic Philanthropies, not bound by Internal Revenue Service restrictions on direct funding for legislative advocacy, provided $26.5 million to the newly created Health Care for America Now (HCAN) coalition.

The Commonwealth Fund, headed by Carter administration health official Karen Davis, a respected researcher, formulated its own detailed and robust proposals and developed key research on many policy priorities. Its "Path to a High Performance U.S. Health System" offered comprehensive recommendations on insurance, payment, and system reforms that resemble in many respects the details and the breadth of the final ACA.[7]

Familiar liberal organizations were also active early, including AARP, the massive senior citizens organization (half of whose members are under age sixty-five and at risk of losing health insurance); Families USA, the savvy consumer advocacy group; the Service Employees International Union (SEIU), the key labor voice promoting reform anywhere and everywhere; the American Cancer Society and other disease organizations; the Center for American Progress, a key progressive policy shop; and many others. Knowing their voices alone were insufficient, these groups formed and joined numerous overlapping coalitions: Divided We Fail, the National Coalition on Benefits, the Partnership to Fight Chronic Disease, the National Coalition on Health Care, the Are You Covered? coalition, Better Health Care Together, the Coalition to Advance Healthcare Reform, the Herndon Alliance, Americans for Health Care, the Healthcare Leadership Council, the single-payer Healthcare-Now coalition, Health Care for America Now, and more.

A few carved out unique and consequential niches.

Health Care for America Now was the most prominent reform coalition during the process. With 142 national organizations, hundreds of state and local groups, and a powerful steering committee including groups such as the AFL-CIO, SEIU, the National Education Association, MoveOn.org, the NAACP, and Citizen Action, HCAN was well financed with more than $51 million from the Atlantic Philanthropies, national labor unions, and other supporters, ensuring significant resources and a loud voice.[8] Many HCAN participants were single-payer advocates who became convinced their preference was not achievable, at least in the 2009 round. They embraced a plan advanced by Yale political scientist Jacob Hacker that proposed a Massachusetts Avenue–like arrangement with a crucial add-on—one insurance option through an exchange had to be a "public-plan option" run by the federal government, paying Medicare rates to hospitals, physicians, and other medical providers and requiring all providers to contract with the plan as a condition to continue their participation in Medicare.[9] HCAN made the public-plan option one of the most compelling controversies in the reform process. By Election Day 2008, HCAN had collected pledges from 140 senators and representatives supporting its principles, including a public option.[10]

The Health Reform Dialogue, the brainchild of Families USA head Ron Pollack, involved America's Health Insurance Plans, the AMA, the Federataion of American Hospitals, the American Hospital Association (AHA), Pharmaceutical Research and Manufacturers of America (PhRMA), SEIU, the Business Roundtable, AFL-CIO, the National Federation of Independent Business (NFIB), and others, eighteen heavy hitters in all. They negotiated for seven months, beginning in the fall of 2008, helped by a professional conflict mediator. In their final agreement, announced in March 2009, they reached consensus on some key principles. The goals were to expand health coverage to all Americans; achieve more effective and efficient care; promote prevention and wellness; and reduce the growth rate for health costs—all of which were contained in the final ACA. Media coverage noted the nonagreement on financing, mandates, and a public-plan option. Because of the lack of an employer mandate and a public-plan option, the SEIU and AFL-CIO refused to sign the final statement. Intending to jump-start congressional consensus, the Dialogue instead gave an early indication of how hard achieving reform would be on the crucial policy controversies. Pollock did persuade some participants (PhRMA, AHA, the Catholic Health Association, and NFIB) to sponsor new TV ads featuring the characters Harry and Louise, sixteen years older. This time, they were back to support undefined national health reform. The ads ran prominently during the 2008 national political conventions and longer. "A little more cooperation, a little less politics," Louise says to Harry, "and we can get the job done this time."[11]

Another hope-triggering sign was the 2007 launch of the Bipartisan Policy Center by four former U.S. Senate majority leaders, Bob Dole (R-KS), Howard Baker (R-TN), George Mitchell (D-ME), and Tom Daschle (D-SD). Mitchell had told Democratic senators at a July 2008 lunch: "I bear a large share of responsibility for the '93–'94 failure—don't repeat my errors."[12] He was determined to help get it done this time, though his personal effort ended prematurely when Obama named him the new Middle East envoy in early 2009. With staff support from Clinton White House health policy chief Chris Jennings and the Bush director of the Centers for Medicare and Medicaid Services Mark McClellan, hopes were high that this group could chart a credible bipartisan pathway to reform. The Bipartisan Policy Center's final June 2009 report, *Crossing Our Lines: Working Together to Reform the U.S. Health System*,[13] found agreement on four key policy areas, most of which found their way into the final ACA. They were preserving and improving quality and value, increasing access to health insurance in a reformed market, promoting individual responsibility, and securing adequate financing. As with the Health Reform Dialogue, there was common ground on key transformation issues and nonagreement on the hot-button controversies.

Between 2007 and mid-2009, much creative, constructive activity got done and helped to mask some high-profile disagreements. The glass was about three-quarters filled; it wasn't until legislation hit the street that the world began to focus on the unfilled quarter.

THE PRESIDENTIAL CAMPAIGN

On health reform, former North Carolina senator and 2004 Democratic vice-presidential nominee John Edwards went first. In February 2007, well before personal scandals eviscerated his reputation, Edwards put forward a bold, comprehensive plan promising universal coverage backed by an individual mandate and a public-plan option, a mandate on employers to cover their workers, and reforms to improve the quality and delivery of medical care. *New York Times* columnist Paul Krugman saluted: "So this is a smart, serious proposal. It addresses both the problem of the uninsured and the waste and inefficiency of our fragmented insurance system. And every candidate should be pressed to come up with something comparable."[14] In the Democratic primary field, the race was on to advance bold and systemic reform.

Because of her unprecedented health reform role as first lady in 1993–94, expectations were high for an audacious and far-reaching plan from the Democratic front-runner, Hillary Clinton. Before settling on one policy, she and her advisors explored alternatives, including health systems in Australia and Switzerland, Senator Ron Wyden's Healthy Americans Act, and more. She embraced the reform proposal developed by the progressive Center for American Progress. "It was always clear we were doing an individual mandate," said one former staffer.

Clinton announced her agenda in three speeches in the summer of 2007, first controlling costs, then improving quality, and finally, guaranteeing universal coverage, the last in mid-September. Her plan, resembling

Edwards's proposal with an individual mandate, received warm praise from Democrats and gave her a boost in Iowa polls. She emphasized what became a Democratic refrain—"If you like the coverage you have, you can keep it." She proposed to pay for the plan, in small part, by taxing the health benefits of those making more than $250,000 a year. She included a tax credit for small businesses, an idea borrowed from Senator Richard Durbin's (D-IL) small business health insurance legislation. She had a fine debate performance in Philadelphia on October 30 until she stumbled badly in response to a question about driver's licenses and undocumented immigrants. Preparing for the next debate in Las Vegas on November 15, she and staffers strategized to put Obama on the defense by attacking his perceived weakness, health care.

Obama released his health plan in late May 2007, months before Clinton, and it fit closely with the Edwards and Clinton positions on expanding coverage, reforming insurance markets, revamping medical care, and promoting prevention and wellness. Two elements stood apart. First, he rejected an individual mandate on adults, favoring one on parents to cover their children. David Plouffe, Obama's campaign manager, writes that the choice was Obama's and contrary to his advisors' advice. He quotes his boss:

> I reject the notion that there are millions of Americans walking around out there who don't want health coverage. They want it but can't afford it. Let's attack costs from every angle, provide incentives for small businesses and families to allow them to provide and buy coverage. I am not opposed to a mandate philosophically. But I don't think we should start there. It could be a recourse if coverage goals aren't being met after a period.[15]

Second, he promised that "the Obama plan will save a typical American family up to $2,500 every year on medical expenditures."[16] The savings would be achieved through investments in information technology, improving the prevention and management of chronic conditions, increasing insurance industry competition and reducing underwriting costs and profits, providing reinsurance for catastrophic conditions, and making health insurance universal. "What we're trying to do," Obama advisor and Harvard economist David Cutler explained, "is to find a way to talk to people in a way they understand."[17] He explained that the $2,500 represented an average family's share of savings in a pie that included the employer's share, plus savings to Medicare and Medicaid, creating a cloudier picture than the specific number implied. While the $2,500 commitment would emerge periodically, it never became a front-burner issue in the primary or general elections. Not so for the individual mandate, which became a heated source of contention once the Democratic primary field had shrunk to Obama and Clinton. An Obama television ad charged:

> Hillary Clinton's attacking, but what's she not telling you about her health care plan? It forces everyone to buy insurance, even if you can't afford it, and you pay a penalty if you don't.[18]

His campaign sent mailings with the same message, provoking Clinton to exclaim at one campaign stop, "Shame on you, Barack Obama!" She then added, "Meet me in Ohio. Let's have a debate about your tactics and your behavior in this campaign."[19]

Obama campaign staff opinions differ regarding the candidate's position on the individual mandate after the primary season concluded in early June. Some believe he knew an individual mandate would eventually become a part of his reform agenda. Others suggest he maintained personal opposition to a mandate throughout the fall campaign. The issue subsided from public view because he and Republican candidate John McCain held the same view. Tom Daschle, Obama's first pick as Health and Human Services secretary, got the first indication of a softening on December 11: "To my pleasant surprise, the president-elect told us, for the first time, that he might be willing to reconsider his thinking on two of the strongest stands he had taken during the campaign: his opposition to requiring everyone to get health insurance, and his refusal to consider any taxation of health care benefits."[20] Obama's first public indication of a changed stance on the individual mandate came in a July 17, 2009, interview with CBS News: "I am now in favor of some sort of individual mandate as long as there's a hardship exemption."[21]

In the summer of 2008, Obama's campaign began preparing for the general election campaign with new personnel, including Clinton campaign veterans. At a meeting on July 2, polling was presented showing Obama and McCain neck and neck. Polling also showed the public's desire for health care reform was murky. A consensus began to form in the room not to emphasize health reform in the fall campaign. Obama himself put the brakes on backing away. "Look," he said, "I want to do health care my first year I'm if lucky enough to be president, and your job is to figure out how to win the issue, and we're going to do it."[22]

A different health policy issue came to the fore in the general election—McCain's proposal to finance his coverage-expansion plan by taxing employer health insurance. The exclusion of employer-provided health insurance from workers' taxable wages is a cherished target of economists, liberal to conservative, as a financing source to pay for universal health insurance and to achieve greater value in the health system. Congress's Joint Committee on Taxation estimated the deduction's cost at $246.1 billion in 2007, making it the single largest federal tax expenditure and the fastest growing.[23] Just cutting it by half could finance robust universal coverage for all uninsured Americans. Harvard health economist Katherine Baicker expressed a prevalent view of economists in testimony before the Senate Finance Committee:

> Most economists would agree that our current tax treatment of health insurance is an important part of the problem, and that reforming that system would be a key component of a broader solution.[24]

More influential than the economists, though, are America's corporate and organized labor communities, rarely on the same side, but united in their opposition to altering the tax exclusion. Corporations do not want to forfeit a key employee benefit, and unions believe their working-class members would be most harmed by elimination or limitation of the exclusion. They were united with the Obama campaign in strident opposition to McCain's plan, which had been crafted by his campaign policy chief and former Congressional Budget Office director Douglas Holtz-Eakin. McCain's plan would have eliminated the exclusion to help finance new $2,500 and $5,000 tax credits for individuals and families to pay for health insurance and would have left existing health insurance markets unreformed without eliminating preexisting-condition exclusions—a basic element in all Democratic plans. It was the proposal to tax health insurance that got the most traction for Obama, and his campaign spent $100 million in ads attacking McCain for the proposal. While the impact of the issue on Obama's dramatic November 4 election is not clear, there is no doubt Obama won the argument with the American people.

Obama's advertising had an impact. A December 2008 poll by the Kaiser Family Foundation found that 73 percent of Americans opposed "taxing all workers with health care benefits."[25] McCain was not the only one who found himself on the wrong side of public opinion on this. Senator Ron Wyden (D-OR) used the exclusion as a major financing source for his "Healthy Americans Act." More importantly, Senator Max Baucus (D-MT), chair of the Senate Finance Committee and one of the biggest boosters of health reform on Capitol Hill, had targeted changes to the tax exclusion as a key financing source for his developing health reform plan. As with the individual mandate, more than a few observers prayed that the new president would change his mind about using the tax exclusion to pay for part of health reform.

Those decisions were for the future. A new president would take office in January 2009 with an electoral mandate and a personal commitment to universal coverage and health reform. The health care stakeholder community was mostly on board, enthusiastically so. A host of 1993–94 veterans was ready to try again, this time determined to get it right because the opportunity would not come again. Democrats had picked up sizable majorities in the House and Senate (looking like fifty-eight or fifty-nine, not sixty). The House and Senate were getting ready.

4. Political Will II— A Health Reform Campaign

Knowledge and strategy would not have led to the Affordable Care Act's passage without the third ingredient, political will—the commitment by political leaders to do what is needed to achieve success. In Washington DC, political will was on display in abundance throughout the process in the White House, the Senate, and the House, for and against passage. It mattered early, it mattered during the process, and in the end, it was indispensable.

THE SENATE MOVES FIRST

In the U.S. Senate, at the start, two figures dominated and used their positions to place health care front and center early, Senator Max Baucus, a moderate Democrat from Montana and the chair of the Senate Finance Committee, and Senator Edward M. Kennedy, a liberal Democrat from Massachusetts and the chair of the Senate Committee on Health, Education, Labor and Pensions (HELP).

If there is an official start date for congressional consideration of health reform, it was June 16, 2008, the day Senators Baucus and Charles Grassley (R-IA) hosted Prepare to Launch: Health Reform Summit 2008 at the Library of Congress on Capitol Hill for 250 congressional members, staffers, and invited outsiders. The session mattered because Baucus's committee holds jurisdiction over Medicare, Medicaid, tax policy, and a lot more, making its deliberations crucial to health reform's success or failure in the Senate. Baucus started the daylong event with a video clip of a countdown leading to a rocket launch. "This will succeed only if we work together and work outside the box, putting political differences aside," he stated. He declared that consensus already existed on six points: covering everyone, revamping payments to reward quality, emphasizing prevention and wellness, expanding health information technology, promoting comparative effectiveness research, and creating an effective pooling of insurance risk.

Grassley, his friend, ally, and the ranking Finance Committee Republican, was also upbeat. "Health care is the number one economic issue in our country, and will be the number one political issue." It will take "real courage," he cautioned, and "compromise." Federal Reserve Board chair Ben Bernanke provided a sense of economic urgency, noting that the share of the federal budget devoted to Medicare and Medicaid had grown from 6 percent in 1975 to 23 percent in 2008 and was heading toward 35 percent by 2025 unless big changes were made.

After a day of presentations and panels, sixteen senators from both parties sat around an open square table talking candidly and openly about the prospects for reform. Though there were no surprises, the mood was upbeat, exemplified by Senator Kent Conrad's (D-ND) comment: "When I came here twenty-two years ago, this is what I thought the United States Senate would be like. . . . I thought the biggest surprise to me was how consistent the recommendations were." Senator Kay Bailey Hutchinson (R-TX) noted, "We all agree . . . doing nothing is not an option." Senator Robert Bennett (R-UT), cosponsor of Wyden's Healthy Americans Act, offered a view from his party: "I think, with a few diehard holdouts, just about every Republican is now willing to accept the idea that every American could be—should be insured."[1]

That day, the Senate seemed all systems go. And Baucus kept at it. As early as 2004, he had bewildered his staffers by talking about doing comprehensive reform, when he was in the minority, right after passage of the 2003 Medicare Modernization Act establishing the Medicare prescription drug program, which he was one of few senior Democratic leaders to support. Over the summer and fall of 2008 he held public hearings, consulted with groups, and insisted on meeting so often with his health staff, led by Liz Fowler, they often would roll their eyes and sigh. Eight days after Obama's election, he issued a health reform white paper on November 12, 2008, detailing his vision for health care reform, the first serious legislative document outlining comprehensive health reform goals and potential pathways to achieve them:

> The policies in this paper are designed so that after ten years the U.S. would spend no more on health care than is currently projected, but we would spend those resources more efficiently and would provide better-quality coverage to all Americans. . . . My door is open and I see partners with "can do" spirits and open minds. I believe—very

strongly—that every American has a right to high-quality health care through affordable, portable, meaningful health coverage. I believe that Americans cannot wait any longer.[2]

What a difference fifteen years seemed to make! Back in 1993–94, the Senate Finance Committee was chaired by New York Democrat Daniel P. Moynihan, a legendary intellect who openly disparaged the Clintons' health reform ambitions, promoting reform of the welfare system instead and worrying about the impact of health system changes on New York's academic teaching hospitals. Moynihan coyly planned to wait until the last moment to cut a deal with Senate Minority Leader Bob Dole (R-KS), but by the time he was ready, the political climate had pushed the Kansan away from the possibility of deal making.

Baucus determined to be different. Not a last-minute savior, he would be the upfront leader who would make it happen—in a bipartisan way. In 2008, it was hard to argue with his logic; few believed Democrats could win sixty Senate seats needed to break a filibuster without Republican crossover votes. The November 4 election seemed to seal the issue as Democrats won a fifty-eight to forty-one majority in the new Senate, with the Minnesota race between Republican incumbent Norm Coleman and Democratic challenger Al Franken heading into an unpredictable recount. Even a win there would leave Democrats one seat short; two members, Senators Kennedy and Robert Byrd (D-WV) were in ill health; and several Democratic Caucus members were considered unreliable on health reform, including Senator Ben Nelson (D-NE), who told leaders early, "You'll get five Republican votes before you get mine." Some Democrats even thought a fifty-eight or fifty-nine vote margin was preferable to sixty—a level triggering unrealistic expectations among the Democratic base.

In the U.S. Senate, the Finance Committee is the big kahuna. Control over money does that to a legislative panel, even when its authority must be shared with the Budget and Appropriations committees. In matters relating to health policy, though, Finance shared jurisdiction with Kennedy's HELP Committee, which had authority over nearly everything else health related, including the Centers for Disease Control and Prevention, the National Institutes of Health, the Food and Drug Administration, and a key law, the 1974 Employee Retirement Income Security Act (ERISA), which sets federal boundaries for employer-provided health insurance. Finance and HELP also share jurisdiction over some key laws, especially the 1996 Health Insurance Portability and Accountability Act (HIPAA), which sets federal standards for health insurance.

Kennedy had served as chair or ranking member of the HELP Committee since 1981—he called his decision that year to become the key Democrat on HELP (then called "Labor and Human Resources") rather than on the Judiciary Committee one of the most important of his legislative career. In 2009, Kennedy was one of three remaining senators who had served in 1965 when legislation creating Medicare and Medicaid had been enacted (the other two were Democrats Byrd and Daniel Inouye of Hawaii). In 1966, he helped to establish the first of a new breed of federally funded community health centers, starting at the Columbia Point housing project in Dorchester. In 1969, at the Boston University Medical Center, he made his first speech calling for national health insurance. He called universal coverage "the cause of my life" and relished the prospect of one more chance that would avoid the errors of 1993–94.

Baucus and Kennedy knew they needed each other, not just because of jurisdiction. Baucus was mistrusted by progressive Senate Democrats, and Kennedy could guarantee their support for almost any deal Baucus approved. Kennedy, by contrast, was not embraced by the moderate-conservatives in the caucus, who wanted Baucus to craft the deal. Together, they could be a powerful team.

On May 17, 2008, Kennedy suffered two seizures at his home in Hyannis Port, Massachusetts. Within days, he was diagnosed with a malignant brain tumor. After his physicians told him he had months to live, he assembled a team of family, friends, and medical experts to choose a different course to give him more time. On June 2, he underwent brain surgery at Duke University Medical Center. He instructed his Senate staff to let nothing slow down preparations for health reform, despite his illness.

To keep HELP in the game with the Finance Committee, and to garner support and momentum for reform, Kennedy's HELP staff, led by his longtime and trusted staff director Michael Myers, worked away from TV cameras. Throughout the summer and fall of 2008, the committee organized roundtables with stakeholders, including physicians, nurses, hospitals, consumers, business, labor unions, health reform coalitions, drug and device makers, think tanks, public health groups, and more. In early fall 2008 the staff launched meetings of stakeholders called the Workhorse Group to push hard for agreements as soon as possible. In a sign of how difficult consensus would be, the Workhorse Group never generated agreement on any specifics.

Before his illness, Kennedy had outlined key strategies he thought crucial for success. First, there should be one bill to serve as the template for all committees, Senate and House. Second, financing health reform needed to be done right away in the new president's budget proposal to be sent to Congress in February 2009 and should be part of the annual congressional budget resolution to be approved in April 2009, keeping open the possibility, if needed, to pass reform using budget reconciliation, which required only fifty-one rather than sixty votes to pass. Despite having used reconciliation themselves to pass prior major legislation, including major tax cuts during the Bush presidency, Republicans were openly furious with suggestions that reconciliation might be used to pass health reform. Third, Republicans needed to be brought on board as rapidly as possible.

Baucus organized the first bipartisan meeting of key senators to discuss reform on November 19, two weeks after the 2008 elections and shortly after the release of his white paper. They met in Senator Kennedy's new Capitol Hill hideaway, room 219, steps away from the Senate chamber, overlooking the Mall, and loaded with Kennedy family mementos, paintings, and photos. Joining Baucus and Kennedy were Senator Chris Dodd (D-CT), the number two Democrat on HELP, Kennedy's designated health reform point person in his absence, and close friend; Jay Rockefeller (D-WV), chair of the Finance Committee's Health Subcommittee; Charles Grassley (R-IA), the Senate Finance Committee's ranking Republican; and Mike Enzi (R-WY), the ranking HELP Republican. The number of participating senators expanded after the first meeting to eleven, hence becoming known as the "group of eleven" or G-11; added were Budget chair Kent Conrad (D-ND), Judd Gregg (R-NH), and Orrin Hatch (R-UT), as well as Majority Leader Harry Reid (D-NV) and Minority Leader Mitch McConnell (R-KY), neither of whom ever showed up, though their key staff always were there to observe.

A pattern emerged in G-11 meetings, late and slow to start, with senators chatting and relaxing before discussion began, sharing stories and information. Baucus would start, expressing hope for a joint statement of some kind. "We'll ask our staffs to explore agreements and disagreements. . . . We hope to have a pathway ready for members in January . . . and keep the White House involved." In every session, Republicans pressed Democrats to commit not to use budget reconciliation and to disavow any kind of public insurance option; Democrats demurred, though Baucus said: "I would hope not to use reconciliation." At the first meeting, a photo was taken of the smiling senators. It was left to staff to sort out and pick up the pieces.

It took time to assemble the first bipartisan meeting of Finance, HELP, and Budget staff to respond to the G-11 members' November 19 directive to prepare a January presentation on areas of agreement and disagreement. The first meeting happened December 3, 2008, and it wasn't small; at least thirty-five staffers were in the room, including Kate Leone and Megan Hauck, the key health staffers for Reid and McConnell, respectively. The meeting tensed as Hauck spoke early: "Look, we know you can do this without us. We can do it together, or we can be part of the loyal opposition. Before that, our members need to know your commitment and the process. We need a commitment—through conference—that you won't use budget reconciliation. We would rather have you break up earlier rather than later."

Democrat staffers, led by Baucus's Liz Fowler, kept trying to draw the conversation to substance, and Republicans, especially Grassley's Mark Hayes and Enzi's Chuck Clapton, kept bringing it back to process and preconditions. It quickly became apparent that these meetings were futile without an agreement on Republican procedural concerns. Democrats were neither able nor willing to unilaterally disavow a key parliamentary device such as reconciliation. Right away, a standstill emerged. Staffers managed to pull together four PowerPoint slides to show the members at their January meeting.

Here's what staffers from both parties agreed to say to the G-11 members on January 21, 2009, about covering all Americans:

- Providing quality, affordable health insurance coverage for all Americans is a bipartisan goal of health reform.
- Successful reform will require shared responsibility by individuals, employers, insurers, health care providers, and government.

    What is the appropriate responsibility of employers to maintain and improve the system?

    What is the responsibility of individuals, and should there be an individual mandate?

    What is the appropriate role for government in coverage reform (e.g., subsidies, public programs)?

- Successful reform will build on, not undermine, the employer-based system.

    How can employer-sponsored coverage be strengthened?

- Americans deserve choice in their selection of health insurance coverage, medical providers, and treatments.

    How can the individual and small-employer markets be reformed to provide better quality, affordable coverage?

What is an appropriate role for public programs in health reform?

How do we determine an appropriate level of coverage and care?

- Coverage reform will be achieved in a fiscally responsible fashion.

After a rambling conversation, Baucus called the session "a good start. We got off on the wrong foot on the SCHIP [the State Children's Health Insurance Program]. I don't want it to continue. We made a mistake on aliens against my better judgment. It poisoned the well in committee." He was referring to the unsuccessful efforts in 2007 and 2008 to reauthorize the State Children's Health Insurance Program (Republicans prefer to call it the *State* Children's Health Insurance Program or S-CHIP, and Democrats prefer *CHIP*, without the *S*). In 2009, Democrats wrote a bill to permit new legal immigrant children to enroll, in spite of strenuous Republican objections. Grassley replied: "Obviously it has not damaged our relationship, or I wouldn't be here. We can talk things out."

Kennedy's heady hopes for a fast and bipartisan start in January came to naught. The sides were not ready, and other pressing issues, such as the collapsing economy, took precedence.

THE HOUSE FINDS ITS FOOTING

The House of Representatives approached health reform more cautiously than did the Senate. Conversations in 2008 with House members and staffers gave mixed signals: *Of course we want to work on this . . . We have to figure out how to do the CHIP reauthorization first . . . We should wait to see what the Obama administration puts on the table.* These were not signs of where the House would end up, only where they began. From Speaker Nancy Pelosi (D-CA) to committee and subcommittee chairs to rank-and-file members and to many staffers, House Democrats had an unquenchable passion for progressive health policy. Nearly eighty members, all Democrats, counted themselves public supporters of a government-run single-payer health system (compared with a half dozen or so in the Senate). The remainder of the caucus had many fervent health reformers with multiple shades of opinion. The Republican Caucus, as well, had members who regarded themselves as specialists in federal health policy reform. Unlike the Senate, though, the culture in the House of Representatives had been far more partisan since 1994—with little genuine collaboration beyond what was necessary.

Among the House health reform advocates, foremost was John Dingell (D-MI), eighty-two years old in 2008, history's longest-serving member and a longtime supporter of national health reform—a position he inherited from his father, also a Michigan congressman, who was the lead House sponsor both of President Harry Truman's health reform plan and of the first bill to establish national health insurance for seniors. Dingell chaired the crucial House Energy and Commerce Committee. Despite his earnest efforts, he had been unable in 1993–94 to bring his large, unwieldy committee to a majority vote on any health reform bill. He showed his renewed passion at a health reform event sponsored by Families USA at the Democratic National Convention in Denver in August 2008. Quoting Alexander Solzhenitsyn, he said, "A man ought not to die like a dog in a ditch." He saw a difference from last time: "The number of opponents has declined but their viciousness has increased." Looking ahead to Obama's first hundred days, he promised: "We're going to make it happen. There are lots of bills pending." He recalled a statement by former Chinese premier Deng Xiaoping: "I don't care if it's a white cat or a black cat; it's a good cat as long as it catches mice." His conclusion: "I will do my best. . . . I'm ready to work my heart out."

Dingell's committee considered much legislation important to the business community beyond health policy, and he encouraged centrist and conservative Democrats to join, especially those who shared his pro-auto-industry environmental views. Because of this, the Energy and Commerce Committee leaned further to the right than the leadership-heavy House Committee on Ways and Means, chaired by Charles Rangel (D-NY), or the more progressive Committee on Education and Labor, chaired by George Miller (D-CA), one of Speaker Nancy Pelosi's closest friends. These were the three House committees that shared jurisdiction on health reform.

An internal Democratic fight over the chairmanship of Energy and Commerce became the first health reform skirmish of the 111th Congress. Second in committee seniority was Henry Waxman (D-CA), then chair of the House Oversight and Government Reform Committee. In November 2008 Waxman announced he would challenge Dingell for the chairmanship of Energy and Commerce. More than health care was at stake—even more contentious was potential climate-change legislation, where the Dingell/Waxman differences were sharp. Pelosi took no public position but privately worked through George Miller on Waxman's behalf. Waxman won a 137–122 secret vote of House Democrats on November 20, 2008.

Many Democratic Senate health staffers felt badly on a personal level for Dingell but thought Waxman would be a more effective committee and House leader on health reform. Waxman had long-serving health staffers, led by Karen Nelson, who were recognized as some of the smartest and most effective staffers on Capitol Hill.

Before health reform, there were other urgent matters to address. First was the deepening international economic crisis that exploded in September with the collapse of the Lehman Brothers firm on Wall Street. In early December 2008, President-elect Obama, Majority Leader Reid, and Speaker Pelosi agreed that an economic stimulus package was needed quickly, in the neighborhood of $500 billion over two years to shock and stimulate the economy away from a looming depression. The legislation would not be financed with new taxes or spending cuts, meaning the so-called pay-go rules would be suspended. Senate, House, and White House leaders also came to see stimulus legislation—known as ARRA, or the American Recovery and Reinvestment Act of 2009—as a way also to jump-start some key and less controversial elements of health reform. The final ARRA price tag was $787 billion, and $147.7 billion of that went to pay for health-related system investments and rescue items, the most important of which included:

- $86.6 billion to help cash-strapped states pay for their shares of Medicaid costs

- $24.7 billion to provide a 65 percent health insurance premium subsidy for the unemployed (known as COBRA subsidies, from the title of the act in which it was created)

- $19 billion to create a national health information technology infrastructure, including a reworking of federal privacy rules relating to the electronic exchange of health information

- $1.1 billion to research the comparative effectiveness of health care treatments

Baucus had suggested at his June 2008 health care summit that health information technology and comparative effectiveness research were two "consensus" matters that all parties agreed should be essential components of health reform legislation. After ARRA's passage, health information technology moved rapidly into deep implementation politics out of the public eye, and a complex and potentially contentious issue was taken off the health reform to-do list. Comparative effectiveness research, by contrast, needed more work in the health reform law and became embroiled in a heated controversy about "death panels" that emerged in the summer of 2009.

Even before the ARRA legislation was finished, the House and Senate completed action on reauthorizing the Children's Health Insurance Program, a key Democratic legislative priority in 2007 and 2008 stymied by President Bush's veto. Needing fewer Senate Republicans to win in early 2009, Democrats advanced a more progressive version than they had pushed in 2007 and 2008 and included expanded coverage for legally residing immigrant children and their parents. This provision had been kept out in 2007–08 to attract Republican support, and while its inclusion pleased the House Hispanic Caucus, it angered many earlier Republican supporters, especially Senator Grassley. The Children's Health Insurance Program Reauthorization Act (CHIPRA) was a proud early deliverable for the new president and the resurgent Democratic majorities in Congress.

In the 1993–94 Clinton health reform process, the three House committees with jurisdiction over health policy matters had been unable and unwilling to coordinate their legislative reform efforts, hindering the ability of the House to produce any health reform bill. Political commentators Haynes Johnson and David Broder described the frustrating situation:

> The president's most important policy initiative was hanging by a
> thread; a historic commitment of the Democratic Party was facing
> imminent defeat; and election disaster was looming. And for almost
> an entire month, committee chairmen and staffers on Ways and
> Means, Energy and Commerce, and Education and Labor used every
> weapon they could find to stake out the widest possible jurisdictions
> for themselves to maintain *future* control of a program that might not
> even pass.[3]

According to key House Democratic staffers, the three committees never made an explicit decision in 2009 to collaborate. It just happened. Tri-Comm, as the three-committee effort became called, started with the reauthorization of the Children's Health Insurance Program in January, went on to the stimulus legislation (ARRA) approved in February, and then moved seamlessly into health reform. As they deepened their work, staffers produced their own black designer tote bags to lug volumes of paperwork from meeting to meeting. The process (as well as the bags) was labeled "Tri-Comm 2009" and was led by veteran staffers Karen Nelson from Energy and Commerce, Cybele Bjorklund from Ways and Means, and Michele Varnhagen from Education and Labor.

When it became clear that the Obama administration would not send a national health reform bill to Congress, the House Committee effort that began with ARRA continued and solidified. The three committee staffs began working on reform right after President Obama signed ARRA into law on February 17, 2009. Multiple sets of meetings every week involved all relevant House staffers, and once a week the meetings involved the three committee and relevant subcommittee chairs. On the night of March 21, 2010, when the House passed the health reform bill, Representative Charles Rangel—Ways and Means chair until his resignation as chair earlier that month—observed, "the word *jurisdiction* was never spoken."[4] House Leaders and key staffers knew that success would require a radically different process from the 1993–94 effort, and they put it in place. It was one of the most tangible lessons from the Clinton failure and a good example of how Congress acted to avoid a repeat.

THE OBAMA ADMINISTRATION MOVES IN

On December 11, 2008, former Senate majority leader Tom Daschle was nominated as President-elect Barack Obama's unsurprising choice to head both the Department of Health and Human Services (DHHS) and the White House Office of Health Reform, with policy expert Jeanne Lambrew as his health reform deputy. In 2008, Daschle and Lambrew cowrote a health reform book—*Critical: What We Can Do about the Health-Care Crisis*—a blueprint for Daschle's ideas, including his big one, a proposal to establish a Federal Health Board, a kind of Federal Reserve for the health system. Combining the two positions in Daschle's hands struck many as another sign of Democrats acting to avoid a repeat of the 1993–94 mistakes, in this instance to avoid the schism between the DHHS and the White House Health Reform Office that had occurred earlier. Daschle had become personally close to Obama, another good sign to keep reform on track. On January 8, the Senate HELP Committee held a laudatory hearing, chaired by Kennedy, at which Daschle's confirmation was considered a sure bet—former Senate majority leader Bob Dole testified to endorse his former colleague.

On February 3, 2009, Daschle withdrew his name from consideration for either position after revelations emerged about personal tax problems that required him to pay the federal government $140,000 in back taxes and interest. It was not until March 2 that Obama nominated another candidate, Kansas Democratic governor Kathleen Sebelius, who waited until April 28 for Senate confirmation. Obama also named former Clinton administration health official Nancy-Ann DeParle as his new White House health care advisor, a position not requiring Senate approval. If reformers needed a reminder that the road to reform would be unpredictable and rocky, this filled the bill.

Daschle's problems exploded as a difference of opinion emerged in the White House among senior Obama advisors on the scope of health reform to be pursued. Vice President Joe Biden, Chief of Staff Rahm Emanuel, and Senior Advisor David Axelrod were joined by skeptics on the president's economic team who believed a drive for comprehensive reform was doomed to replay the calamitous consequences of the Clinton fiasco and would distract the administration from working on fixing the economy. For Emanuel, it was not abstract—he had served as a key political aide in the Clinton White House and witnessed the results of health reform overreaching. With Daschle gone from the scene, there was no effective counterweight, except the president himself. In February 2009, for the second time—the first was in July 2008 after the Democratic primary season—Obama declared comprehensive health reform a top administration priority, overruling his key aides.

On February 23, the president hosted a White House "Fiscal Responsibility Summit" providing a public demonstration that any reported rift between health care and economic policy was false. Office of Management and Budget director Peter Orszag made the case:

> So, to my fellow budget hawks in this room and in the rest of the country, let me be very clear: Health care reform is entitlement reform. The path to fiscal responsibility must run directly through health care. We also must recognize that reforms to Medicare and Medicaid will only succeed in the context of slowing the overall growth rate of health care costs. Improving the efficiency of the health system so that we get better results for less money is therefore not just or even primarily a budget issue. It would also provide direct help to struggling families, since health care costs are reducing worker's take-home pay to a degree that is both underappreciated and unnecessarily large. And for many states, health care is increasingly crowding out other priorities like higher education, which, in turn, is leading to higher tuition and painful cutbacks at state universities. All of this is why the president has said, time and again, that he is committed to reforming the health system this year.[5]

A few days later, on February 26, Obama showed he meant it when Congress and the public saw his initial fiscal year 2010 budget proposal to Congress, which included a ten-year $634 billion reserve fund as a "down payment" on financing health reform. White House officials said the $634 billion would be about half the cost of an estimated $1.2 trillion price tag over ten years. His proposal would cap itemized deductions for the wealthiest Americans, lower Medicare payments to private Medicare Advantage insurance plans, raise premiums for higher-income Medicare drug plan enrollees, and more. Although the idea to cap deductions was shot down on Capitol Hill at the speed of sound, the other proposals found their way into the final version of the ACA. Obama's larger purpose was to demonstrate a public and tangible commitment to pay for reform and a willingness to take criticism for putting real ideas on the table. Though he would not file his own bill, he showed an early, meaningful commitment to get reform done. This was more than lip service.

Obama put his next public foot forward on March 5, 2009, hosting a White House health reform summit for about 150 lawmakers (from both parties), patients, physicians, nurses, and health industry leaders. His message was clear: "The status quo is the one option that is not on the table." At the final session, Senator Kennedy made an emotional and surprise appearance, wowing the audience and declaring himself a "foot soldier" in the drive for universal coverage. "This time we will not fail," he assured the audience.

Seated in the room were many power brokers whose participation meant the difference between success and failure. One of them, labor leader Dennis Rivera of the Service Employees International Union (SEIU), began conversations with Jay Gellert of the managed care company Health Net and George Halvorson of the Kaiser Foundation Health Plan on what the health industry could do together to restrain rising health care costs. Karen Ignagni, from America's Health Insurance Plans (AHIP), joined the process, as did Pfizer chief Jeff Kindler, David Nexon of the medical-device trade group AdvaMed, and Richard Umbdenstock of the American Hospital Association (AHA). Nancy-Ann DeParle, from the White House, persuaded the American Medical Association to participate. To avoid publicity, they met at a local hotel and not at the White House, with some administration officials making cameo appearances for encouragement.

Key health industry leaders representing AdvaMed, AHIP, AHA, AMA, the Pharmaceutical Research and Manufacturers of America (PhRMA), and SEIU gathered at the White House on May 11, 2009, for an announcement of their breakthrough: "Over the next 10 years—from 2010 to 2019—they are pledging to cut the rate of growth of national health care spending by . . . over $2 trillion," President Obama declared.[6] Afterward, the industry leaders emphasized the wording of their letter: "We will do our part to achieve your administration's goal of decreasing by 1.5 percentage points the annual health care spending growth rate—saving $2 trillion or more."

AGREEMENTS, DEALS, AND LACK THEREOF

Max Baucus was pleased and perplexed to see deal making on health reform financing done by the White House without him. "If you've got savings," he told the six groups shortly after their announcement, "I want them." Baucus's health team, led by Liz Fowler, an attorney with a PhD and lengthy Capitol Hill experience, had already been analyzing the economic performance of all health industry sectors to evaluate how much each could be pressed to contribute to paying for reform; in 2009, she hired a former Wall Street analyst, Tony Clapsis, to perform detailed financial analyses of each sector. Finance Committee staffers—sometimes with White House participation and sometimes without—began meetings with drug companies, insurers, hospitals, device makers, home health companies, hospices, and others to hammer out detailed concessions from each industry to pay for as much of the health reform tab as possible. All participants rejected the word *deal* to describe their deals.

The first, with PhRMA, announced on June 20, 2009, also was the most controversial. The White House, Team Baucus, Team Kennedy, and the drug industry all wanted to avoid a replay of 1993–94, when drug companies spent millions for a fierce anti-reform advertising assault. Not involved or invited to the discussions was the House of Representatives, whose leaders wanted price controls and other drug company requirements that would have been deal breakers. The industry originally offered $45 billion to $50 billion in savings over ten years while DeParle for the White House suggested $120 billion. In the agreement, the industry ceded $80 billion over ten years in rebates, assessments, and contributions and in return got commitments from the administration and Baucus to resist measures opposed by the industry, such as permitting reimportation of drugs from outside the U.S. The deal and the negotiators came under quick attack from numerous quarters, including the House leadership, who demanded details. Critics contrasted the behind-closed-doors negotiations with candidate Obama's commitment to broadcast health reform negotiations live on C-SPAN. Even the White House pulled back, referencing an agreement "reached between Senator Max Baucus and the nation's pharmaceutical companies." It was not until early August that the administration acknowledged its role in the negotiations.[7] Around the same time in early August, the industry announced plans for a $150 million advertising campaign to support reform.

Though critics on the right and the left used the agreement as an easy target just as congressional committees were beginning to debate proposed health reform legislation, the deal turned a potentially fatal reform opponent into a crucial reform supporter. Given the slender margin by which the final ACA was approved in March 2010, it is hard to imagine a successful legislative outcome had the pharmaceutical industry been on the other side. Some questioned the value of the industry's bland pro-reform advertising campaign, though few doubted the industry's potential as a full-throated adversary.

The second agreement, announced on July 8, 2009, by Vice President Joe Biden, involved $155 billion in Medicare and Medicaid payment reductions to hospitals over ten years. The American Hospital Association, the Federation of American Hospitals, and the Catholic Health Association were the industry parties. AHA is the United Nations of U.S. hospitals and had an automatic seat; FAH was headed by Chip Kahn, a former high-level Republican congressional staffer and former insurance industry lobbyist (he was a seasoned dealmaker and Democrats appreciated the symbolism of having him on their side); the Catholics were the firmest reform supporters of any hospital industry group, for reasons of faith more than dollars and cents. The industry, Team Baucus, and administration leaders met at least ten times, in Baucus's and other Senate Finance offices and in the White House Roosevelt Room. At White House sessions, Chief of Staff Rahm Emanuel and others would drop by or wander through.

The hospitals had done financial modeling and concluded that if the percentage of insurance coverage for all Americans could grow from the current 83 percent level to 95 percent, then hospitals could withstand Medicare payment reductions because revenues generated by the expanded coverage would exceed the losses. The White House thought new revenues would exceed $250 billion over ten years, Senate Finance modelers thought about $200 billion, and hospitals pegged the number at $170 billion. All sides agreed on reductions of $155 billion as long as coverage would reach the 95 percent threshold as determined by the Congressional Budget Office (CBO). Thus, 95 percent became the overarching target in writing the coverage titles of the legislation (Titles I and II). Then all sides had to agree on how to achieve $155 billion. In spite of hopes for cutting-edge delivery-system reforms, about two-thirds of the savings came from straight rate reductions; savings from reforms such as reducing preventable readmissions and hospital acquired infections were small. Negotiations were rocky until the final hours, and Baucus's OK was uncertain. He never showed up at the July 8 announcement with the vice president and hospital leaders. No matter, the deal was done and hospitals, a huge player, were on board.

The medical-device industry was less experienced in high-stakes negotiations than hospitals and drug companies. Its trade association, AdvaMed, had signed the $2 trillion letter to be helpful. Its savings ideas—working with the AMA to reduce overused procedures and improving the design of devices to reduce errors—scored no savings. Baucus's staff proposed $60 billion in ten-year savings or payments. The industry's position was zero, countering that they would end up absorbing the impact of cuts to their primary customers—hospitals, nursing homes, labs, and physicians providing imaging services—through increasing price pressures and reduced demand. While a few companies were willing to support some assessment, the industry as a whole strongly resisted any industry-specific tax. Industry leaders also believed the Finance Committee's bipartisan Gang of Six (Baucus, Grassley, Kent Conrad, Jeff Bingaman, Mike Enzi, and Olympia Snowe) would veto a fee because both Grassley and Enzi were opposed. When the Gang's talks ended in mid-September without resolution, Baucus recommended $40 billion in industry assessments. In the November-December negotiations among Democrats on a final Senate bill, the assessment dropped to $20 billion as a concession to Senators Evan Bayh (D-IN) and Amy Klobuchar (D-MN), who demanded the reduction as a condition for their votes.

Discussions between the Senate and the insurance industry proceeded without White House participation. Though the industry is perceived as a monolith, its players are diverse, reflected in the widely varying effects that different kinds of cuts and savings would have on different companies, and making negotiations difficult. Some thought failure was inevitable: "Karen [Ignagni, of America's Health Insurance Plans] was never going to get the negotiation she wanted. The Democrats understood there had to be a villain here. From a populist standpoint, you can't not have them as a villain, unless you've got real bipartisanship. I don't think it was ever possible," concluded one source. The industry proposed administrative simplification as a way to save dollars, but the CBO said such measures would not produce scorable federal budget savings, so that didn't help. AHIP was prepared to negotiate as much as $80 billion in Medicare Advantage reductions, but Finance Committee staffers wanted at least parity with savings agreed to by the hospital industry, $155 billion. By late July, the parties stopped meeting. Attacks on the insurance industry by House and White House leaders were escalating. In August, with funds from large insurers, including Aetna, CIGNA, Humana, UnitedHealthcare, and WellPoint, AHIP began secretly funneling financial support to the U.S. Chamber of Commerce to bankroll its major advertising campaign against reform, done in the name of small business. In all, AHIP gave $86.2 million to the Chamber, well more than half the business group's available money to attack the Democrats' reform agenda.[8] Within five days in October, AHIP, the Blue Cross and Blue Shield Association, and insurance giant WellPoint—the most antagonistic of the largest companies to reform— each released actuarial studies claiming huge premium increases resulting from the pending Senate Finance health reform bill. From then on, any collaboration with insurers was off, and so were the gloves.

REPUBLICANS—CURRENT AND FORMER

On April 28, 2009, Republican senator Arlen Specter from Pennsylvania shocked the nation by announcing he was switching to the Democratic Party to keep alive his 2010 reelection hopes. Suddenly, a sixty-vote Democratic Senate majority was not only reachable but certain—Minnesota Senate contender Al Franken had been certified as the winner in his razor-thin win over Republican Norm Coleman in January and March—only a final decision by the state's Supreme Court remained (it came on June 30). Most Senate Democrats said they still wanted a bipartisan health bill, but after April 28, they no longer needed one.

By spring 2009, Senate Democrats and Republicans interested in health reform had spent lots of time romancing each other. Baucus and Grassley had cohosted the health reform summit in June 2008; their respective health policy staffers worked together, met with stakeholders together, shared drafts and more under the assumption that they were in this together; indeed, Grassley's team authored many provisions that remained in the final ACA, such as the Physician Payments Sunshine Act in Title VI. Senate Finance and HELP Committee hearings showed both policy disagreements and a continuing desire for bipartisanship. Kennedy and Orrin Hatch (R-UT) talked regularly by phone. Ron Wyden (D-OR) had lured eight Republicans as cosponsors of his Healthy Americans Act. Beginning in November 2008, the bipartisan group of key senators and staff known as G-11 began meeting regularly to figure out how to move from talk to action.

Things began getting in the way. In the Senate, Republicans insisted on guarantees that Democrats would not use budget reconciliation rules to pass health reform with fifty-one votes—something Democrats said they did not want to do, and would not do unless faced with Republican obstruction. The disagreement was never settled. In January 2009, Democrats moved ahead with the Children's Health Insurance Program Reauthorization Act (CHIPRA), signed into law by President Obama on February 4,

2009. The inclusion of coverage for legally residing immigrant children and their parents angered Republicans, especially Grassley, who had supported the Democratic bill in 2007 and 2008 against their own party's president.

In December 2008, Senate and House Democrats began working with the Obama transition team to write a large spending package to stimulate the nation's economy away from the feared depression. The final legislation (ARRA, the American Recovery and Reinvestment Act) included $787 billion in spending and tax cuts ($285 billion), came on the heels of the controversial 2008 bill to rescue the nation's banking industry, and was approved with zero Republican votes in the House and three in the Senate (one belonging to Specter). As partisan recriminations volleyed back and forth, prospects for bipartisanship began to evaporate, and Republicans proved they could hold their beleaguered minority together. That was the public and the private message of Mitch McConnell and John Boehner, the respective Senate and House minority leaders.

In April 2009, Republican communications and message impresario Frank Luntz distributed a twenty-eight-page memo outlining suggested words and themes Republicans should use to stand their ground in the coming health care debate. Here is a sample:

WORDS THAT WORK: THE PERFECT PLATFORM FOR
HEALTHCARE REFORM

As a matter of **principle**, Republicans are firmly **committed** to providing **genuine** access to **affordable, quality** healthcare for **every**
American. The time has come to create a **balanced, common sense**
approach that will **guarantee** that Americans can receive **the care
they deserve** and **protect** the **sacred doctor-patient relationship**. We
will oppose any **politician-run system** that **denies you the treatments
you need, when you need them.**"[9]

In the House, the stimulus experience was a continuation of a fifteen-year hyperpartisan environment. House leaders on both sides of the aisle readied for health reform in separate camps, convinced from the start that bipartisan agreement was inconceivable. In the Senate Finance Committee, the Baucus and Grassley teams worked collaboratively to ready their bipartisan effort, believing it would succeed and trump all other efforts.

In the Senate HELP Committee, there also was a history of bipartisan bills engineered by the acknowledged master, Senator Kennedy. Without his daily and fully engaged presence, the committee members taking leadership roles—Chris Dodd (D-CT), Tom Harkin (D-IA), Barbara Mikulski (D-MD), Jeff Bingaman (D-NM), and Patty Murray (D-WA)—could not replicate his magic. At the staff level, dozens of bipartisan meetings on coverage, delivery-system reform, and prevention were held between March and May of 2009. To Republican staffers, it seemed Democrats were going through the motions for appearance's sake; to Democratic staffers, it seemed Republicans did not have a coherent stance and could not agree to anything. Kennedy had wanted a health reform bill ready for the day after President Obama's inauguration, followed by a multicity presidential tour. The economy, CHIP, stimulus, and the budget got in the way—and Kennedy kept pushing for action. By May, the bipartisan staff meetings petered out as HELP Democratic members and staff, led by health policy director David Bowen, focused on writing and readying their own bill. Moving a bill early was a critical lesson Democrats took from the 1993–94 failure and time was believed to be running out. .

The so-called G-11 bipartisan meetings of senior senators continued through the spring without any decisions of consequence. Once HELP Committee Democrats began writing their bill, Baucus reconstituted G-11 as a purely Senate Finance group comprising himself, Jeff Bingaman, Kent Conrad, Mike Enzi, Charles Grassley, Orrin Hatch, and Olympia Snowe, the moderate Republican from Maine. The group again became a Gang of Six on July 22, 2009, when Hatch decided he had had enough and announced his withdrawal: "Some of the things they're talking about, I just cannot support. So I don't want to mislead anybody," he told reporters.[10]

No matter, assumed Baucus, as long as he held on to his key partner, Grassley, who stated on June 14, 2009, on Fox News his views on an individual mandate: "When it comes to states requiring it for automobile insurance, the principle then ought to lie the same way for health insurance, because everybody has some health insurance costs, and if you aren't insured, there's no free lunch. Somebody else is paying for it. So I think individual mandates are more apt to be accepted by a vast majority of people in Congress."[11] Three months later in September, his views had shifted: "Individuals should maintain the freedom to choose whether to purchase health insurance coverage or not."[12] What happened? Many cite the angry town meetings in August where conservatives calling themselves tea party activists dominated more than forty sessions that Grassley had attended across Iowa. Some suggest he feared a primary challenge from the right in his 2010 election campaign. Others believe pressure from party leaders Mitch McConnell and Jon Kyl (R-AZ) was critical. Others suggest he just got increasingly uncomfortable with the direction and cost of the emerging plan—all three Republican "Gang members" were uncomfortable with the proposed new fees on drug and medical-device makers as well as on insurance companies. They also doubted Baucus's ability to defend any deal they might negotiate as pressure from progressive Democrats would push the legislation to the left once it was out of the Finance Committee.

For a period, there was a split between a minority of Senate Republicans who wanted serious engagement and bipartisanship on health reform versus Republicans who believed Democratic overreaching on health care could produce a replay of the stunning Republican takeover of the House and Senate in November 1994 in the wake of the Clinton health reform collapse. In mid-July, South Carolina Republican senator Jim DeMint said on a widely reported conference call with conservative activists: "If we're able to stop Obama on this, it will be his Waterloo. It will break him."[13]

Between May and December 2009, the policy and political perspectives among Republicans merged. The last Republican moderate, Olympia Snowe, joined the opposition in early December. The policy-oriented Republicans concluded, as Hatch had done in July, that the Democrats' reform designs—with mandates on individuals, tax increases, plus new requirements on states and employers, Medicaid expansions, expensive subsidies—was a bridge too far for them and especially for the party's hardening base. The more politically oriented Republicans wondered what had taken them so long.

MARKUP MASH-UPS

In every one of the five congressional committees with health reform jurisdiction, staffers worked around the clock to draft legislation for the formal committee proceedings, called "markups," where any committee member could propose additions, deletions, and changes to the underlying bill. Months of expert advice, stakeholder input, member and staff requests, data analysis—it all boiled down to legislative language hammered out by the professional committee staff and their respective drafting experts from the Senate and House Legislative Counsel's Offices. Drafts were shared, torn apart, and redone, and redone, and redone. The revision process can go on forever, until the member in charge blows the whistle signaling time is up.

If there is a single image from the HELP Committee health reform markup process in the minds of Democratic staffers, it is this: twelve Democratic senators, all HELP Committee members with staff, about forty in all, crowded into Senator Kennedy's Capitol hideaway office, working their way through yet another health reform policy decision. Senator Chris Dodd, assuming the chair's role for his best friend in the Senate,

Ted Kennedy, gets a call on his BlackBerry cell phone. He retreats to the small side room, where Kennedy had a bed for rest. Some minutes later, he returns and resumes his chair duties with his upbeat manner, skillfully leading the meeting to a consensus. Only later did we learn the subject matter of the interruption—a family member had called with news that his sister was dying of cancer. Dodd had other troubles on his mind during the arduous five-week stretch of formal legislative markup proceedings—the longest markup of a bill in the committee's history and among the longest in the Senate's history. The committee Dodd actually chaired, Banking, had a white-hot financial regulatory reform agenda to address; Dodd was facing the bleakest election prospects of any sitting senator; and he was keeping to himself his own medical diagnosis of prostate cancer. Day after day after day, he sat through a determined campaign by Republican members to derail the bill and never stopped smiling and encouraging everyone to move forward.

The HELP markup lasted fifty-six hours, stretching across twenty-three sessions over thirteen days between Wednesday, June 17, and Wednesday, July 15. The proceedings were held in the historic, high-ceiling Russell Building Senate Caucus Room (renamed the "Kennedy Caucus Room" in September 2009), the scene of Senate hearings on the sinking of the *Titanic* (something Democrats were urged not to mention for fear of inspiring parallels), the announcement of the presidential candidacies of John and Robert Kennedy, the Senate Watergate hearings, the Supreme Court confirmation hearings of Clarence Thomas, and more. Of the 788 amendments submitted, three-quarters were filed by the ten Republican members. Senator Tom Coburn from Oklahoma, proud of his nickname, "Dr. No," filed 332 of them. In all, 287 amendments were formally considered, and 161 Republican amendments were adopted in whole or in revised form.

House Democratic leaders had insisted that at least one Senate committee begin markup before any of the three House committees did so, as a sign of seriousness and commitment. HELP was more ready than Finance, which was tied up in Gang of Six talks and stakeholder financial negotiations. Because of HELP's jurisdictional limits—the committee's bill could not touch Medicaid, Medicare, or taxes to pay for coverage expansions—the HELP proposal had big gaps that the Republicans exploited to characterize the bill as half baked. As the first health reform bill out of the box, a lot was in need of refinement as members, staff from both parties, experts, stakeholders, and others explored the bill for flaws and needed improvement. The legislation got its final vote on July 15 and survived the markup without serious damage and, most importantly, with all thirteen

Democrats united. Some votes on amendments were bipartisan—such as requiring members of Congress and their staffs to obtain health insurance through the new exchanges (called "gateways" in the HELP version). Most were party line, thirteen to ten—and the HELP Committee met its obligation to move a bill forward. As opposed to Baucus, who sought bipartisan agreement upfront, Kennedy and Dodd believed it was most important to create forward momentum and hope that deal making with Republicans would gel later. They moved it. As a result, health reform was no longer hypothetical—it was happening.

Two days after the HELP Committee began its markup, the chairmen of the three House committees unveiled their unified legislative health reform proposal. It was a full plan distinctly to the left of the Senate's direction—financed significantly with new taxes on millionaires and including a requirement on most employers to cover their workers or pay a hefty assessment to the federal government. It included a robust public-plan option to be offered in the new insurance exchange, which, unlike anything in the Senate versions, would be a single federal entity, not a state-by-state amalgam. The proposal emerged from an intense collaborative effort by members and staff of the three key House committees. The plan was for each committee to do its own separate markup, then to reconsolidate the three bills into one under the aegis of the House Rules Committee and then to bring the full reform package before the full House.

The liberal-dominated Education and Labor Committee, chaired by Pelosi ally George Miller (D-CA), went first, starting on the afternoon of July 15, just hours after the HELP Committee finished its marathon. They finished by Friday the 17th, approving twenty-one of forty-two amendments considered. One advanced by Dennis Kucinich (D-OH) would permit states to establish their own single-payer health systems; it passed twenty-seven to nineteen, with thirteen Republicans joining fourteen Democrats in support, mischief making by the minority. Next went the Committee on Ways and Means, chaired by Charles Rangel (D-NY), not nearly as liberal as Education and Labor, but heavily Democratic dominated. Ways and Means started on July 16 and finished on July 17, considering and defeating all twenty-three proposed amendments and approving the measure by a vote of twenty-three to eighteen.

The Energy and Commerce Committee's markup started the same day as Ways and Means. Similarities end there. On the committee were thirty-six Democrats, chaired by the canny Henry Waxman (D-CA), and twenty-three Republicans; Democrats could lose up to six votes and still prevail on any issue. The thirty-six Democrats included seven "Blue Dogs," a House caucus of fifty-four moderate to conservative Democrats who characterize themselves as committed to national and financial security and who prefer bipartisanship and compromise over ideology and party discipline. In May, two months before the July health reform markup, Waxman had pushed through his committee comprehensive climate-change legislation, which triggered the same sharp partisan divide as health reform, and he prevailed by splitting the Blue Dogs on his committee. Leading to the health reform markup, the Blue Dogs knew if they stayed united they had the balance of power. They would not be fooled again. They used their leverage for several purposes: to weaken the public-plan option, to equalize Medicare rates of payment between rural areas and the rest of the nation, to reduce the number of businesses that would pay penalties under the employer mandate, to produce a plan that relied less on Medicaid, and to bring the total ten-year cost of the bill to under $1 trillion—even though their other priorities all increased the cost of the legislation.

Representative Mike Ross (D-AR) was the Blue Dogs' health policy leader, and on July 21, he brought the Energy and Commerce markup to a halt when it became apparent all committee Blue Dogs would stick together. On July 30, the committee reconvened and approved changes that reduced the total cost of the legislation by about 10 percent, primarily by limiting subsidies for uninsured persons, exempting more small businesses from the payroll tax, and changing the public option to resemble the HELP Committee's version by paying higher-than-Medicare rates to medical providers—all to the chagrin of House progressives. House leaders also committed to delay any vote by the full House until at least September. With those commitments, four of the seven Blue Dogs, including Ross, voted for the bill, which was approved thirty-one to twenty-eight. All three House committees had approved their version, and HELP made four. Only Senate Finance was left to act.

Senate Majority Leader Reid paid attention to the evolving health reform process and rarely interfered, trusting his committee chairs to do their jobs. On Tuesday, July 7, 2009, he broke his pattern, weighing in with Baucus, his Finance Committee chair. As reported by *Roll Call*, "Reid told Baucus that taxing health benefits and failing to include a strong government-run insurance option of some sort in his bill would cost ten to fifteen Democratic votes; Reid told Baucus that several in the Conference had serious concerns and that it wasn't worth securing the support of Grassley and at best a few additional Republicans."[14] Ever since the release of his health reform white paper in November 2008, Baucus had made known his intention to use changes in the tax treatment of health insurance as his major financing source to pay for reform. Reid's directive, backed by the White House and supported by the House, was motivated in part by the seating of Minnesota's Al Franken, the Democrats' elusive sixtieth vote, meaning that Republicans were no longer needed to pass a bill. This directive, though, left Baucus's plan with a gaping financial hole. Baucus was criticized in many quarters for not moving faster and for spending too much time wooing Republicans in his Gang of Six. But after the loss of the tax exclusion as a funding source, his team struggled for weeks to find an alternative way to finance reform. By the end of July, Grassley and Snowe were still in play, while Enzi was considered a lost cause. Continuing the Gang of Six was convenient cover for a staff scurrying to find an alternative financing plan.

In August, many town meetings attended by senators and representatives from both parties featured large crowds and shouting matches over health reform—with the news media focusing on the minority of events, scenes, and moments with the greatest theatrical value. The many town meetings that did not include disruptions or angry outbursts were unreported by the national media. The process had the unexpected effect of solidifying both parties in their support for or opposition to reform.

Also, in late August, Senator Kennedy passed away, fifteen months after his diagnosis in May 2008. The emotional memorial service at the JFK Library in Boston, his funeral in the Mission Hill neighborhood of Boston, and related events further solidified the resolve of many Democratic members to win reform as a tribute to their late friend and colleague. "Do It for Ted" buttons began to appear as a message to Democrats. Days before his passing, Kennedy sent a letter to Massachusetts governor Deval Patrick and legislative leaders asking them to approve legislation to permit the governor to name an interim appointment to his seat until a special election could be held. In September, Patrick named former Kennedy aide and Democratic National Committee chair Paul Kirk as the new sixtieth Democratic vote.

The town meeting uproar convinced President Obama it was time to play the presidential card of a joint address to both houses of Congress. His forty-seven-minute September 9 address was well received, boosting favorable poll numbers, though it was most memorable for an outburst from Representative Joe Wilson (R-SC)—"You lie!"—in response to Obama's statement that the bill would not provide insurance coverage for undocumented aliens. That controversy distracted attention from one line in the address of particular concern to key Democratic House and Senate members and staffers alike: "Add it all up, and the plan I'm proposing will cost around $900 billion over ten years."[15] In spite of public perception to the contrary, the president never submitted his own plan, and the $900 billion ceiling would require a plan with significantly thinner subsidies than either the House or HELP Committee versions already approved. His February 2009 budget submission estimated that reform would cost about $1.2 trillion over ten years, so this was a substantial reduction. House leaders were particularly distressed. "Nine hundred billion," mused one House staffer. "Is that net or gross?" It was an offhand comment, though of critical importance—because $900 billion in gross spending would give Congress far less spending flexibility than $900 billion in net spending. Obama never clarified, though the final ACA price tag of $940 billion was in *net* spending.

From where did the $900 billion ceiling come? Over the summer and into August as the Senate Finance process dragged on, Obama's team had worked up its own health reform legislation to have in reserve if needed. In that plan, the total cost was less than $900 billion and the president used $900 billion to provide some "breathing room," according to an administration source. The new ceiling also had the collateral effect of killing any chance to include a fix of the costly Medicare physician-payment problem as part of the main health reform bill.

Under increasing pressure from Reid and Obama, on the Tuesday after Labor Day, Baucus sent a proposal to the other five Gang of Six members, asking them for support, ideas, and modifications. He got no response from the three Republican participants and proceeded to turn the proposal into the chairman's mark, or recommended legislation, for Senate Finance Committee consideration.

Between 10 a.m. on September 22 and 2 a.m. on October 16, the Senate Finance Committee debated amendments to Baucus's health reform proposal, advanced by the chairman alone, with no support from Grassley or Enzi and only ambivalence from Snowe. Unlike the other four committees, the Finance Committee does not give its twenty-three members or anyone actual legislative language. Instead, the committee considers a "conceptual draft" of plain-text language to be converted to legislative form after the markup is completed. On Capitol Hill, the Finance Committee is legendary for plowing through complex issues quickly—if necessary by turning up the heat in the room to make members uncomfortable. The Baucus plan cost less than the House or HELP plans, covered fewer uninsured, and provided less generous subsidies to purchase coverage—and it may have been the only plan that could survive a Finance markup. The CBO determined that the Baucus mark was fully paid for and that it would bend the health care cost curve in years ahead.

In all, 564 amendments were offered to the 223-page summary document, and 135 were considered over eight days of sessions, the longest Finance Committee markup in twenty-two years. The plan contained no public option, offering instead support for hypothetical nonprofit health insurance cooperatives proposed by Conrad. An amendment by Charles Schumer (D-NY) to add a public-plan option was voted down ten to thirteen, with Baucus, Conrad, and Blanche Lincoln (D-AR) joining all ten Republicans. Another amendment offered by Schumer and Olympia Snowe to sharply reduce penalties related to enforcement of the individual mandate—including eliminating any penalty in the first year—was adopted, much to the alarm of the health insurance industry. While not touching the health insurance tax exclusion, the plan proposed a new "Cadillac" tax on high-cost health insurance policies, a proposal advanced by John Kerry (D-MA) that drew immediate fire from organized labor. The final vote in committee was fourteen to nine, with Snowe the only Republican to vote with Democrats. At the end of the markup, health reform was as controversial and partisan as ever. Still, five of five committees with jurisdiction had acted. Health reform had never gotten so far in seventy-five years.

ON THE FLOORS

Two out of three House committees had approved the original House health reform legislation essentially intact, with only minor changes, while the third, Energy and Commerce, had made major adjustments—on the public-plan option by delinking provider payments from Medicare, on employer responsibility by exempting more employers from any fee, on increasing Medicare payments to rural areas, and more. Because the final vote in the full House of Representatives was expected to be close in spite of the Democrats' eighty-one-seat numerical advantage over the Republicans, the Energy and Commerce version held the day. Sufficient votes were not there for the original version.

After an excruciating process to line up a majority, Speaker Nancy Pelosi and her team delivered a 220-to-215 win on late Saturday evening, November 7, 2009, with 1 lone Republican voting yes, and 39 Democrats voting no. To achieve the win, the Speaker was compelled to allow a vote on a strict antiabortion amendment that prohibited any plan operating in any new health insurance exchange from offering abortion coverage, except through a separate payment; pro-choice Democrats had wanted at least one plan covering abortions and at least one that did not. The amendment succeeded by a 240-to-194 vote, and provided Pelosi with the needed votes of pro-health-reform Democrats who were also pro-life, especially their leaders, Bart Stupak (D-MI) and Brad Ellsworth (D-IN).

House Leaders and staff had begun readying the final House version—called the Affordable Health Care for America Act—after Energy and Commerce finished its work in late July (it held a final mop-up markup session in mid-September). By the time Senate Finance finished its markup on October 16, House leaders were already counting noses for a final vote. The House had four principal committees involved: Energy and Commerce, Ways and Means, Education, and Labor, plus the House Rules Committee. The Senate had only two—Finance and HELP. While the House started with a single merged bill, Senate Finance and HELP had not. Most of the titles in the two Senate bills were clearly within the jurisdiction of one committee or the other, easing the task—though not so for Title I, which dealt with the controversial issues of insurance-market reform, individual and employer responsibility, exchanges, premium subsidies and cost sharing, and more.

The Senate "merger meetings" were held in the vice president's office in room 201 of the Dirksen Senate Office Building. A large oval wooden table sat about twenty, with lots of space around the borders of the room for more. Attending were a throng of Finance and HELP staffers led by Liz Fowler and David Bowen, drafters from the Senate Legislative Counsel's Office, a cadre from the administration that included White House health czar Nancy-Ann DeParle plus HHS health reform coordinator Jeanne Lambrew, and Majority Leader Harry Reid's key staff. In this phase and in this room, Reid was fully in charge, chiefly represented by his health aide, Kate Leone. It was an endless process of editing, reviewing, changing, over and over, for weeks—lists containing hundreds of action items were exhausted, only to have an equally long list emerge a day or two later. This is where the essential language and structure of the Patient Protection and Affordable Care Act, or PPACA, was shaped.

Slowing down Senate and House Democrats at every turn was the unavoidable need for budget scores on every section from the Congressional Budget Office. While CBO analysts worked double and triple overtime to produce credible estimates, congressional staffers seethed at their pace. When scores came back with disappointing results, staffers hurriedly reworked policies to achieve more favorable estimates that could survive public scrutiny. Often, House and Senate staffers clashed with CBO officials over who had been first in line to get an estimate. When the CBO released a health report on a non-Democratic-directed topic, as it did on October 9, 2009, on medical-liability reform, Senate staffers cursed loudly at the CBO's sense of priorities.[16]

While drafting and policy fine-tuning were under way in room 201, Reid worked to find the sixty votes needed simply to allow Senate debate to begin. On Thursday, November 19, he unveiled his "merged" legislation along with a CBO score showing a ten-year price tag of $848 billion, along with $130 billion in deficit reduction. His version included a public-plan option permitting states to choose to opt out; he included a "Cadillac" excise tax on high-cost health insurance plans, a new Medicare payroll tax on affluent Americans, and an allowance for exchange plans to include abortion coverage as long as no federal dollars were used to pay for the procedure. On late Saturday, November 21, he got the go-ahead, a vote of sixty to thirty-nine to allow the Senate to begin debating his proposed health reform bill, the minimum necessary to proceed on the Senate floor. Yet a vote to proceed did not assure a vote for final passage. As they voted, a cadre of Democrats made clear, publicly and privately, they would vote for a final bill only if significant changes were made. After a break for Thanksgiving, health reform would reach the Senate floor for the first time.

A team of staffers from Finance, HELP, and the majority leader's office set in place an extensive operation to manage the Senate floor process. More than fifty staffers were divided into four groups, with war rooms and operations plans—the floor team, the media team, the members team, and the stakeholders team. Each prepared to engage the Republicans, manage the message, and keep members and key supporting organizations informed on an up-to-the-minute basis. It turned out to be completely unnecessary. On the floor, Republicans and Democrats engaged in little more than message management. Republicans had their themes and talking points—Medicare cuts, new taxes, the individual mandate, Medicaid, CLASS, and more—and only few of the hundreds of amendments filed ever saw the light of day. At one point, the debate ground to a halt for nearly a week over a procedural disagreement regarding Senator Byron Dorgan's (D-ND) amendment to allow the reimportation of prescription drugs.

For Harry Reid, though, the time was not wasted—it was precious time to do what was necessary to assemble sixty votes needed for final passage. Statements from Senators Ben Nelson (D-NE) and Joe Lieberman (D-CT) made it clear that Reid's plan to include a public option would forfeit their two essential votes. In early December, Reid designated Chuck Schumer (D-NY) as his lead negotiator to meet in Kennedy's former hideaway office with nine other members; the total group comprised five progressives and five moderates. Most other Democratic members were angered not to be included, fearing the loss of an inside opportunity to shape the final version. Ahead of time, Schumer met to strategize with the other liberals, Sherrod Brown (D-OH), Russ Feingold (D-WI), Tom Harkin (D-IA), and Jay Rockefeller (D-WV).

Schumer opened: "Here's the ticktock." Nelson and Snowe were meeting with President Obama to gauge which one would be vote number sixty. The public-plan option would have to go. The question was what progressives would get in place of it, because, Schumer said, "Any move away from that is big for us and we need something big in return." There were two items on his list: allowing uninsured adults between the ages of fifty-five and sixty-four to be able to buy into Medicare, and imposing tougher measures against the insurance industry. For three days, the five of them negotiated with Tom Carper (D-DE), Blanche Lincoln (D-AR), Mark Pryor (D-AR), Mary Landrieu (D-LA), and Ben Nelson. Lieberman had been invited as one of the moderates but only sent staff. The ten members met, accompanied by twenty-five staffers, and agreed on a package of tough insurance reforms, a limited Medicare buy-in for those fifty-five to sixty-four years old, and a new national nonprofit insurance plan to be offered in all state exchanges. Reid walked in to congratulate the participants: "The distance we've traveled this past week is amazing. The best is, all ten of you agree on every line." His sentiment did not apply to the eleventh member, Senator Lieberman, who was not in the room but who quickly announced he would not support any version of a Medicare buy-in, removing that option—which he had endorsed as the Democratic vice-presidential nominee in 2000—from consideration. The majority leader had no choice but to drop the Medicare buy-in that progressives had wanted so badly.

The final negotiation involved Senator Nelson, a participant in the Schumer meetings who had his own list not discussed in the ten-member meetings. Key was his insistence either that Medicaid expansion be voluntary for states or that the federal government pick up all state costs related to it—a request Reid met for Nebraska only, a deal that became known as the "Cornhusker kickback." Nelson also demanded and won stronger language on abortion than the Reid version after tense negotiations with Senators Barbara Boxer (D-CA) and Patty Murray (D-WA). All the other Democratic members got items from their wish lists: Landrieu won special Medicaid payments for Louisiana (dubbed the "Louisiana purchase") plus coverage for foster children until age twenty-six; Lincoln won the elimination of any employer penalty for noncoverage of workers during new-employment waiting periods; Rockefeller got more money for the Children's Health Insurance Program; on and on, for all sixty Democrats. Altruism and self-interest were both on abundant display—the Senate at work. All the changes that Reid, Baucus, and Dodd agreed to were consolidated into one single amendment, called the Manager's Amendment, which was added to the legislation as a new Title X. It made reading the actual legislation messy—anything in the first nine titles might be amended in Title X. It was OK, they thought, because it would all get cleaned up in a final process merging the Senate and House bills.

The final Senate vote was called at 7 a.m. on December 24, 2009. Senator Bernie Sanders (I-VT) gave Democrats heart palpitations by arriving at nearly the last moment to cast the final vote. Majority Leader Reid unintentionally blurted out "no" and corrected himself to say "yes." Senator Robert Byrd shouted from his wheelchair in the chamber, "Mr. President, this is for my friend Ted Kennedy. Aye." Staff were ordered to put "pens down" over the holidays and to be ready to start nonstop negotiations with the House on a final bill beginning right after New Year's Day.

A FAUX CONFERENCE AND PING-PONG

When both the Senate and the House have approved broad and complex legislation, the usual process is to organize a bipartisan conference committee to meld two bills into one and then to bring the merged product back to both chambers for an up-or-down vote. Like nearly everything else about health reform, the final stages of the process were not normal. Because Senate Republicans were determined to do anything they could to defeat the legislation, or to slow it down if they could not stop it, they made clear they would act to slow down the forming of a conference committee. It was clear they could do so, delaying the process by weeks or even longer. As a result, Senate and House Democratic leaders decided to bypass the conference route and instead negotiate a merged version among the Senate and House Democratic leaders and staff, and then have the final merged bill approved in the exact form in each chamber—a process referred to as legislative ping-pong.

Beginning Wednesday, January 6, 2010, an army of House, Senate, and administration staffers began working to merge all the common elements of the House and Senate bills. At Reid's insistence, the first meetings were held at the White House and the adjacent Eisenhower Executive Office Building to emphasize that this was the administration's moment to take ownership. Numerous items had been included in either the House or the

Senate bill that were never intended for inclusion in a final law—that's the usual process. Senator Kennedy, after once graciously agreeing to accept an objectionable amendment to a bill he was carrying on the Senate floor, remarked to his aide, David Bowen: "That amendment is going no further than the Ohio clock," referring to the elegant eleven-foot timepiece that has graced the corridor outside the Senate chamber since 1817. One advantage of the conference process—faux or real—is the opportunity to delete unsavory items and then blame the other chamber, a bicameral and bipartisan practice.

Marching orders were issued by White House chief of staff Rahm Emanuel right after New Year's Day. A staff steering committee with members from all key Senate and House committees, leader offices, and the administration would manage the process. Twelve subgroups were created: Coverage, Medicaid and CHIP, Medicare, Fraud-Abuse-Transparency, Abortion, Prescription Drugs, Geographic Equity, the CLASS Act, Comparative Effectiveness, Workforce, Revenue, and Immigration. Others quickly cropped up. The directive was to wrap up each issue quickly, with everything done and sent to the CBO by Friday, January 15, and with action in the House by Friday the 22nd and action in the Senate by Friday the 29th. The mission for the Senate participants, according to HELP staffer Mark Childress, was "to find what we can agree to with the House that will not lose us sixty votes. And there's no new money to add." Reid's health aide Kate Leone added, "Don't get kicked around by those House bullies."

There is a saying among House Democrats: "In the House, the Republicans are our opponents and the Senate is our enemy." It's understandable. Every year, the House sends hundreds of approved bills to the Senate, where they die from inaction. When the Senate does act, often the margin of approval is so slender that the Senate compels the House to take its version or nothing. That dynamic also played out in early 2009 involving large portions of the American Reinvestment and Recovery Act (ARRA, the stimulus bill). Although the meetings in the early weeks of January 2010 involved only Democratic staffers, the animus of many House staffers was palpable as they chafed against the "We have no room to move" message and attitude they perceived from Senate staffers. While less controversial titles and sections were resolved smoothly and quickly, others dragged.

Many meetings at the White House during the week of January 11 involved President Obama himself, who cleared whole days on his calendar to wrap up the process. In one tense meeting on Friday the 15th, sometime past 1 a.m. the president stood up, announced that his participation was clearly not helping, and that he was leaving, available to be called—but leaving. Into the weekend, progress was slow, with important issues not yet resolved. Among Senate staffers, concerns were raised that some concessions already made to House negotiators would result in the Senate's falling short of the sixty votes needed to secure passage of the agreed-upon deal.

The January 19 special election in Massachusetts to fill the unexpired term of Senator Kennedy was only an occasional sidebar conversation. Members and staffers had heard that the Democratic candidate, Attorney General Martha Coakley, was doing poorly. There was a sense of hurry in the legislative negotiations, though unrelated to the special election. The surprising win of Republican state senator Scott Brown to fill the seat was a bona fide game changer in the sense that Democrats would no longer have sixty votes once Brown was seated, and, since Brown indicated he would not vote for the Democrats' health bill, the process as envisioned in early January became inoperative.

Many observers viewed the vote as a referendum by Massachusetts voters on national health reform. Yet polls indicated that more than half of Brown's own voters supported the Massachusetts health reform law, on which the national reform was based. Anger at the Massachusetts state government for recent tax increases and other foibles, an unprepared and poorly performing Democratic candidate, an asleep-at-the-wheel national and state party structure, and a likable moderate in Scott Brown, who was surprisingly adopted by tea party activists across the nation, seemed at least as important as any judgments by the Massachusetts electorate of national health reform. Whatever the reason, the damage was done, and health reform, for the moment, was off the tracks.

BYRD BATHS, END GAMES, AND A SIDECAR

The Thursday before the Massachusetts election, Ron Pollack, from Families USA, circulated a memo proposing a two-track strategy if the Democrats lost their sixty-vote margin in the Senate. Track one would have the House approve the Senate-enacted PPACA bill with no changes—requiring no further Senate action to send the legislation to the president's desk, and thus no sixty-vote hurdle. Track two would require the House and Senate to approve a separate bill making agreed-upon amendments to the larger Senate bill, and using the budget reconciliation process, which requires only fifty-one Senate votes for passage. The Senate-House budget resolution adopted in April 2009 had already left the door open for the use of reconciliation; though no one could have foreseen these circumstances, the decision to leave the option available, long advocated by Senator Kennedy, was prescient. It would surely involve numerous traps and pitfalls. Yet, importantly, from the get-go on the evening of January 19, there was a path—not pretty or appealing or easy—yet a path to achieve national health reform.

On the night of January 19, the president met with Reid and Pelosi in his office to talk strategy, and the Speaker forcefully told them there was no way she could round up enough votes in the House to pass the Senate bill. Later in the week, though, in a meeting with Emanuel and others, she derided White House–generated incremental ideas—expanded coverage for children or seniors or catastrophic coverage—as "kiddie care." Thus began a two-month process that seemed to evoke Elisabeth Kübler-Ross's five stages of grief—denial, anger, bargaining, depression, and acceptance.[17] House Democrats had to move through a painful, courageous process to accept the necessity of voting for the Senate bill, with only limited changes permissible in the reconciliation bill, often referred to as the "sidecar." Had the tables been turned, and the Senate been confronted with the imperative to enact the House health reform bill in toto, it is inconceivable that reform would have passed.

Once Pelosi and her key lieutenants, including Majority Leader Steny Hoyer (D-MD) and Majority Whip James Clyburn (D-SC), accepted the path, they moved methodically and relentlessly to win over a majority of House members one by one. Senators, uncharacteristically, kept their mouths shut. Options were suggested to make the process easier for House members, including having the Senate vote on the reconciliation sidecar before the House adopted the Senate's PPACA bill, and having the House approve the Senate bill without a formal roll-call vote through a House process known as "deem and pass." These and others tactics were rejected by Senate parliamentarian Alan Frumin, an obscure official reluctantly thrust into the public spotlight. Reid helped Pelosi by producing a letter signed by more than fifty-one Senate Democrats committing to vote for the sidecar as negotiated—a letter never released publicly. Once engaged, Pelosi would not let the matter die: "We will go through the gate," she told a January 28 news conference. "If the gate is closed, we will go over the fence. If the fence is too high, we will pole-vault in. If that doesn't work, we will parachute in. But we are going to get health care reform passed."[18] This was pure political will personified.

President Obama stepped into the process in new ways. On February 22, he released the President's Proposal, a list of policy initiatives to address key inadequacies in the Senate's PPACA bill approved on Christmas Eve. Some thought Obama was advancing a new bill, but it was a laundry list for the sidecar. It included

- eliminating the Nebraska Medicaid deal known as the Cornhusker kickback;
- closing the Part D "doughnut hole" faster and more completely than done in the Senate bill;
- improving affordability provisions for insurance subsidies, which were much weaker in the Senate than in the House bill;
- expanding provisions to fight fraud, waste, and abuse; and
- raising the income threshold for the so-called "Cadillac" excise tax on high-cost health insurance policies so fewer would be affected by it, and delaying implementation until 2018.

Except for the fraud and abuse sections, all were included in the final reconciliation bill.[19] The fraud and abuse provisions were ruled out of order by the Senate parliamentarian.

Later that week, the president hosted a daylong bipartisan health reform summit televised at the Blair House, across from the White House. The summit, which involved leaders from both chambers, served several purposes: first, it distracted attention and bought time while Pelosi and Reid worked through the mechanics and politics of their final legislative moves; second, it allowed the president to claim the high ground by engaging in pointed public dialogue with his fiercest Republican critics; and third, it gave the president a response to complaints that he had not met his promise to engage in televised negotiations.

The insurance industry also played an inadvertent supporting role in aiding final passage. In early February, the giant for-profit Anthem Blue Cross plan in California (part of the WellPoint network) announced rate increases for its individual policyholders as high as 39 percent, triggering headlines and expressions of outrage across the nation and throughout Capitol Hill. It was the first time that rate increases in one state's individual market had become a national controversy. "WellPoint" became a rallying cry for Democrats and, in their off-the-record comments, an unbelievable gift. Just when most observers thought health reform dead, a major insurer's enormous rate increase threw cold water on claims that reform itself was driving premium hikes. WellPoint had invested millions in defeating California governor Arnold Schwarzenegger's health reform plan in 2008; it was the most virulently anti-reform of the major insurers, engaging in especially aggressive medical underwriting and policyholder rescissions across the nation; so the fact that it was WellPoint in this position was a source of glee to White House and Capitol Hill staffers.

The Senate reconciliation rules did not permit changes to be made to the PPACA bill in the sidecar regarding abortion coverage, because any changes would have had trivial budget consequences, so President Obama issued a presidential executive order to appease Congressman Stupak and his small group of allies whose votes were, in the end, critical to success. The abortion controversy triggered a sharp dispute between Catholic bishops who opposed the bill and Catholic nuns, especially those who were leaders of the Catholic Health Association, a network of Catholic hospitals. At the signing ceremony on March 23, Sister Carol Keohane was the only nonpublic official to receive one of President Obama's signing pens.

Pelosi achieved her winning margin only in the final hours of House deliberations on March 21, 2010, by a final vote of 219 to 212 after a day of hostile tea party demonstrations around the Capitol. Shortly thereafter, the House approved the reconciliation sidecar.

The Senate followed up that week to act on the sidecar. Its rules are stricter than those in the House, due to the efforts of the late Senator Robert Byrd (D-WV), a former majority leader, who objected in the 1970s to the use of the budget reconciliation process to pass all kinds of legislation outside the normal Senate process. As a result, the only matters that can be included in a reconciliation bill are those having a direct and substantial impact, positive or negative, on the budget. Any senator can challenge any item or portion of any item as a violation of the Byrd rule. Senate parliamentarian Frumin rules on challenges in a process called the Byrd bath; items removed in the process are called Byrd droppings. The Democrats' fear was that if any significant changes were made, then the House might not have the votes to pass a revised version. For this high-stakes process at the end of March, Democrat staff budget experts, led by Senator Conrad's staff director, Mary Naylor, prepared diligently to face off with their Republican counterparts in behind-closed-doors proceedings that had the aura of a courtroom in which Frumin acted as judge and jury.[20] On all major challenges, he ruled for the Democrats and their carefully drafted revisions, agreeing with only two minor Republican objections. After the Senate approved the sidecar by fifty-six to forty-three on March 26, the House held one final vote to approve the bill.

President Obama signed the Affordable Care Act into law at the White

House on March 23 and signed the sidecar one week later. It was a few days more than nineteen months since Max Baucus had hosted the Health Reform Summit at the Library of Congress.

.   .   .

Political will is the determination to see a matter through regardless of the firestorm, regardless of the advice of allies, friends, media figures, and others who say stop. At various points along the way to passage, President Obama, Speaker Pelosi, Majority Leader Reid, and Chairmen Waxman, Baucus, and Dodd each had their moments when the process could have died or suffered irreparable harm:

- In the 2008 presidential campaign in July, candidate Obama overruled most of his advisors' advice to downplay health reform.

- In February 2009, when Vice President Biden, Chief of Staff Emanuel, Senior Advisor David Axelrod, and most White House advisors wanted to scuttle comprehensive reform, President Obama said no, ordering its inclusion in his first budget proposal to Congress.

- In June–July 2009, when the Senate HELP Committee was mired in the longest legislative markup in the committee's history and the CBO scores looked dismal, Senator Dodd kept committee Democrats united to be the first congressional committee to act.

- In July 2009, when Energy and Commerce chair Waxman faced a revolt by Democratic Blue Dogs on his committee, he made key concessions to keep the reform process on track.

- In August 2009, when the tea party movement was transforming the health reform debate into a culture war, and Chairman Baucus was mired in Group of Six negotiations, and Emanuel again was looking to scale back the plans, Obama once again committed to staying the course and teeing up an address to a joint session of Congress.

- In October and November 2009, Speaker Pelosi and her team worked tirelessly to win a majority of votes in her chamber for the House health reform bill.

- In November and December, when Majority Leader Harry Reid had zero margin for error, he brought along sixty out of sixty Democratic senators to fashion a final Senate bill that could be enacted.

- And in January through late March 2010, when the results of the Massachusetts special election caused most of Washington DC and the nation to believe comprehensive reform was dead, White House advisors were hard at work preparing incremental fallbacks and Obama and Pelosi pushed back hard to stay the course to final passage of two complementary laws.

Moments after the House vote on March 21, 2010, Obama told reporters: "This is what change looks like."[21] He could have added: "This is what political will looks like." Because that's what it took.

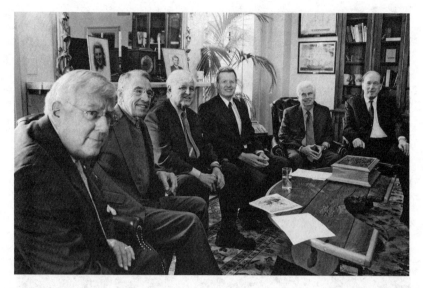

Senator Edward M. Kennedy (D-MA) is flanked by Senate colleagues during a November 19, 2008, Capitol Hill meeting to discuss national health reform. *From left:* Senators Mike Enzi (R-WY), Charles Grassley (R-IA), Kennedy, Max Baucus (D-MT), Christopher Dodd (D-CT), and Jay Rockefeller (D-WV). (Photo by Mark Wilson/Getty Images)

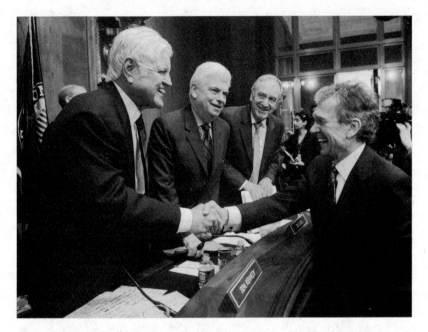

Edward M. Kennedy (D-MA), *left,* chair of the Senate Health, Education,
Labor and Pensions Committee, along with Christopher J. Dodd (D-CT)
and Tom Harkin (D-IA), congratulate Tom Daschle, President-elect Barack
Obama's nominee to run the Department of Health and Human Services, after
committee's hearing on Daschle's nomination in early January 2009. Daschle
promised Republicans that the new administration would not try to ram a health
care overhaul through Congress under expedited budget procedures. (Photo by
Scott J. Ferrell/Congressional Quarterly/Getty Images)

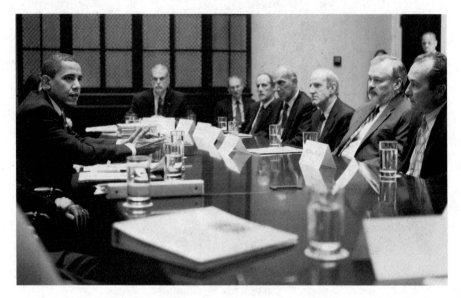

President Barack Obama, *left*, conducts a meeting in the Roosevelt Room at the White House on May 11, 2009, with health care stakeholders who promised to do their part to save $2 trillion in health spending over ten years. (Official White House photo by Pete Souza)

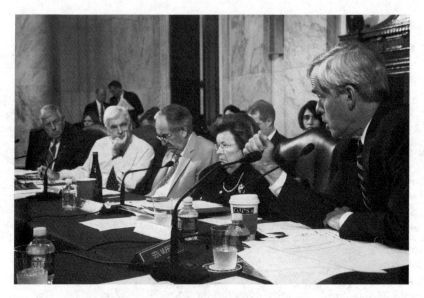

Senator Jeff Bingaman (D-NM), *right*, discusses health reform legislation with Senate Health, Education, Labor and Pensions Committee colleagues. *Seated from left:* ranking Republican Mike Enzi (R-WY), acting chair Christopher J. Dodd (D-CT), Tom Harkin (D-IA), and Barbara A. Mikulski (D-MD). (Photo by Ryan Kelly/Congressional Quarterly/Getty Images)

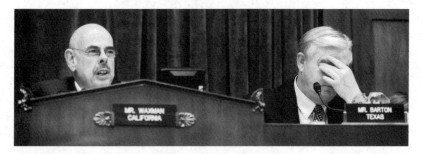

Representative Joe Barton (R-TX), *right*, ranking member of the House Energy and Commerce Committee, reacts to a comment by committee chair Henry Waxman (D-CA) that members should not make plans before 1 a.m. as the committee was expected to vote on amendments to its health care bill into the wee hours of the night. (Photo by Linda Davidson/*Washington Post*/Getty Images)

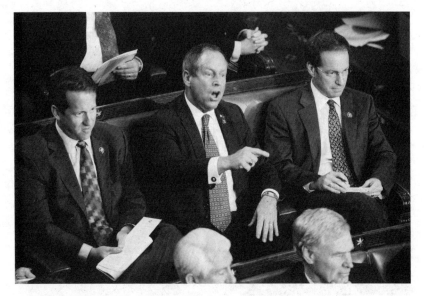

Representative Joe Wilson (R-SC), *center*, shouts "You lie!" as President Barack Obama addresses a joint session of Congress at the Capitol on September 9, 2009. Obama urged passage of his national health care plan, the centerpiece of his domestic agenda. (Photo by Chip Somodevilla/Getty Images)

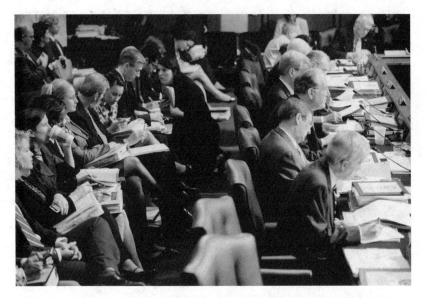

Members of the Senate Finance Committee meet to debate the health care bill. Behind them, the aides pass notes to the senators and constantly check their BlackBerry phones. (Photo by Sarah L. Voisin/*Washington Post*/Getty Images)

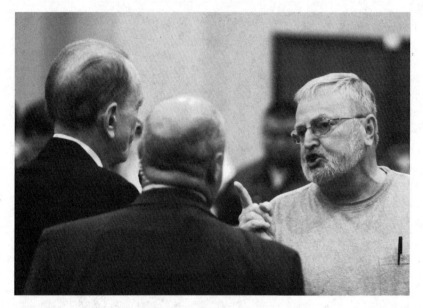

Senator Arlen Specter, *left*, listens as an unidentified man shouts at him during a town hall meeting on August 11, 2009, in Lebanon, Pennsylvania. (Photo by Chris Gardner/Getty Images)

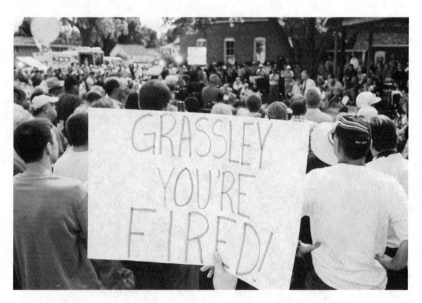

A woman holds up a "Grassley You're Fired" sign during Senator Charles Grassley's town hall meeting on health care reform in Adel, Iowa, on August 12, 2009. (Photo by Bill Clark/*Roll Call*/Getty Images)

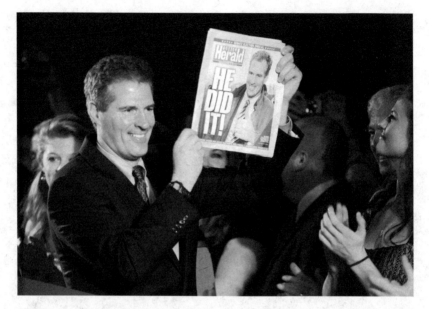

U.S. Senator-elect Scott Brown displays a special edition of the *Boston Herald* after winning the Massachusetts U.S. Senate seat on January 19, 2010. Brown, a Republican, defeated Democrat Martha Coakley in a special election to fill the seat of late Edward M. Kennedy. (Photo by Robert Spencer/Getty Images)

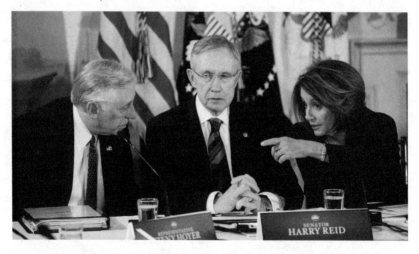

Senate Majority Leader Harry Reid, *center*, listens to House Majority Leader Steny Hoyer, *left*, and House Speaker Nancy Pelosi during a bipartisan summit on health care with President Barack Obama in Washington on February 25, 2010. Obama urged lawmakers to find ways to overhaul the health care system, saying Congress couldn't afford to ignore one of the "biggest drags" on the U.S. economy. (Photo by Shawn Thew/*Bloomberg*/Getty Images)

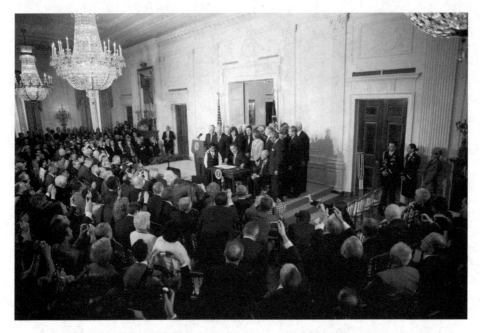

President Obama signs the Patient Protection and Affordable Care Act into law on March 23, 2010. (Official White House photo by Lawrence Jackson)

PART II

Policies—Ten Titles

. . . . .

Just as a book has chapters, a play has acts and scenes, and a baseball game has innings, so too does a federal law have titles, each with its own purpose, shape, identity, history, assumptions—data-based and otherwise— and curiosities. Some fit comfortably into the whole act or statute, and some stick out at an odd angle. Some may look pretty darn appealing during markup or floor consideration and then take on a ghastly appearance once implementation time rolls around. One senior House staffer likened the Affordable Care Act (ACA) to a garden packed with a wide array of plants. Some will grow grand and plentiful as intended, some will never grow at all—unexpectedly or as intended—while others will grow in surprising ways, better or worse than expected. Some are artificial, planted purely for visual effect. And as in all other gardens, tending, cultivation, and weeding come with the terrain.

The garden metaphor has a useful point. Those who get into the ACA find that there is a lot in it. Throughout the health reform prelude and process, many hundreds of intriguing ideas were advanced to improve the nation's health care system, and a large number of them found their way into the final ACA. Few found a place in the law as extensive and robust as their principal proponents would have preferred, but still, many provisions involving access, quality, and cost control found a place. Becoming part of the ACA provides no guarantee of successful implementation, though getting into the law is an essential precondition for any provision to have a chance at success.

The core premise of this book, and of this second part, is that the law itself, beyond the process controversies and the noise, matters, and that a full appreciation or condemnation demands familiarity with the ACA as a statute. It is broad, complex, intricate, varied, and challenging. It contains far more than most people appreciate, much of it surprising and more than a small amount with a bipartisan pedigree. Whether one wants it implemented in toto or repealed in full, those opinions need to be tested in the context of a robust understanding of this extraordinary law.

The ACA has ten parts, or titles. Within each title are subtitles, and within each subtitle are sections—487 of them, including 35 health-related sections in the Health Care and Education Reconciliation Act (HCERA, also known as the reconciliation sidecar)—signed into law on March 30, 2010, one week after the signing of the PPACA, and making amendments to the base law. Here is the structure with the number of sections in parentheses and a brief description:

Title I: Quality, Affordable Coverage for All Americans (65) deals with expanded private health insurance coverage and regulation of the private health insurance market.

Title II: Role of Public Programs (42) expands and reforms public coverage in Medicaid and the Children's Health Insurance Program.

Title III: Improving the Quality and Efficiency of Health Care (98) improves the quality and efficiency of medical care delivered to all Americans and makes changes to Medicare.

Title IV: Prevention of Chronic Disease and Improving Public Health (27) creates new initiatives and programs to prevent injury and disease and to improve public health systems.

Title V: Health Care Workforce (53) increases the numbers and improves the quality of health professionals in the United States.

Title VI: Transparency and Program Integrity (50) provides new tools to combat fraud and abuse in public and private health insurance, discloses health industry financial information to the public, protects elders from abuse, and improves nursing home quality.

Title VII: Improving Access to Innovative Medical Therapies (6) creates a new pathway for the production and sale of generic-like biologic pharmaceuticals, also called biosimilars, in the United States.

Title VIII: Community Living Assistance Services and Supports—CLASS Act (2) sets up a new voluntary public program to provide financial support to disabled persons to help them live independently in their communities and homes.

Title IX: Revenue Provisions (20) pays for about half the cost of expanded coverage in Titles I and II.

Title X: Strengthening Quality, Affordable Health Care for All Americans, the so-called Manager's Amendment (89), makes amendments to Titles I through IX.

Finally, the Health Care Education and Reconciliation Act of 2010 (35) makes amendments to the previous ten titles. Changes made in the HCERA are described and discussed in the chapter on Title X for convenience's sake even though it is a separate, stand-alone law. A reminder about terminology: the Patient Protection and Affordable Care Act (PPACA) refers to the legislation approved in the U.S. Senate on December 24, 2009, and in the House of Representatives on March 21, 2010, and signed by the president on March 23, 2010. The HCERA was approved in the House and Senate on March 25, 2010, and signed by the president on March 30. The term *Affordable Care Act*, or *ACA*, refers to the original PPACA statute as modified by the HCERA.

Before diving into Title I, it may be helpful to understand the big-picture money flows to get a sense of how the ten titles connect and relate to each other. Table 1 presents three sets of data: first, the numbers of uninsured Americans who are projected to be insured by 2019 through the ACA; second, the projected gross federal expenditures associated with each title; and third, the projected gross savings or revenues associated with each title. All estimates for Titles I through VIII were generated by the Congressional Budget Office (CBO) in its final report on the impact of the ACA; all estimates related to Title IX were generated by the Joint Committee on Taxation (JCT). The CBO and JCT are the official, nonpartisan scorekeepers for Congress on all legislation with federal budgetary impacts.

What does the table tell us? First, thirty-two million uninsured Americans are projected to be covered by 2019; half of them will obtain private coverage made possible under Title I, and half are projected to obtain coverage through the Medicaid expansions in Title II. Second, unsurprisingly, the most expensive ACA titles are the two associated with the major coverage expansions; the $54 billion in ten-year expenses in Title III reflects costs to close the Medicare prescription drug "doughnut hole" and the addition of clinical preventive services as a new benefit for all Medicare enrollees. Third, most of the savings and revenues to finance the cost of the ACA are related to the new revenues in Title IX and to the Medicare savings in Title III; most of the revenues in Title I are associated with the individual- and employer-responsibility provisions, and the revenues in Title II mostly apply to new fees for prescription drugs related to Medicaid as well as hospital payment reductions in the Disproportionate Share Hospital program. It is important to keep in mind that these are gross, not

TABLE 1. Affordable Care Act impacts, 2010–2019

ACA title	Newly covered lives (in millions)	Projected expenses (in billions of dollars)	Projected revenues and savings (in billions of dollars)
I. Private coverage	16	509.0	80.6
II. Medicaid/CHIP	16	458.8	52.7
III. Delivery reform and Medicare	—	54.0	449.9
IV. Prevention	—	18.0	0.8
V. Workforce	—	18.2	—
VI. Transparency/fraud	—	2.8	7.0
VII. Biological similars	—	—	7.0
VIII. CLASS	—	—	70.2
IX. Revenues	—	—	437.8
Interactions and indirect tax effects	—	—	77.6

SOURCES: Titles I–VIII, Congressional Budget Office, March 20, 2010, ACA/HCERA estimate; Title IX, Joint Taxation Committee, March 20, 2010, ACA/HCERA estimate.

net, estimates and thus do not equal the $940 billion net cost estimated by the official scorekeepers.

One other important caveat, discussed in more detail later on: usually the scorekeepers are wrong and usually, though not always, in the same direction—overestimating costs and underestimating savings and revenues. It is not malice or incompetence—it's the inherent difficulty in making ten-year estimates with so much uncertainty, and the institutional caution that estimators bring to their responsibilities. In 1967, the House Ways and Means Committee estimated that the new Medicare program, enacted in 1965 and launched in 1966, would cost the federal government $12 billion in 1990; the actual cost came to $110 billion. Even though the CBO did not exist in until 1974, the erroneous original Medicare estimate is among the most well known in the history of federal financial estimating. The determination to avoid similarly directed estimating errors is a driving institutional imperative for the CBO and the JCT.

Still, the numbers provided a badly needed starting benchmark, and for our purposes here, they provide a useful introductory window into the world of the ten titles of the Affordable Care Act.

5. Title I—The Three-Legged Stool

Thank you, Senators Dorgan and Conrad and Representative Pomeroy, for your hard work toward health care reform. It is unfortunate that members of our community and Blue Cross Blue Shield have focused their efforts on misinforming the public and attacking our delegation. A recent mailing by BCBS warned that health care reform would increase premiums. Without reform my insurance increased at a double percentage rate last year and will again this year.

My son has hemophilia, a bleeding disorder that requires lifelong treatment with high-cost clotting medications that allow the blood to clot and prevent painful and life-threatening bleeds. The House passed a health care bill with a public option and which would eliminate lifetime caps on health insurance benefits. In the Senate version, existing plans are exempt from the elimination of lifetime caps or spending limits on benefits. Once they are met, the provider no longer provides coverage, ever.

By 12, my son reached his lifetime cap. We obtained a second policy at a substantial expense. He has used $1 million of this $2 million cap, and will cap out in 3 years or less. His clotting medication costs $30,000 per month. Dosage and cost increase with growth. If lifetime caps are not increased or eliminated, my son will not receive quality and life-sustaining care.

Blue Cross is unwilling to increase the $2 million caps established in the 1970s, though health care costs have risen and individuals with chronic conditions such as hemophilia, cancer, cystic fibrosis, spinal cord and brain injuries face these unreasonable limits. When Congress returns to deliver a final health care bill, it is essential that lifetime caps be eliminated in all plans.

BRENDA NEUBAUER, letter to the editor,
Bismarck Tribune, North Dakota, December 28, 2009

TITLE I: QUALITY, AFFORDABLE HEALTH CARE FOR ALL AMERICANS

Like many other parents of children with chronic and disabling illnesses, Brenda Neubauer is a tenacious advocate for her son, Jake. When she realized that health insurance coverage for Jake would hit a lifetime cap by the time he was sixteen, she contacted her U.S. senator, Byron Dorgan (D-ND), for help. Dorgan was surprised to learn that insurance companies would limit coverage for individuals who had paid premiums in good faith. In 2008, along with Senator Olympia Snowe (R-ME), he filed legislation to prevent any health insurer from imposing lifetime limits less than $5 million and increasing over several years to $10 million. Representative Anna Eshoo (D-CA) filed a companion bill in the House.

Brenda Neubauer was not working alone; the National Hemophilia Foundation formed a Raise the Caps Coalition with about forty organizations, including AARP, the American Heart Association, the Autism Society of America, the Epilepsy Foundation, the National Organization for Rare Disorders, and more. There are hundreds of disease-specific organizations across America; collectively, they are indefatigable advocates for their respective concerns. The Caps Coalition retained an actuarial consultant to gauge the financial impact of creating a national minimum on benefit caps of $5 million and $10 million, estimating that a $5 million floor would increase premiums between 0.6 and 0.8 percent, and that further raising the cap from $5 million to $10 million would increase premiums by an additional 0.1 percent. They also estimated national savings to Medicaid of $11 billion over ten years by implementing such a cap.[1]

It seemed a simple and straightforward issue in reforming the nation's health insurance market. As was true with every other element of the ACA, it turned out not to be simple at all.

Dorgan's aides contacted Senate committee staffers involved in writing health reform legislation to get a limit on lifetime limits on the radar screen. Looking at the issue and the Dorgan bill, Senate Health, Education, Labor and Pensions (HELP) staffers decided to go further and eliminate lifetime caps entirely. Also, insurance experts suggested that companies could circumvent the outlawing of lifetime caps by imposing annual caps instead, which many plans already did, separately or in addition to lifetime limits. The HELP Committee's first bill included the elimination of annual limits as well.

The House also banned lifetime and annual limits in its legislation, with a key difference. In his presidential campaign, Barack Obama repeatedly emphasized, when talking about health reform, "If you like what you have, you can keep it." This concept boiled down to one word, *grandfathering*, meaning that new insurance-market rules would not be applied to existing insurance policies. The House loosely applied grandfathering and did not apply it at all to the elimination of lifetime or annual limits—so everyone would be included in the new rules. The Senate made a stricter grandfathering interpretation: the Senate bill eliminated lifetime and annual caps on all plans—except for those affected by grandfathering—

thus excluding from the protections nearly all health insurance policies currently held, including Brenda Neubauer's.

There was another issue. As the Senate assembled its final health reform bill in late 2009, the Congressional Budget Office, Congress's nonpartisan budget scorekeeper, advised that eliminating lifetime caps would not significantly raise health insurance premiums, but that eliminating annual caps prior to 2014 would. So the final Senate PPACA bill, passed on Christmas Eve, eliminated lifetime caps in 2010 for all but grandfathered plans, eliminated annual caps after 2014, and gave the secretary of health and human services the ability to restrict "unreasonable" annual caps before 2014—something the CBO suggested would not trigger an adverse estimate.

In January 2010, as Senate and House members and staff negotiated a final bill, senators became concerned about the impact of grandfathering and limiting the availability of reforms in the law they were promoting proudly to the public. House Speaker Nancy Pelosi and others pressed the administration and senators on this potential public relations disaster.

The final version of the ACA, as amended by the Reconciliation Act, eliminates lifetime caps in all plans—including grandfathered plans—effective September 2010, for all "essential health benefits" specified in the law. Beginning in 2014, annual limits will be prohibited for all group coverage and for all individual plans bought after March 23, 2010. Prior to 2014, as defined by the HHS secretary in regulation, annual limits are prohibited if they are lower than $750,000 before September 2011, $1.25 million between then and September 2012, and $2 million between then and January 2014.

In short, Brenda and Jake won. Welcome to Title I of the ACA—where *nothing* is easy.

UNDERSTANDING TITLE I

Title I, called Quality, Affordable Health Care for All Americans, is the part of the ACA that regulates private health insurance, expands private health insurance to many uninsured Americans, provides subsidies to help many Americans afford the cost of private health insurance, establishes new state health insurance "exchanges" to make it easier for individuals and some businesses to buy coverage, requires most individuals to purchase insurance and many businesses to pay when they don't provide coverage, and more. The other major title involved in coverage expansion is Title II, which expands eligibility for state Medicaid programs, as explained in the next chapter. The CBO estimates that both titles will, by 2019, cover an additional thirty-two million currently uninsured Americans, sixteen million in Title I and another sixteen million in Title II, and leaving about twenty-three million uninsured. Depending how implementation goes, many more may be covered or many fewer. Title I provisions are estimated to have a gross cost of $540 billion between 2010 and 2019 according to the CBO, and Title II will cost $434 billion.[2] These two titles account for more than 90 percent of all new spending in the law.

Title I has seven subtitles, organized in a reasonably understandable way.

Subtitle A establishes improvements, new rules, and new benefits for most Americans with private health insurance, mostly taking effect in 2010 and 2011.

Subtitle B creates new programs and requirements to improve coverage and the health insurance system in 2010 and 2011.

Subtitle C implements major health insurance market reforms in 2014, such as guaranteed issue and the banning of medical underwriting, with the most extensive changes affecting the individual and small business health insurance markets.

Subtitle D establishes new health insurance exchanges in states beginning in 2014 to help individuals and businesses find coverage.

Subtitle E creates premium and cost-sharing subsidies in 2014 to help Americans buy private coverage and to support small businesses with a new tax credit beginning in 2010.

Subtitle F sets standards for individual and employer responsibility for health insurance coverage beginning in 2014.

Subtitle G protects employees against various forms of discrimination, sets forth rules about implementation, and more.

Let's review the major provisions in each of the seven subtitles in order. There are many. Numbers in brackets [ ] indicate the cost or savings to the federal treasury of each section as estimated by the CBO. A plus sign (+) means the provision costs billions (B) or millions (M) and a minus sign (−) means the section is projected to reduce federal costs by the indicated amount. The number in parentheses ( ) indicates the section in the law.

Subtitle A: Immediate Improvements in Health Care Coverage for All Americans focuses on changes that Congress wanted to happen quickly in 2010 or 2011. Title I's biggest elements don't take effect until 2014, including major health insurance market reforms, the health insurance exchanges, the individual mandate, and the insurance subsidies. Congress wanted to include reforms that could start earlier and put all of these provisions into Subtitles A and B. Relevant sections are identified in parentheses—where there are two section numbers, the first refers to the section in the ACA and the second refers to the section in the Public Health Service Act; if there is only one number, it refers to the ACA section number. Subtitle A's key changes include:

- A prohibition on lifetime and annual benefit caps by insurers—though the restrictions on annual caps don't take full effect until 2014 (sections 1001/2711).

- A prohibition on an insurance industry practice known as "rescissions," which a company uses to cancel someone's coverage after the individual files a claim because of an alleged error or misstatement on a coverage application. Rescissions connected with fraud or deliberate misrepresentations by a policyholder are permitted (sections 1001/2712).

- A requirement that all insurance policies must cover clinical preventive health services with an A or B rating from the U.S. Preventive Services Task Force (more on this in Title V, discussed in chapter 9) and must provide these services without cost sharing (sections 1001/2713).

- A rule that insurers and plans must allow parents to keep their adult children on their health insurance plans until the son or daughter reaches age twenty-six (sections 1001/2714).

- New standards that insurers must follow to provide enrollees with a clear and understandable summary of benefits and coverage not exceeding "4 pages in length" and not including print "smaller than 12-point font" (sections 1001/2715).

- A rebate to consumers if an insurer spends less than 85 or 80 percent of premium dollars on medical-related expenditures, plus mandatory reporting to the HHS secretary and the public on each insurer's "medical loss ratio" (sections 1001/2718).

- New national standards for internal and external appeals for consumers to challenge an insurer's coverage determinations and claims decisions (sections 1001/2719).

- Patient protections including choice of primary care providers, coverage of emergency services, and access to pediatric and obstetrical and gynecological care (sections 1001/2719a).

- New grants to states to establish or expand offices of health insurance consumer assistance to help consumers file appeals and respond to complaints [+$30M] (section 1002).

- An annual public review by states of "unreasonable increases in premiums for health insurance coverage" plus grants to states to help them establish or strengthen these review processes [+$250M] (section 1003).

Subtitle B: Immediate Actions to Preserve and Expand Coverage doesn't sound different from Subtitle A. The main difference is that Subtitle A helps those who already have insurance, while Subtitle B is directed at system improvements to help uninsured persons or specific groups. Like Subtitle A, most of these provisions take effect in 2010 and 2011. There are four key sections:

- Creation of a $5 billion program (until 2014) to provide health insurance for high-risk uninsured individuals who have pre-existing conditions that block them from obtaining coverage. The U.S. Department of Health and Human Services calls this the Pre-Existing Condition Insurance Plan. The program may be run through existing state high-risk pools where states are willing [+$5B] (section 1101).

- Establishment of a program to subsidize employer and union plans that cover early retirees between ages fifty-five and sixty-four. DHHS calls this the Early Retiree Reinsurance Program, and $5 billion is provided through 2014 [+$5B] (section 1102).

- Development by DHHS of a new Internet portal for individuals and businesses to find coverage options for themselves and their workers. The site launched in 2010 at http://www.healthcare.gov/ (section 1103).

- New "administrative simplification" standards for the electronic exchange of information to simplify and reduce the paperwork and clerical burden on patients, providers, and insurers, effective January 2, 2013 [−$11.6B] (section 1104).

Subtitle C: Quality Health Insurance Coverage for All Americans launches dramatic health insurance market reforms taking effect on January 1, 2014, in the individual and group insurance markets in states; some changes also will affect employer self-funded plans regulated by the U.S. Department of Labor. Major provisions include the following:

- New rules affecting the individual and group insurance markets in all fifty states. These include no discrimination or preexisting-condition exclusions based on health status (permitted within specified limits for tobacco use, age, and wellness program participation), guaranteed availability and renewal of coverage, no discrimination in issuing insurance based on health status, required inclusion of specified "essential health benefits" in policies, and required coverage for individuals participating in clinical trials (sections 1201/2701–08).

- A definition of *grandfathering*—the right to maintain most coverage that was in effect before the ACA's enactment—detailing which provisions apply and which do not (section 1251).

Subtitle D: Available Coverage Choices for All Americans establishes a new marketplace called the American Health Benefit Exchange in each state, through which individuals and businesses may purchase coverage beginning in 2014, and sets new rules for all insurance plans offering coverage through these new state-based entities. Key provisions include the following:

- A definition of a "qualified health plan," meaning a health insurance plan eligible to be offered through an exchange (section 1301), and a list of "essential health benefits," to be defined by the HHS secretary, that must be provided in all insurance policies except for grandfathered plans. Among these benefits are:

  ambulatory patient services

  emergency services

  hospitalization

  maternity and newborn care

  mental health and substance abuse services including behavioral health treatment

  prescription drugs

  rehabilitative and habilitative services and devices

  laboratory services

  preventive and wellness services and chronic disease management

  pediatric services, including oral and vision care (section 1302)

- "Special rules" relating to the coverage and noncoverage of abortion services in qualified health plans (section 1303).

- Establishment of exchanges by January 1, 2014, by each state or by the HHS secretary when a state fails to act (sections 1311 and 1321).

- Definitions of "qualified individuals" and "qualified employers" eligible to obtain coverage through an exchange (section 1312). (The section specifies that, beginning in 2014, this will be the only health insurance coverage option available to members of Congress and their personal staff.)

- Creation of new Consumer Operated and Oriented Plans (CO-OPs) to provide nonprofit, member-run health insurance options in states or groups of states (section 1322).

- Allowances for states to create alternative programs to cover eligible individuals and businesses as long as a program covers at least the same number of persons, provides all "essential benefits," and costs the federal government no more (sections 1311 and 1332).

- Provisions permitting states to jointly offer coverage and mandating the creation of at least two new multistate plans to be offered through all fifty state exchanges (sections 1333 and 1334).

- Establishment of reinsurance and risk adjustment so that insurers, in the early years of each exchange, do not suffer financial harm if their plans attract a high number of expensive, high-risk individuals [+$106B] (sections 1341, 1342, and 1343).

Subtitle E: Affordable Coverage for All Americans establishes premium tax credits and cost-sharing protections for exchange policies sold to income-eligible individuals and families to make the purchase of insurance affordable for those with insufficient incomes. Key sections include the following provisions:

- Premium tax credits and maximum premium contributions for eligible individuals and families with incomes up to 400 percent of the federal poverty level (up to about $88,000 for a family of four in 2010), and a requirement that participants contribute between 2 and 9.5 percent of income [+$350B including the cost of section 1402] (section 1401).

- Reduced cost-sharing for individuals enrolled in qualified health plans, based on income. The maximum out-of-pocket limits ($5,950 for individuals and $11,900 for families) are reduced to one-third for those between 100 and 200 percent of the federal poverty level, to one-half for those between 200 and 300 percent of the FPL, and to two-thirds for those between 300 and 400 percent of the FPL (section 1402).

- Establishment of a new tax credit for eligible small businesses that provide health insurance to their workers, limited to 35 percent of the employer's contribution, rising to 50 percent beginning in 2014 [+$37B] (section 1421).

Subtitle F: Shared Responsibility for Health Care defines the responsibilities of individuals and employers in the new market that begins in 2014. Key elements include:

- "Individual responsibility," requiring most individuals to maintain minimum essential health insurance coverage or face a tax penalty of $95 or 1 percent of income in 2014, $325 or 2 percent of income in 2015, and $695 or 2.5 percent of income in 2016 (whichever is higher). Families will pay half the penalty amount for uninsured children, up to a $2,250 family cap. Exceptions include religious objectors, incarcerated individuals, those who cannot afford coverage, taxpayers with incomes below the filing threshold, those who have received a hardship waiver, and those uninsured for fewer than three months [–$17B] (section 1501).

- A "free rider" provision requiring employers with two hundred or more employees to automatically enroll new full-time employees in coverage and requiring employers to notify workers about exchanges, especially when the employer does not offer coverage or pays less than 60 percent of the total cost of benefits. Larger employers (fifty or more employees) with workers who obtain exchange premium subsidies will be assessed between $2,000 and $3,000 for each worker. No penalties are assessed on firms with fewer than fifty full-time workers [–$52B] (sections 1511, 1512, and 1513).

- A "free choice" voucher allowing any worker whose premium for employer coverage would cost between 8 and 9.8 percent of income to buy insurance through an exchange and to use the employer contribution to lower the cost (section 1515).

Subtitle G: Miscellaneous Provisions prohibits discrimination against individuals or organizations that do not support assisted suicide (section

1553); prohibits the HHS secretary from limiting access to health care services (section 1554); guarantees that no individual, business, or insurer must participate in any federal program created under the Act (section 1555); changes the Black Lung Benefits Act (section 1556); protects individuals against discrimination on the basis of sex, race, national origin, disability, or age in health programs or activities (section 1557); and prohibits any employer from firing or discriminating against any worker because the employee received a premium tax credit (section 1558).

THE STRUGGLE OVER HEALTH INSURANCE

In 1993, Deborah Stone wrote a classic article called "The Struggle for the Soul of Health Insurance."[3] In it, she described two competing values undergirding disagreements about the U.S. health insurance system. She called one value the *solidarity principle*—the view that health insurance exists to protect all of us from the impact of high medical expenses, that insurance actualizes the communitarian ideal that we look out for each other, and that payments made today for someone else will benefit us when we need support tomorrow. The competing value is *actuarial fairness*—the notion that we want to share risks and premiums only with those we consider like us, however we may define "us." So if I don't smoke, I might prefer not to be lumped in a pool with smokers; or if I watch my diet, I don't want to be pooled in with obese folks suffering from chronic illness. It can be helpful not to think about this as right versus wrong or good versus bad; these are different values and worldviews. In truth, many of us carry a little bit of both inside ourselves. The ACA deliberately seeks to move the U.S. health system toward the former ideal and away from the latter. At a deeper level, this explains why so many Americans who embrace the actuarial fairness value hate the new law, and why many who embrace the solidarity principle are so disappointed because it did not go nearly far enough.

Health insurance in the United States began in the 1920s as a hospital- or physician-organized nonprofit venture in the communitarian mode for those who could afford to buy it. Premiums were "community" rated, meaning that everyone paid the same regardless of age, infirmity, or whatever else. Blue Cross and Blue Shield plans were organized to take all comers, charging everyone the same premium, and many states granted licenses to Blue plans with an explicit requirement that they play that role—as insurers of last resort. In the 1940s, for-profit commercial health insurance plans entered state markets and honed the actuarial fairness value into actuarial accounting—charging older applicants and enrollees more than younger ones, charging more to those with preexisting conditions or refusing to write them coverage at all, organizing books of business to favor newer, younger, and healthier blocks of enrollees.

Over many years, there have been limited assaults on actuarial fairness at the federal level—most prominently, passage of the Health Insurance Portability and Accountability Act (HIPAA) of 1996, which set national standards mostly for group coverage, as well as significant and widely varying actions by states. Still, the fundamental privilege of insurance companies in most states to write policies under their own rules has been their right for as long as commercial health insurance has been written. The ACA, specifically Title I, if implemented as written, will turn this paradigm upside down. The law's changes to the business of health insurance will transform carriers from private, profit-making enterprises into near-public utilities. While not without limits—there are no price regulations, for example—the transformation represents the most thorough industry reform in history.

The most fundamental changes in insurance markets will not happen until 2014. Still, Subtitles A and B include a lengthy set of policy and program changes taking effect in 2010 and 2011. In part, these provisions reflect political lessons learned from the experience of the 1988 Medicare Catastrophic Coverage law, which was repealed in 1989 before any of the reforms actually took effect. Among the key changes that were already effective or nearly so by 2011 were

- ending lifetime benefit limits and curtailing annual limits;
- prohibiting preexisting condition requirements in private insurance plans for children;
- permitting parents to keep adult children on their health insurance plans until age twenty-six;
- establishing new high-risk pools to provide a coverage option for adults with preexisting conditions prior to implementation of guaranteed issue in 2014;
- creating new standards for consumers to appeal insurance company coverage denials;
- prohibiting the practice of "rescissions," when insurers cancel coverage retroactively;
- making available new small business tax credits to help employers pay for insurance;

- setting limits on insurers for how many premium dollars can be spent on nonmedical expenses—so-called medical loss ratios;

- launching a new national consumer website with public and private health insurance options;

- making subsidies available for employers and unions that provide insurance coverage for early retirees; and

- requiring insurers to cover preventive services without cost sharing.

These "early deliverables" are among the most significant federal interventions health insurance regulation ever made. Still, they pale in comparison with the changes scheduled for 2014.

THE THREE-LEGGED STOOL

Understanding the profound changes mandated by Title I requires understanding three essential components, each interrelated like the legs of the three-legged stool. Take any one or two away, and it falls over. The three legs are insurance-market reforms, an individual mandate, and insurance subsidies. We'll look at each in turn.

The First Leg—Insurance-Market Reform

Since the development of health insurance in the United States in the 1920s, regulation of it has been a chore for states—except when the federal government chooses to step in. In 1945, Congress passed the McCarran-Ferguson Act, which categorizes the business of insurance as interstate commerce subject to federal regulation and oversight. Because the federal government in 1945 had not been regulating insurance prior to this, and because the industry preferred state regulation, the practice was "deemed" to states as long as the feds chose to stay out. Whenever they desire, the federal government has the undisputed right to intervene as it has done occasionally. Besides the HIPAA law, it has passed laws addressing mental health parity, genetic nondiscrimination, Medicare supplemental insurance policies, and other issues.

Health insurance comprises several distinct markets, with important differences. The basic markets cover individuals, small groups, large groups, and the self-insured. Let's take them in reverse order. Most large corporations in the United States do not buy health insurance for their workers; they self-insure their workers and usually pay a third-party administrator (often a large insurance company) to run their plan for them, and they buy stop-loss insurance in case their medical costs run too high in any given period. Self-insured plans are not subject to any state regulation and are overseen with a light touch by the U.S. Department of Labor. Other large employers purchase traditional insurance from carriers; states regulate these policies lightly. Small businesses, generally with fifty or fewer workers, purchase insurance from carriers, and these policies are subject to much tougher oversight by states. Finally, individuals who cannot obtain coverage through a group plan and but who can afford the premiums will buy coverage in the individual—or nongroup—market. The insurance-market changes required by the ACA affect individual coverage the most, then small-group, then large-group, and then self-insured plans the least.

For the most part, the federal government grants states wide latitude in going tough or light on regulating health insurers. A few states have banned practices such as preexisting-condition exclusions and medical underwriting and have narrowed the differences in how premiums are set for different groups, while most states tread lightly or not at all, especially in the volatile market for individual (or nongroup) coverage. Some states aggressively protect consumers from insurer underwriting practices, while others mostly monitor the actuarial soundness of their companies—the essential function of insurance regulation. The result is a patchwork of regulation exemplified by comparing New York State and Pennsylvania.

In the early 1990s, New York State imposed new rules in its state-licensed markets, including strict community rating in its individual market so that premiums cannot vary except by geography—not by age, medical status, or gender. Also, all insurers selling individual coverage are subject to "guaranteed issue," requiring them to sell policies to all comers. In Pennsylvania, by contrast, insurers may refuse to write coverage, and they may charge higher premiums based on age, gender, health status, smoking status, or whatever else the insurer chooses. In New York, individual coverage is available for anyone, and it is highly expensive, resulting in a tiny market for individual coverage. In Pennsylvania, individual premiums are more affordable and more consumers purchase individual coverage—though buying insurance is much more expensive for older consumers and for those with chronic medical conditions.

The insurance-market reforms in Title I, especially reforms in Subtitles A and C, move the nation's individual health insurance markets much closer to the New York model and away from the Pennsylvania brand, though not quite as far in some important respects as in others.

The cornerstone requirement, effective in all states beginning January 1, 2014, is "guaranteed issue"—insurers must sell a policy to any qualified applicant. Medical underwriting—the practice of covering, or refusing to cover, someone or pricing premiums based on the applicant's medical history—will be outlawed. Insurers will be allowed to vary premiums within a geographic region by just three categories—how old the applicant is (older participants must pay no more than three times the premium of the youngest participants; the current practice in most states is much higher), whether the applicant uses tobacco products, and whether the applicant is part of an employer or insurer program that rewards enrollees for participating in certain wellness activities.

The new rules do not regulate the premiums that insurers charge. Premium price controls were not included in the ACA. Instead, the law requires insurers to spend at least eighty or eight-five cents of every premium dollar on medical costs and to refund the difference to policyholders (80 percent of the premiums for small employer groups and individuals; 85 percent for large employer groups). Also the HHS secretary, along with state governments, has new authority to review "unreasonable increases" in premiums, though not to restrain or overrule premium increases unless the state permits such limits.

So insurance-market reform, particularly in the individual coverage market—and especially guaranteed issue—is the first essential leg of the reform stool. When guaranteed issue is imposed in a market—guaranteeing consumers the right to purchase coverage whenever they need it—many persons with chronic illness and high medical costs will sign up for coverage right away, and many younger, healthier individuals will defer buying coverage until they need it. This results in a spike in premiums, which then causes younger, healthier consumers to opt out, further increasing premiums, triggering an insurance cycle known as a death spiral. This dynamic can be seen in New York State, where guaranteed issue was implemented in the early 1990s and the individual market dropped from 752,000 covered lives in 1994 to approximately 34,000 in 2009 as younger and healthier enrollees dropped coverage.[4] In the 1990s, Kentucky, New Hampshire, and Washington implemented guaranteed issue in their individual markets and then repealed the new rules following large premium increases. Besides New York, only Maine, Massachusetts, New Jersey, and Vermont instituted full guaranteed issue and kept it in place despite the spike in individual insurance premiums that followed.

Guaranteed issue alone creates problems—and needs the other two legs of the stool.

The Second Leg—Individual Responsibility

All other advanced nations around the globe require their residents to obtain and pay for health insurance coverage, whether in public systems in Canada and Great Britain or in private systems in Switzerland and the Netherlands. Voluntary systems create a "free rider" problem, as some take advantage of services and benefits without contributing. In the United States, a mandate on individuals to purchase health insurance first became a serious topic of discussion during the 1993–94 Clinton reform period when moderate Republicans, led by Senator John Chafee (R-RI) advanced the idea. It was known as "Chafee-Dole" because Senate Republican leader Bob Dole (R-KS) wanted his name included as a leading supporter. Conservative health economist Mark Pauly is credited with first developing the idea in the U.S. health policy context in the 1980s.[5] The conservative Heritage Foundation began promoting the idea in the late 1980s.[6] While the idea never attracted a groundswell of support in either political party, a number of Senate Republicans signed on to it as an alternative to the Clinton proposal, only to turn against the idea in 2009–10.

Although the idea periodically reappeared—prominently, Senator John Breaux (D-LA) advanced it in the late 1990s—it was the signing of the 2006 Massachusetts health reform law that put the individual mandate front and center. Even though Massachusetts had a lower level of uninsurance pre-reform than the nation as a whole, its ability to implement the mandate with minimal political opposition and overt Republican support suggested the basis for a national health reform compromise. Even Senator Charles Grassley (R-IA), the ranking Republican on the Senate Finance Committee and a backer of the individual mandate in 1993–94, publicly endorsed the idea until tea-party-led town meetings in August 2009 deepened a growing political polarization. By September, he publicly changed his position to oppose an individual mandate.

The rationale for an individual mandate—or individual "responsibility," in its polite form—was embraced by a wide swath of the health policy community, including insurance companies, business organizations, medical provider groups, and think tanks. A portion of the political left slowly embraced the concept—as long as a "public option" was included as one coverage choice for those subject to the mandate. For the insurance industry, the only way to achieve guaranteed issue was by tying it to an effective individual mandate—and their key word is *effective*, meaning substantial. For insurers, an effective mandate penalty needed to be close to the actual cost of buying insurance; otherwise, many would pay the penalty instead of obtaining coverage. Even though Massachusetts lowered its overall uninsurance rate from 8–10 percent to between 2 and 3 percent, an estimated sixty thousand to eighty thousand persons chose to pay the penalty instead of buying coverage. In the Senate Finance Committee markup in September–October 2009, Senators Olympia Snowe (R-ME) and Chuck Schumer (D-NY) successfully amended the Finance bill by eliminating any penalty in the first year and lowering it substantially in subsequent years—a change that alarmed insurers, leading them to release a series of actuarial analyses predicting an explosion in premiums if the current version prevailed. By March 2010, sentiment had shifted to higher penalties in order to persuade the CBO to estimate that the law's coverage provisions would lead to at least 95 percent coverage of all Americans.

In Massachusetts, the penalty started small in 2007, the loss of the state personal income tax exemption, or about $220. In 2008 and beyond the penalty rose to no more than half the cost of the most affordable insurance plan, about $900, and rising annually thereafter. In Massachusetts, the mandate penalty applies only to adults, not to children, while the ACA includes penalties on parents for noncoverage of their children.

The ACA mandate is written to work this way: beginning in 2014, every citizen and legal immigrant must have health insurance that meets the law's minimum standards or face a penalty when filing taxes for the year. In 2016, when fully implemented, the fine will be 2.5 percent of income or $695, whichever is higher. (In 2014, the penalty is 1 percent of income or $95, and in 2015 it is 2 percent or $325.) Cost-of-living adjustments will be made annually after 2016. The penalty for uncovered children is one-half the adult penalty up to 2.5 percent of income or the adult penalty times three. If the least inexpensive policy available would cost more than 8 percent of one's monthly income, no penalties apply, and hardship exemptions will be permitted for those who cannot afford the cost. Also, there is no penalty for a spell of uninsurance of less than three months.

There are also exemptions for those with religious objections, as well as for those who participate in an established "health care sharing ministry," a nonprofit cooperative where members share the cost of each other's medical expenses. How did this latter provision happen? The Christian Care Ministry—which runs a network called "Medi-Share"—reached out to Senate staffers and convinced us it was a legitimate, albeit unorthodox, coverage alternative for people of faith that would otherwise be forced out of business by the mandate. The exemption got into the original HELP bill markup in June 2009, got tightened along the way so that new entities could not use it as a loophole, and stayed.

TABLE 2. Individual-mandate penalties

Year effective	Tax penalty (in dollars)	Percentage of income
2014	95	1.0
2015	325	2.0
2016	695	2.5
2017 and beyond	695*	2.5

* Plus inflation index

Opposition to ACA on the basis of the individual mandate was slow to emerge, to the surprise of members and staffers. Many other issues drew heavy fire—the public option, the employer mandate, budget reconciliation, the revenues needed to pay for reform, and so much more. In the final months of the legislative process, Republican state attorneys general began threatening to sue against the ACA on constitutional grounds, targeting the individual mandate. Two groups of attorneys general did file separate legal actions shortly after the ACA's signing along with other groups. Senate staffers anticipated a constitutional challenge and, taking the advice of constitutional scholars, included as the first part of the individual mandate section—1501(a) in Title I—congressional findings that declared the ACA's constitutionality.[7] The argument rests on two forms of constitutional authority: first, the power to regulate interstate commerce (Congress declared the business of insurance as interstate commerce in the 1945 McCarran-Ferguson Act); and second, the power to tax and spend for the general welfare. Others disagree, and the final verdict seems likely to come from the U.S. Supreme Court.[8]

The ACA does not contain a common legislative device known as a "severability clause," which declares the intent of Congress that if one provision of a law is declared unconstitutional, then the rest of the law will still stand, and some have questioned why. There is an answer. The House had included a severability clause in its health reform legislation approved in November 2009, putting the matter in play when the House and Senate would later merge their respective bills. By the late fall, Senate Republicans had begun to argue against the constitutionality of the individual mandate as a talking point against reform, and Democratic staffers decided to leave out severability to deprive Republican senators of a talking point against the law—Republicans would claim that the inclusion of severability showed the Democrats' lack of confidence. Unfortunately for Democrats, the January 19 Massachusetts special Senate election ended the merger process, and Democrats could not insert a severability clause through the reconciliation sidecar because the provision would have no fiscal impact. If there is such a thing as "congressional intent," the intent was to deprive Republicans of a talking point on the Senate floor, and then to insert severability in the final legislative stage.

Although Massachusetts is not representative of the nation as a whole, it has demonstrated that implementation of an individual mandate is feasible and can address the issue of adverse selection triggered by guaranteed issue, even if imperfectly. There was, though, an additional problem. How could a mandate to purchase coverage work when the price of health insurance was well beyond the financial capacity of most uninsured persons?

The Third Leg: Insurance-Purchase Subsidies

Guaranteed issue eliminates most discrimination in insurance markets and requires an individual mandate to prevent individuals from waiting to buy coverage until they need medical care. An individual mandate addresses selection problems created by insurance reform and requires subsidies to make the purchase of insurance affordable for those who otherwise could not afford it. Creating a workable subsidy structure was one of the most important and difficult policy challenges in crafting health reform.

There are two parts to subsidies, each equally important: premium reductions and cost-sharing reductions. Premium subsidies are needed so that the cost of purchasing health insurance does not take too much out of a family's household budget. It's not good enough, though, to reduce premiums to an affordable level if the coverage requires co-payments, deductibles, or co-insurance that prevents individuals and families from obtaining necessary medical care. Both elements are important, and both are addressed in Subtitle E of Title I of the ACA.

The subsidies are scheduled to take effect in 2014 at the same time as the major insurance-market reforms, the exchanges, and the individual mandate, all by design. Uninsured persons with incomes below 133 percent of the federal poverty level (that is, up to $14,404 in annual income for an individual and $29,327 for a family of four in 2010) will be eligible for Medicaid in all states beginning at the same time. All other individuals and families who cannot get insurance through their employers or other sources will be allowed to purchase coverage through a new state exchange; and those with incomes between 133 and 400 percent of the federal poverty level will be eligible for premium and cost-sharing subsidies (up to about

TABLE 3. Premium and cost-sharing subsidies under the ACA

Income		Required premium contribution		
Income as percentage of poverty level	Annual amount (in dollars)	Percentage of income	Monthly amount (in dollars)	Actuarial value of coverage
Family of four				
133–150	29,547–33,075	3.0–4.0	74–110	94
150–200	33,075–44,100	4.0–6.3	110–232	87
200–250	44,100–55,125	6.3–8.1	232–372	73
250–300	55,125–66,150	8.1–9.5	372–524	70
300–350	66,150–77,175	9.5	524–611	70
350–400	77,175–88,200	9.5	611–698	70
Individual				
133–150	14,512–16,245	3.0–4.0	36–54	94
150–200	16,245–21,660	4.0–6.3	54–114	87
200–250	21,660–27,075	6.3–8.1	114–182	73
250–300	27,075–32,490	8.1–9.5	182–257	70
300–350	32,490–37,905	9.5	257–300	70
350–400	37,905–43,320	9.5	300–343	70

SOURCE: January Angeles, "Making Health Care More Affordable: The New Premium and Cost-Sharing Credits" (Washington, DC: Center for Budget and Policy Priorities, May 19, 2010).

$42,000 for an individual and $88,000 for a family of four). Individuals or families who are eligible for Medicaid or Medicare or offered employer coverage will not be able to obtain premium subsidies unless the employer coverage would cost them more than 9.5 percent of their income. Table 3 shows the level of premium and cost-sharing subsidies for an individual and for a family of four.

The table shows that, for example, a family of four making about $55,000 would pay 8.1 percent of the cost of premiums, or about $372 per month for family coverage. Individuals making about $16,000 a year would pay 4 percent of their income for premiums, or $54 per month.

The subsidies to reduce cost sharing apply to those with family incomes below 250 percent of the federal poverty level. The far-right column in table 3 is labeled "actuarial value of coverage." *Actuarial value* in health insurance refers to the average portion of the total cost of covered benefits paid by a health insurance plan. For families and individuals with incomes over 250 percent of the FPL, the actuarial value is set on average at 70 percent, with enrollees, *on average*, paying the other 30 percent in the form of co-payments, deductibles, or co-insurance (the combination will vary widely by insurer and, thus, so will the real risk faced by enrollees). Enrollees can buy more comprehensive coverage but will have to pay the difference themselves. Like the premium credits, the cost-sharing credits are "progressive" in that they provide the greatest assistance to those with the lowest incomes. So a family of four with a $30,000 income is liable for 6 percent cost sharing, and a family of four with a $54,000 annual income is liable for as much as 27 percent.

How should one judge these subsidy levels? First, they are not cheap—the Congressional Budget Office estimates they will cost about $337 billion over six years, 2014 through 2019. When combined with the cost of risk adjustment and reinsurance, the total cost is estimated at $464 billion over the six years—cheaper, though, than the cost of subsidies in the health reform bill passed by the House of Representatives in November 2009, estimated at $602 billion for seven years, 2013 through 2019. The cost of subsidies in the HELP Committee bill marked up in July 2009 was estimated at $723 billion over eight years, 2012 through 2019. So the cost of subsidies went from $723 to $602 to $449 billion as the legislation progressed.

How did that happen? In several ways: the start date was pushed from 2012 in HELP to 2013 in the House to 2014 in the final Senate version, lowering costs a lot; second, the generosity of the subsidies was reduced; and third, the actuarial values of the insurance policies—meaning the level of required consumer cost sharing—was reduced a lot, *increasing* the cost to consumers. Why? It was done to reduce the total cost of the legislation to the federal government. In his September address to Congress, when President Obama set a $900 billion limit on the ten-year cost of a bill, that pressured both Chambers to lower the generosity of premium and cost-sharing subsidies. Financial assistance in the ACA was limited to hold down the bill's total cost. The result is sizable though not overly generous premium subsidies as well as cost-sharing subsidies and protections that will leave many lower-middle-income individuals and families at risk of significant expenses when they suffer illness or injury.

Further, during the ten-year window from 2010 to 2019, subsidies will increase each year but will probably not match the overall rate of growth in health insurance costs, exacerbating affordability challenges. Beginning in 2020, the annual increases are pegged to the rise in the consumer price index, which nearly always rises at a rate well below that of health insurance premiums and medical inflation. This formula likely guarantees a further and growing affordability gap for consumers receiving premium and cost-sharing subsidies through state exchange policies. This was done to achieve a favorable budget score from the CBO for the second decade of the law between 2020 and 2029. It is one of the significant pieces of unfinished business in the ACA.

THE EXCHANGE

Before health insurance exchanges become a reality in all fifty states in 2014, it's easy to visit one or two well before the 2014 implementation. Massachusetts's Commonwealth Health Insurance Connector Authority can be found at http://mahealthconnector.org/ and the Utah Health Exchange can be found at http://www.exchange.utah.gov/. Some businesses in Massachusetts can purchase health insurance in a matter of minutes using the Connector website. That is what an exchange does— it provides an organized marketplace to buy health insurance. It can be run by a government agency or a nonprofit or a for-profit group (see, for example, http://www.ehealthinsurance.com/). It can act like a virtual "yellow pages," just giving individuals information about options and access to purchase, or it can act as an advocate and agent for consumers, setting standards that insurance companies must meet in order to get listed on the site. One key power of the exchange will be the ability to include or not include insurers, because the premium and cost-sharing subsidies will guarantee a substantial marketplace for individual coverage at least.

What can an exchange do with the power of exclusion? It can protect safety-net providers by requiring health plan administrators to contract with them. It can promote more integrated delivery systems that deliver comprehensive care services. It can pressure plans to reduce their administrative costs and lean on them to keep premiums lower than they might otherwise be. The exchange needs to be careful in using this power. Too much pressure may result in a significant shrinking of the choice of plans within it, lessening the entity's clout and ability to deliver a better deal for individuals and small businesses. The state exchanges will have guaranteed participation by lower-income individuals eligible for subsidies, but they will attract businesses and higher-income individuals only by offering meaningful value and choice. Achieving both the business and social objectives is a challenging balancing act, one that will play out differently state by state and market by market.

The exchange idea is not new; the Clinton health plan proposed regional "health alliances" that would act as purchasing pools for businesses and individuals—powerful alliances that would have claimed a state's entire health insurance market except for Medicare. Though that plan crashed, the idea lived on. Early in the new century, the conservative Heritage Foundation proposed a health insurance exchange to the Washington DC city government and received a mixed response. When it learned that Massachusetts Republican governor Mitt Romney wanted private-market ideas to expand health insurance, it fed him the idea and he bit, adding an exchange in his first proposal released in 2004. The Massachusetts legislature liked the idea too, just not enough to give Romney naming rights, so it changed the name to the Connector. It is close to the same thing, though the Connector has more regulatory power than Romney and Heritage preferred. Along with the individual mandate, it was a key and bipartisan idea from Massachusetts that had bipartisan legs for a national reform plan.

Under the ACA, every state may organize its own exchange to meet basic federal standards, but if a state fails to begin establishing one by the end of 2012, then the secretary of health and human services will step in to do it using federal authority. The House, in its reform plan, wanted a single federally run exchange, and President Obama preferred the House version in the House-Senate negotiations just prior to the January 19, 2010, Massachusetts special election. Because changes to the exchange structure were ruled by the Senate parliamentarian in the March 2010 reconciliation debate to have no significant budget impact, the Senate version and language remained.

Insurance companies that want to participate in an exchange need to meet a series of statutory requirements and be designated a "qualified health plan." Many plans will want to do this because the only way consumers can obtain premium and cost-sharing subsidies will be with policies obtained through their state exchange. The CBO estimates by 2019 there will be about twenty-five million Americans obtaining insurance through exchanges, about nineteen million of them with subsidies. The prior individual, or nongroup, market will still be around, though it will shrink substantially as many of its participants move to the exchanges. Insurers who participate will be required to offer coverage at these actuarial-value levels:

bronze	60 percent
silver	70 percent
gold	80 percent
platinum	90 percent

What differentiates one category from the next is no mystery. Bronze means lower premiums with cost sharing averaging as high as 40 percent of the cost of services, platinum means higher premiums with cost-sharing averages at 10 percent, and gold and silver are in between. Subsidized premiums and cost sharing are pegged at the silver level. As mentioned, the exact structure of the cost sharing (deductibles, co-insurance, and co-payments) will differ widely from plan to plan. A catastrophic-coverage level—with more cost sharing than bronze—must be offered to individuals under age thirty and to those exempted from the individual mandate penalty because of unaffordability or hardship. State exchanges also must set up a SHOP (Small Business Health Options Program) plan to help small businesses find affordable coverage; they are allowed to combine this with individual coverage. The SHOP model was taken from bipartisan legislation filed by Senator Richard Durbin (D-IL) to help small businesses and bring them into the health reform fold.

Subtitle D of Title I, the exchange section, provides several forms of flexibility. For example, the HHS secretary may provide start-up loans to establish member-run, nonprofit health insurance cooperatives, an idea advanced by Senator Kent Conrad (D-ND) as an alternative to the public-plan option. States may establish "basic health programs" for lower-income persons, as Washington State did with its Basic Health plan, Senator Maria Cantwell's (D-WA) idea. States can obtain waivers for up to five years to try an entirely different model as long as it covers at least as many persons, provides basic benefits and cost protections, and costs no more than the ACA formulation, an idea championed by Senators Ron Wyden (D-OR) and Bernie Sanders (I-VT), though no state can obtain a waiver from this section before 2017.

This subtitle also addresses an especially controversial health reform issue—abortion. Section 1303, Special Rules (Senate staffers, unlike House staffers, did not want to use the word "abortion" in the title), requires that no federal dollars can be used, directly or indirectly, to pay for abortion services. States may go further and prohibit any coverage of abortion in any qualified health plan offered through their exchange—an incentive for conservative states to set up their own exchanges rather than having the federal government do so. Also, health plans may determine whether or not to provide coverage for abortion services, as long as funds for the service are segregated.

WHO IS LEFT OUT?

The ACA is often characterized by its cheerleaders as "universal health insurance." Not quite. The CBO estimates that by 2019, if fully implemented, the United States will have 23 million non-elderly uninsured persons; the chief actuary for the Centers for Medicare and Medicaid Services makes a more precise estimate of 23.6 million. Without the ACA or other changes, the CBO says the United States would otherwise have 54 million uninsured, and CMS says 56.9 million. Pretty close. Who are the 23 to 23.6 million who will not be covered?

For the most part, they fit into three categories, roughly equal in size, though substantial uncertainty resides in these estimates. One big group is undocumented immigrants (a.k.a. illegal aliens) who are ineligible for Medicaid or exchange subsidies or even unsubsidized private coverage through an exchange. The second group includes lower-income persons who will be eligible to enroll in state Medicaid programs and will not do so. There are millions in this category today and there will be many more in the future; how many depends on how aggressive state governments choose to be in finding and signing them up—some states have long used their enrollment procedures to discourage eligible individuals and families from signing up for coverage. Under the ACA, hospitals, health centers, and other medical providers will be able to sign up these low-income persons when they seek care, so their failure to enroll will not prevent them from obtaining care when needed. The third group consists of individuals who are unable to find affordable coverage options available to them and those who choose to pay the individual mandate penalty rather than sign up for coverage—it is their choice under the law. In Massachusetts, this group comprised an estimated 52,956 persons in 2008.[9]

The third group illustrates why the term *individual mandate* is a bit of a misnomer. For example, in Switzerland, under that nation's individual health insurance mandate, uncovered individuals, when identified, are enrolled automatically in coverage and sent a bill, which the government makes sure is paid. The ACA's individual mandate is less a mandate than a tax penalty for not buying coverage when required to do so. That is why the term *individual or personal responsibility* is more accurate than the term *individual mandate*.

EMPLOYER RESPONSIBILITY

"Shared responsibility" was the essential political mantra of Massachusetts health reform. Every major party—government, consumers, insurers, medical providers, and business—had to assume new responsibilities to achieve the goals of reform. The responsibilities of business, in particular those of businesses that did not provide insurance coverage to their workers, was a contentious topic. The final result in Massachusetts was an annual assessment of $295 per uninsured worker on businesses with ten or more workers that do not make a "fair and reasonable" contribution to providing their employees with health insurance.

Requiring all or most employers to provide worker health insurance has been a standard feature in universal coverage schemes since President Richard Nixon's 1973 plan. It was a central feature of the 1993 Clinton reform plan and a core element in the Obama, Clinton, and Edwards presidential campaign health platforms. It is also a feature opposed strenuously by Republicans and many conservative Democrats, and more so by business organizations such as the U.S. Chamber of Commerce, the National Federation of Independent Business and industry-specific trade groups such as the National Restaurant Association and the National Retail Federation.

The House of Representatives reflected this polarization, though Democrats had enough of a majority to include in its health reform bill a robust "pay or play" obligation on employers to pay at least 8 percent of total payroll on employee health insurance or pay the difference to the federal government. It was not just a political obligation—it was an important part of the House's health reform financing plan, with $135 billion in employer contributions over ten years. It was also a core element of the policy structure to make employers less likely to stop offering coverage to workers because of the fees they would otherwise have to pay. Policy experts and the CBO advised that a failure to include employer responsibility would trigger a massive dropping of insurance by businesses, something that would sharply increase the cost of any plan.

A House-like structure was inconceivable in a Senate which had zero Republican support for an employer mandate and a bevy of moderate Democrats unwilling to go there. An alternative approach was needed—not just to produce revenue but also to disincentivize employers who might drop worker health insurance and encourage their employees to enroll in subsidized exchange plans. The CBO backed up the fear with warnings about its scoring of any plan that failed to keep employers in the health insurance game.

Back in 2004, the Massachusetts state government began producing an annual report detailing by name employers that had fifty or more workers obtaining public forms of health insurance coverage through the state. The report showed that the cost to the state to provide coverage for these workers amounted to $805 million in 2009.[10] The listed companies were not struggling small businesses, but major corporations, including universities, hospitals, retailers, and even state and local governments. Would it be possible, Senate staffers wondered, to frame an assessment based not on a firm's failure to offer coverage but instead on a firm's reliance on public funds to finance part or all of its workforce's health insurance needs?

Senate HELP Committee Democrats were intrigued by the idea—dubbed the "fair-share assessment" on employers—until unions and the Center on Budget and Policy Priorities, a liberal think tank, sharply objected that the scheme would open workers receiving public insurance to discriminatory treatment by their employers; the matter was dropped in favor of a $750 hit on employers with at least twenty-five workers for each uncovered full-time employee and $375 for each part-timer. Though HELP discarded the "fair share" idea, Senate Finance staffers Liz Fowler and Yvette Fontenot in the summer of 2009 decided it might be a workable approach in their committee, where discussions among the bipartisan Gang of Six were still proceeding. Even Republicans Chuck Grassley and Mike Enzi expressed openness for an assessment on employers whose workers obtained public health insurance support as opposed to an assessment on employers for not covering their workers.

Though the Gang of Six broke up in mid-September without a deal, Baucus included the idea in the plan he brought before the full Finance Committee in mid-September. The chairman's mark included a section titled Required Payments for Employees Receiving Premium Credits, which required all employers with more than fifty workers to pay a $400 annual fee for each employee who receives a tax credit for health insurance through a state exchange. This reframing of employer responsibility survived the Finance markup. The downside was that the proposal brought in only $23 billion in revenue as opposed the House-generated revenue of $135 billion.

Reid included the Baucus formulation in the merged health reform bill he advanced in November, and it survived intact in the final Senate PPACA approved on December 24, 2009, after negotiations with the Business Roundtable and the Center on Budget and Policy Priorities. It was expected to be controversial in the House-Senate negotiations, and no final deal was reached prior to the January 19 Massachusetts special election. The final reconciliation sidecar bill modified the employer-responsibility provisions by substantially increasing the assessment: a business that employs at least fifty workers and that offers coverage but has at least one full-time employee receiving the premium assistance tax credit will pay the lesser of $3,000 for each employee receiving a tax credit or $2,000 for each of the full-time employees, for an estimated ten-year revenue of $52 billion. This tougher standard is a key reason why the CBO estimates that only 3 million workers with employer health insurance—out of an estimated 162 million—will drop coverage and move to exchange plans by 2019.

This structure is certain to be controversial as 2014 draws closer. The principle of employer responsibility for worker health insurance coverage, albeit in a limited and unorthodox form, has been incorporated into federal law via the ACA.

IMMIGRANTS

It was the most dramatic moment of President Obama's September 9, 2009, address to a joint session of Congress to promote national health reform. It followed a month of tense and confrontational town meetings across the nation where self-described "tea party" activists opposing health reform and the Obama agenda shouted down members of Congress and reform supporters. In his address, Obama said: "There are also those who claim that our reform effort will insure illegal immigrants. This, too, is false. The reforms—the reforms I'm proposing would not apply to those who are here illegally."

"You lie!" shouted South Carolina Republican congressman Joe Wilson.

"That's not true," Obama responded.

Section 1312 of the ACA (Title I, Subtitle D) settles the matter:

RESIDENTS.—If an individual is not, or is not reasonably expected to be for the entire period for which enrollment is sought, a citizen or national of the United States or an alien lawfully present in the United States, the individual shall not be treated as a qualified individual and may not be covered under a qualified health plan in the individual market that is offered through an Exchange.

Because subsidies can be obtained only through enrollment in a qualified health plan, undocumented (or "illegal") aliens are ineligible for financial support and ineligible to enroll in an exchange plan even without subsidies. Individual insurance markets outside exchanges are expected to continue in smaller form as a pathway for these residents to purchase individual coverage. An estimated twelve million undocumented aliens were living in the United States in 2006, and 60 percent have no health insurance, according to the Pew Hispanic Center.[11] The most likely sources of care for undocumented aliens are community health centers and hospital emergency departments; the ACA doubles federal support for federally qualified community health centers (and greatly expands financing for the National Health Service Corps, which provides medical personnel for many health centers), thus enhancing their ability to provide medical treatment to this population. Excluding undocumented immigrants from purchasing even unsubsidized coverage through an exchange seemed overkill and unwise policy to some Democratic members and staffers, House and Senate; but given the continuing controversy, it was judged an unwinnable political issue.

For legally residing immigrants, the ACA represents real improvement. In 1996, President Clinton signed federal welfare reform legislation into law, establishing a five-year waiting period before newly entering legal immigrants could obtain health coverage through a state Medicaid program. The ACA does not change that requirement. However, there is no parallel waiting period for enrollment and subsidies in qualified health plans through state exchanges, providing a new coverage pathway for legal immigrants. This is a meaningful and positive change for this population.

So the bottom line on the ACA and immigrants is mostly the status quo for undocumented immigrants and significant improvements for legal immigrants.

THE PUBLIC-PLAN OPTION

A contentious issue not included in the final ACA, though it played a marquee role in the national debate, is the public option, or public-plan option. Were it included, it would be in Subtitle D. The idea is straightforward: in addition to an array of private health insurance choices, each exchange would offer an additional choice, a federally sponsored health insurance plan.

The idea goes back at least to 1991 in a paper written by Karen Davis of the Commonwealth Fund (then at Johns Hopkins University),[12] and it has been advanced by various sources in intervening years.[13] In 2007, Yale political scientist Jacob Hacker developed an updated version of the idea in his "Health Care for America" proposal.[14] His plan caught the attention of progressives seeking a health reform platform with a greater chance of success than the single-payer/Medicare for All approach. Activists launching the Health Care for America Now coalition saw the public option, properly structured, as a gradual and sure-footed path to a form of single payer. Opponents from the insurance industry, Republicans, and others had the same vision—only to them, it was a nightmare.

The power of the public option, in its pure form, is about money. The Hacker plan proposed to pay physicians, hospitals, and other providers at Medicare rates of payment, and required all Medicare providers, especially physicians, to participate in the public plan as well. Generally, though not everywhere, Medicaid pays providers the least, private plans pay the most, and Medicare is in the middle, closer to Medicaid than to private reimbursement rates. The Hacker arrangement would have enabled the public plan to charge premiums far less than what private plans charge and, with a guaranteed broad base of participating providers, might have provoked a massive exodus from existing insurance plans into the new public-plan option. The Lewin Group, a health consulting firm owned by the giant insurer United Healthcare, estimated that a public plan tied to Medicare and open to all comers (something never envisioned in congressional reform plans) could attract as many as 131 million enrollees within a ten-year span, about 119 million of whom would drop existing private coverage to enroll in the public plan.[15] While Lewin was criticized for some of its assumptions, no one disagreed that a wide-open, Medicare-linked public option would be a major game change dwarfing most other impacts of the ACA. The only difference was whether one loved or hated that outcome.

If insurance companies had been alone in opposing the public plan, it may well have made its way into the ACA. That was not the case. Hospitals, physicians, a host of other provider groups, and most business organizations adamantly opposed the public option. In particular, hospitals and physicians in the central and mountain states informed senators and representatives that their Medicare payment rates were especially low when compared with those of other states—creating an even wider gap between Medicare and private payment rates in those parts of the nation—and that a public plan tied to Medicare would be financially disastrous for them. A host of plains states Democrats, including liberals such as Iowa's Tom Harkin, made clear in the spring of 2009 that they could support only a public option that paid providers at negotiated private rates, not Medicare. The Lewin Group had estimated that a public plan tied to private rates would attract only 12 million from existing private coverage as opposed to 119 million under the Medicare version. The CBO, in its analysis, estimated that a public-plan option not tied to Medicare and limited to exchange-eligible individuals and businesses would attract between 2 and

3 million enrollees—from game change to nearly inconsequential. Public-option opponents still feared that a weakened public option, once enacted, could be expanded by a future Congress, a possibility that explains progressives' continuing attachment to the concept.

Still, the Democratic Party's progressive wing, including House members, organized labor, and the well-financed and organized Health Care for America Now coalition, staked much of their commitment to reform on the inclusion of a public option. Indeed, for many progressives, including those in Congress, the public option was their essential justification for supporting the process and moving away from a single-payer plan. Others considered the public option debate a significant distraction from issues such as the affordability of insurance subsidies; one thing all sides would agree on was that the public option debate generated enormous attention throughout the process.

The HELP Committee, in its June–July 2009 markup, was the first to advance a scaled back, non-Medicare-linked public option, designed by Senators Sheldon Whitehouse (D-RI), Sherrod Brown (D-OH), and Kay Hagan (D-NC), called the Community Health Insurance Option (CHIO). Most observers seemed to miss the significance of the delinking to Medicare, thus sustaining the public option debate as one of the most contentious and publicized in the process. When the House Energy and Commerce Committee stalled in its deliberations in late July over many issues including the public option, the Democratic Blue Dogs agreed to a scaled-back public option modeled on HELP's CHIO in their deal with chair Henry Waxman to move the bill out of committee. In November, the House-approved health reform legislation included a CHIO-like public option.

Senator Max Baucus included no public option, CHIO or otherwise, in his mark for the Senate Finance Committee, only Senator Conrad's idea to encourage private and nonprofit health insurance cooperatives. Senators Jay Rockefeller (D-WV) and Charles Schumer (D-NY) proposed amendments to add a CHIO-like public option, and both failed, with Baucus, Conrad, and Blanche Lincoln (D-AR) voting no. When Majority Leader Harry Reid advanced his November version of health reform—merging the Senate Finance and HELP bills—he surprised many by including the CHIO, modifying it to permit states to decline the option if they so chose. If it was going to be dropped, he would not be the one to do it and would give his progressive members a fighting chance. As he worked to acquire sixty votes to pass the PPACA in the Senate in December, Senators Ben Nelson (D-NE) and Joe Lieberman (I-CT) declared they would not vote for any bill containing a public-plan option. After several days of mulling the inclusion of a Medicare buy-in for those aged fifty-five to sixty-four, the idea was dropped in order to achieve the needed sixty votes. All that was added was a requirement for the development of multistate, nonprofit private plans to be offered in all states, facilitated by the federal Office of Personnel Management, which runs the health insurance program for federal workers.

As the reconciliation option emerged in February 2010 as the path to bring health reform to closure in the wake of the Democrats' loss of their sixty-vote majority in the Senate, public-plan advocates made one last push for inclusion, because reconciliation rules allowed legislation to pass with only fifty-one Senate votes. House Speaker Pelosi declared that proposal a nonstarter, and Senator Rockefeller, a public-plan diehard, publicly renounced the suggestion, ending the conversation.

The idea of a public plan in the exchanges is not dead. It could be added at any point in the future depending on the success or failure of the ACA coverage structure and the future political makeup of the House and Senate. In the wake of the Republican takeover of the House in January 2011, it is moribund for the foreseeable future.

ADMINISTRATIVE SIMPLIFICATION

One of the most noted inefficiencies in the U.S. health care system is the enormous paperwork and bureaucratic burden, estimated to consume as much as 24 percent of all U.S. health spending.[16] The noted health economist Henry Aaron made this comment about the system's complexity:

> I look at the U.S. health care system and see an administrative monstrosity, a truly bizarre mélange of thousands of payers with payment systems that differ for no socially beneficial reason, as well as a staggeringly complex public system with mind-boggling administered prices and other rules expressing distinctions that can only be regarded as weird.[17]

The 1996 Health Insurance Portability and Accountability Act (HIPAA) included provisions on administrative simplification designed to reduce the bureaucratic burden on providers and on the larger health care system. As a result of these provisions, new rules were written, but positive results were difficult to see. One explanation is that the HIPAA standards were voluntary for many providers and were implemented sporadically without achieving visible savings. Since HIPAA's passage, the development of new health information technologies (HIT) has accelerated dramatically.

Additionally, the American Recovery and Reinvestment Act of 2009 (a.k.a. the stimulus act) included a $19.2 billion investment to create a national HIT infrastructure but neglected to address administrative simplification. Also, on their own initiative, Utah and Massachusetts established their own process and standards for uniform administrative transactions, demonstrating both feasibility and real savings.

Section 1104 of the ACA, its drafters having learned from HIPAA's shortcomings, takes a new and more aggressive run at establishing and enforcing new standards. It sets firm deadlines and targets for the HHS secretary to devise uniform operating rules, and requires compliance with these new rules by all health insurers, with financial penalties for noncompliance levied by the Treasury Department.

Will it work this time? The CBO believes so, which is why it credited administrative simplification with $20 billion in federal budget savings between 2010 and 2019. Some suggest the cost savings could be substantially higher once the system is fully operational. Currently about 14 percent of physician-practice revenue is swallowed by claims-management processes alone. A variety of sectors—insurers, physicians, hospitals, and others—as well as Senate, House, and White House policy makers concurred that these provisions were important and necessary, and a potential game changer. These provisions received no public attention during the lengthy and contentious health reform debate. Many are hopeful that they may be among the ACA's most signal accomplishments.

.   .   .

If this survey of the policy changes brought about by Title I seems overwhelming, rest assured, there is much more embedded in the title. For example, mental health advocates praise the ACA because it extends mental health parity requirements to millions of insured Americans who were unprotected prior to passage—mental health parity requires that benefits for mental illness and substance abuse be on a par with benefits for other illnesses.[18] Similarly, substance abuse experts view the law as groundbreaking for its required coverage of addiction treatment and prevention.[19] Women's health advocates celebrate the ACA for eliminating sex discrimination against women who have always had to pay higher premiums than men simply because they get pregnant.[20]

If implemented as designed, Title I will alter the structure and operation of private health insurance in the United States in fundamental ways and transform relationships among insurers, states, the federal government, and consumers. Its effects will vary state by state, market by market, and in many cases, household by household. Its impact will benefit many consumers and disadvantage others. It will be challenging to differentiate between the real effects of the ACA and the dynamics of insurance markets always in flux. Because so many changes will be happening at once, understanding the real effects of the varied elements will be even harder. The only certainty is that health insurance in the United States will never be the same.

6. Title II—Medicaid, CHIP, and the Governors

Yes, there are thirty-one million Americans who are going to
have health insurance, fifteen million of whom are delegated into
Medicaid, the most dysfunctional delivery system that exists in
the American health care system.

SENATOR RICHARD BURR (R-NC), December 21, 2009

The other important stat is the fact that half of the expansion
in health care benefits that is occurring under this bill is under
Medicaid, probably the worst health care program in America.

SENATOR ROBERT CORKER (R-TN), December 14, 2009

And that is our answer? Move fifteen million more Americans
into Medicaid. . . . That is not reform to health care. That is
banishing people to a substandard system as compared to what
the rest of the system is and then feeling good about it. That is
not reform. That is discrimination.

SENATOR TOM COBURN (R-OK), December 7, 2009

The fact is, this bill would consign sixty million Americans to a
health care "gulag" called Medicaid. I say that because, although
Medicaid provides what some people would say is coverage, it
certainly doesn't provide access.

SENATOR JOHN CORNYN (R-TX), December 6, 2009

When Medicare first passed, it didn't cover individuals with
disabilities or individuals with end-stage renal disease. Now
it does. Similarly, Medicaid evolved to allow States to cover
additional services such as home- and community-based care.
Now, both Medicare and Medicaid are indispensable elements
of the social contract of the United States.

SENATOR JOHN KERRY (D-MA), December 18, 2009

TITLE II—THE ROLE OF PUBLIC PROGRAMS

In four weeks of Senate debate on the PPACA through December 2009, it is easy to find statements by Republican senators disparaging the Medicaid program. Far more difficult is finding statements from Democratic senators either supporting or defending the program that provided health insurance protection—including the Children's Health Insurance Program (CHIP)—to an estimated 60.4 million Americans in 2010, now the nation's largest health insurance program (by contrast, Medicare had an estimated 46.8 million enrollees in 2010).[1] If the ACA is implemented as written, that number is projected to grow by 21.8 million to 82.2 million by 2019.[2] Through the ACA, Congress has enacted the most thorough revamping of Medicaid in its history, and there was no Democratic senator who articulated a vision—or even just an explanation—of what was being done and why.

Though the Medicaid expansion drew little public attention or controversy—except for Senator Ben Nelson's Nebraska deal—during the legislative process leading to passage of the ACA, directing 16 million Americans with incomes at or below 133 percent of the federal poverty level into this program is among the most consequential policy decisions in the law. Title II represents a revolution in the nature and structure of Medicaid as it has been known since 1965, as for the first time it becomes the health insurance program for nearly all low-income Americans; for the first time, there will be uniform eligibility across the nation, a single way to calculate income, and these rules will also apply to the state exchanges and eligibility for premium subsidies. Medicaid is a domain where differences divide Democrats and Republicans sharply, though not as much as may appear from each side's rhetoric. While Republicans often castigate the program, eliminating it is nowhere on their real, as opposed to rhetorical, to-do list.

The growth and importance of Medicaid in the U.S. health care system would surprise those who created it along with Medicare in 1965. Then, it was referred to as the bottom layer of a three-layer cake, including Medicare Part A hospital services and Medicare Part B physician services. Despite widespread public perception, it was not set up to serve all the poor, just some of them, principally poor children and their mothers who received public assistance. It was a policy afterthought. The definitive book on the legislative enactment of Medicare barely mentions Medicaid by name.[3] The notion of Medicaid as a program covering all low-income persons in America was never even contemplated. This is where the program now is heading under Title II of the ACA, and it is only a part of a brewing revolution in the program.

UNDERSTANDING MEDICAID

Medicaid and CHIP are the nation's key public health insurance programs for about sixty million low- and lower-income Americans. While the programs cover approximately 15 percent of the U.S. population, Medicaid and CHIP cover more than 40 percent of low-income Americans, 24 percent of African Americans, 23 percent of Hispanics, 53 percent of low-income children, and 41 percent of all U.S. births—as well as 20 percent of Americans living with severe disabilities, 44 percent of persons living with HIV/AIDS, and 65 percent of nursing home residents. That's quite a program to be called a "gulag."

There are four major groups covered by Medicaid and CHIP: fully 50 percent are children, and 25 percent are their adult parents; another 15 percent are low-income disabled persons; and 10 percent are poor seniors. Here's a big surprise: the 25 percent of enrollees who are elderly or disabled account for 68 percent of total Medicaid spending. Here's another surprise: about 18 percent of Medicaid enrollees are so-called dual eligibles, enrolled in both Medicaid and Medicare, both senior and disabled; this 18 percent of enrollees accounts for 46 percent of Medicaid spending.[4]

Unlike Medicare, which is a 100 percent federal health program, Medicaid is a shared responsibility project between the federal governments and the states. This is a legacy part of the program. Medicaid's roots are in public assistance, or "welfare," which was always a state and local responsibility with federal financing. For many years, Medicaid was managed as a subset of state public-assistance agencies because it was seen as a welfare and not a health program. While the federal government pays the lion's share of Medicaid costs (between 50 and 75 percent in 2011 for traditional Medicaid depending on a state's per capita income and between 65 and 85 percent for CHIP), state governments feel burdened and beleaguered by their share, particularly by the annual increases in their costs as medical inflation grows faster than overall inflation and faster than state revenues in most years; in addition, states have less taxing capacity than does the federal government, and forty-nine face balanced-budget requirements.

The federal government pays its share and sets rules that states must follow to qualify for federal reimbursement. Participation by state governments in Medicaid is voluntary—any state can drop out if it wishes to do so, but it must drop out of everything. Arizona took the longest time to decide whether to participate, joining in 1981, fifteen years after the program's creation. These days, though they legally can, states have not felt it is a realistic option to drop out because Medicaid has become such an integral and essential part of their health systems—though in the wake of the ACA, some states mulled over the option. States must pay their share and administer the programs according to federal rules or obtain waivers granting them some flexibility. Governors are the most vocal and involved state officials in Medicaid and—when they agree among themselves—the most influential state voice on Medicaid policies in Washington DC through their lobbying organization, the National Governors Association (NGA).

Medicaid's defenders, and there are many, note that the program is a major engine for state economies, the largest source of federal financial support to states, and a funding source for millions of health care jobs as well as the essential health care safety net for America's neediest and most vulnerable. Medicaid is an insurance program without deductibles, without co-insurance, and with minimal co-pays, something that triggers middle-class resentment, though for individuals and families with no economic resources, cost sharing often results in patients obtaining no services and delaying medical treatment until their conditions get worse and more costly to treat. Families and advocates have spent many years improving their Medicaid programs—they are fiercely protective of what they have built.

Another reality of Medicaid is that demand for it spikes when states have the least fiscal leeway, during economic downturns. During national disasters, including the September 11, 2001, terrorist attack in New York City and Hurricane Katrina in Louisiana and Mississippi in 2005, Medicaid played a vital role in enabling families to survive and states to respond. To governors and state legislatures, though, the burden of paying their share of Medicaid costs, including anticipated costs associated with the ACA, leads to disinvestment in other vital state needs such as public education, transportation, economic development, housing, environmental protection, and everything else a state does. Governors dismiss the economic-development benefits of Medicaid, seeing other opportunities for those same dollars in sectors that could provide an equal or better return on investment. The essential federal-state partnership that is Medicaid is a source of strength and weakness. Its strengths include a relentless culture of innovation in fifty state laboratories, where innovators' ideas can catch on quickly across borders. A key weakness is the varying commitments by states to making the program a real source of meaningful coverage for the low-income populations within their borders. Some states seek to make enrollment as easy as possible to cover needy persons, while other states make enrollment as difficult as possibilities to manage their budgets.

Another prominent criticism of Medicaid is the low rate of reimbursement paid to hospitals, physicians, and other providers, generally lower than any of the major payers. Many complain that to make up for losses from Medicaid, hospitals, physicians, and other providers demand higher payments from private insurers, pushing non-public health insurance premiums higher. Others assert that the low reimbursement leads to low provider participation, leaving Medicaid enrollees with restricted access to medical providers. These critics note that Medicaid on average pays physicians only 72 percent of what Medicare pays physicians—and Medicare rates are also well below private-payer reimbursement rates. But that 72 percent average masks a revealing variability among the states: eleven states actually pay more than 100 percent of Medicare rates, twenty-one states pay between 85 and 99 percent, seven states pay between 70 and 84 percent, and only eleven states pay less than 70 percent, according to data between 2003 and 2008. That last set of eleven, though, includes California, Illinois, Indiana, Michigan, New Jersey, New York, and Ohio, skewing the overall average downward significantly.[5] Further, access problems confront Medicaid enrollees in nearly all fifty states, regardless of reimbursement levels, suggesting other causes beyond reimbursement for the poorer access by Medicaid enrollees to medical providers.

UNDERSTANDING TITLE II

Title II mandates the most comprehensive and far-reaching set of changes to Medicaid since its establishment in 1965. There is a saying in Medicaid circles: "If you've seen one state Medicaid program, you've seen one state Medicaid program." States have substantial discretion to fashion eligibility and benefits to their liking. Engineered primarily by David Schwartz of the Senate Finance Committee along with Andy Schneider and Tim Westmoreland of the House Energy and Commerce Committee, Title II of the ACA, if implemented as designed, will change this perception and reality. In addition to a huge eligibility expansion, greater uniformity and federal direction will result in a more national program for the populations that depend on it. Title II has forty-two sections included within its twelve subtitles. Here is a brief overview of each subtitle, followed by an explanation of the most important and controversial sections.

> *Subtitle A: Improved Access to Medicaid* sets a new national income standard for Medicaid eligibility for all individuals and families with incomes below 133 percent of the federal poverty level (FPL) and establishes financing terms for the expansion populations between the federal and state governments.

Subtitle B: Enhanced Support for the Children's Health Insurance Program extends the life of CHIP and increases federal financial support to states.

Subtitle C: Medicaid and CHIP Enrollment Simplification streamlines and simplifies enrollment in Medicaid and CHIP to make it easier for individuals and families to enroll and requires a single enrollment process for both programs and for insurance coverage within state exchanges.

Subtitle D: Improvements to Medicaid Services addresses freestanding birth centers, hospices, and family-planning services.

Subtitle E: New Options for States to Provide Long-Term Services and Supports provides new options for states regarding home- and community-based services for those in need of long-term services and support, as well as new client protections.

Subtitle F: Medicaid Prescription Drug Coverage increases the drug manufacturers' required rebates for outpatient prescription drugs to help pay for the ACA.

Subtitle G: Medicaid Disproportionate Share Hospital (DSH) Payments reduces federal DSH payments by $14.1 billion over five years, beginning in 2014, as Medicaid and exchange expansions take effect.

Subtitle H: Improved Coordination for Dual Eligible Beneficiaries establishes a new federal Coordinated Health Care Office to improve care and services to elderly and disabled individuals dually enrolled in Medicare and Medicaid.

Subtitle I: Improving the Quality of Medicaid for Patients and Providers sets new requirements to improve the quality of care delivered to Medicaid enrollees.

Subtitle J: Improvements to the Medicaid and CHIP Payment and Access Commission strengthens the capacity of the newly formed Medicaid and CHIP Payment and Access Commission to advise Congress on ways to improve the programs.

Subtitle K: Protections for American Indians and Alaska Natives adds new protections, especially regarding cost sharing, for American Indians and Alaska Natives.

Subtitle L: Maternal and Child Health Services makes programmatic improvements such as early-childhood-visitation programs.

Key Sections of Title II

Following are descriptions of key Title II sections, including the CBO's estimated costs in brackets. A plus sign (+) means the section will cost the federal treasury billions (B) or millions (M) and a minus sign (–) means the provision will save federal dollars.

- Eligibility: In all states by 2014, Medicaid will be open for all individuals not previously eligible—chiefly non-elderly, non-pregnant, childless adults—with household incomes at or below 133 percent of the federal poverty level (that is, up to $14,404 for a single adult in 2010, $29,327 for a family of four). Actually, because the first 5 percent of every enrollee's income is not counted, the new national eligibility standard will be 138 percent. States may implement these changes before 2014. Income eligibility for Medicaid will be determined by a new uniform national standard called "modified adjusted gross income"—the same standard to be used by health exchanges to determine eligibility for subsidies for individuals and families with incomes between 134 and 400 percent of the federal poverty level [+$434B] (section 2001, Subtitle A).

- Federal payments to states: The federal government will pay states for the costs of services to newly Medicaid-eligible individuals at these rates: 100 percent in 2014, 2015, and 2016; 95 percent in 2017; 94 percent in 2018; 93 percent in 2019; and 90 percent thereafter. For states that have already expanded coverage to the new populations, additional federal support will be phased in so that by in 2019, the "expansion states" will receive the same payment as other states for the newly eligible. A $200 million "special adjustment" is provided for states that have experienced a major statewide disaster. Only Louisiana meets the threshold as of the signing of the ACA (section 2001, Subtitle A).

- CHIP: All states must maintain their CHIP eligibility levels at least through September 30, 2019. Between 2016 and 2019, states will receive a 23 percent increase in their CHIP federal matching rate (currently between 65 and 83 percent), capped at 100 percent (section 2101, Subtitle B).

- A Community First Choice Option establishes an optional state Medicaid benefit, beginning October 1, 2011, to provide community-based attendant services and support for Medicaid beneficiaries with disabilities who otherwise would require care in a hospital, nursing home, or intermediate care facility for the mentally retarded [+$6B] (section 2401, Subtitle E).

· Drug rebates: The drug manufacturer's required rebate for brand-name outpatient prescription drugs will increase from 15.1 to 23.1 percent, and for generics from 11 to 13 percent. All additional revenues generated will be used to help pay for the ACA, generating $38 billion over ten years [–$38.1B] (section 2501, Subtitle F).

· Disproportionate Share Hospital Payments: Medicaid DSH payments to hospitals that provide greater than average medical services to Medicaid, CHIP, uninsured, or other low-income patients will be reduced by $14.1 billion over five years beginning in 2014. No state will receive less than 35 percent of its 2012 allotment [–$14B] (section 2551, Subtitle G).

· Dual Eligibles: "Duals" are individuals enrolled in both Medicaid and Medicare—one of the most expensive groups of enrollees in both programs, including senior citizens with low incomes and disabled persons under age sixty-five who meet the standards for both programs. This section directs the HHS secretary to establish a federal Coordinated Health Care Office within the Centers for Medicare and Medicaid Services to integrate benefits for dual eligibles and to improve coordination between the federal and state governments for them (section 2602, Subtitle H).

· Quality of Care: These sections aim to improve quality for Medicaid and CHIP patients and providers, including establishing new adult health quality measures [+$300M] (section 2701); prohibiting Medicaid payments for services related to health-care-acquired conditions such as infections (section 2702); allowing states to enroll Medicaid beneficiaries with chronic conditions in a "health home" to provide care coordination by a health team [+$700M] (section 2703); creating a demonstration project to study bundled payments for hospitals and physicians (section 2704); creating a demonstration project to test new payment structures for safety-net hospitals (section 2705); and creating a demonstration project to allow pediatric providers to be paid as "accountable care organizations" similar to the Accountable Care Organization demonstration in Medicare in Title III (section 2706).

THE NUMBERS GAME

From the beginning of the congressional health reform process in 2008, Democratic policy makers saw expanding Medicaid for all low-income persons as part of the overall strategy. The earliest official indication of this came in Senator Max Baucus's health reform white paper, issued in November 2008:

> Medicaid is a vital source of coverage for low-income Americans, but existing state Medicaid programs have not reached everyone living below the poverty level. The Baucus plan aims to solve that problem by extending Medicaid eligibility to every American living in poverty. . . . Providing Medicaid to everyone below the poverty level is both consistent with the original intent of Medicaid, and the easiest and quickest way to provide insurance to those living in poverty. Building on the existing Medicaid program is also efficient.[6]

If there was disagreement among those paying attention in 2008 and early 2009, it was not whether to use Medicaid; rather, it was how far up the income ladder to go. In his white paper, Baucus proposed a ceiling at 100 percent of the federal poverty level, while some suggested 133 percent (the existing federal standard for children under age six and for pregnant women), while others, including Families USA and community health centers, pushed for 150 percent or even higher. The insurance industry—America's Health Insurance Plans and the Blue Cross Blue Shield Association—agreed that those under 100 percent of the federal poverty level should go into Medicaid because that low-income population's needs—heavy mental health and substance abuse, for example—were not something they felt competent to address, because state Medicaid agencies had a lengthy history serving them, and because this population had no money to pay premiums. Above 100 percent, they preferred that eligible individuals obtained private coverage through state exchanges. Most provider organizations such as hospital and physicians also preferred keeping Medicaid at 100 percent of the federal poverty level because state Medicaid programs paid them less than the private plans that would operate in state exchanges. Of the Republicans who negotiated with Baucus on health reform, two Gang of Six members, Charles Grassley (R-IA) and Olympia Snowe (R-ME), did not object to expanding Medicaid to everyone at 100 percent of the federal poverty level or lower, while Mike Enzi (R-WY) preferred expanding it only to those under 50 percent of the federal poverty level and giving others up to 100 percent of the FPL a choice between Medicaid and private coverage.

Further, if Medicaid eligibility were expanded to 133 percent of the FPL, the Republicans wanted to give enrollees a choice of enrolling in Medicaid or the exchange; the conservative position was to move as many persons as possible into private coverage through exchanges.

The decisions to go higher than 100 percent of the federal poverty level in the Senate and the House were driven by dollars. The Congressional Budget Office, the nonpartisan congressional advisory body, estimated much higher costs to cover individuals through an exchange rather than through Medicaid because the latter pays medical providers much less than private insurers can get away with and because Medicaid administrative costs are much lower. In the early summer of 2009, when Senate Majority Leader Harry Reid and the White House pressured Baucus to abandon plans to tighten the federal health insurance tax exclusion as a financing source, Senate Finance leaders and staff scrambled to find new revenues and to hold down costs—moving from 100 to 133 percent of the FPL for Medicaid eligibility was one important step in that direction. Why not 150 percent? Finance officials knew there were existing Medicaid populations at 133 percent of the FPL, including children up to age six and pregnant women, while there were none at 150 percent of the FPL—it would be a more difficult and complex change. Further, governors and some Democratic senators felt going higher than 133 percent of the FPL was a line they were not willing to cross: 133 was it.

The key moment for House leaders came in September 2009, when President Obama set a $900 billion limit on the total price tag for health reform in his joint address to both houses of Congress. House leaders had planned on a 133 percent FPL threshold, and the Obama spending limit persuaded them to move to 150 percent of the FPL to drive down further the cost of their legislation. In the January 2010 House-Senate dialogues, House leaders pushed for the 150 percent FPL limit, though Senate negotiators emphasized they would not have sixty votes for that level of Medicaid eligibility. After the Massachusetts special election, when the Senate bill became the path to a bill signing, the issue dropped off the table. The final number was 133 percent.

Who gets paid what. The next set of politically charged numbers—even more than the eligibility percentage—involved the portion of the cost of Medicaid expansions that would be covered by the federal government and the portion to be financed by states. The base level of federal financial participation (through a formula known as the Federal Medical Assistance

Percentage, or FMAP) is currently between 50 and 75 percent, depending on a state's per capita income; the lower the income level, the higher the FMAP. So in Connecticut, a high-income state, the federal government pays 50 cents for every dollar the state spends on an allowable Medicaid service; and in Mississippi in 2011, it was 74.7 cents, so every dollar of state spending draws 74.7 cents in federal reimbursements. For the Children's Health Insurance Program (CHIP), the range is between 65 and 85 cents, again based on per capita income. To some, the arrangement seems like a good deal for states, though one would never know it by talking with governors and state legislators who complain that their obligation to balance their state budgets (in forty-nine of the fifty states) and their limited taxing capacity (along with their unwillingness or inability to raise taxes) result in Medicaid obligations that trigger severe fiscal distress, especially during downturns.

When the nation's governors are united, they are a potent political force. That was less true in 2009 among the twenty-eight Democratic and twenty-two Republican governors. To speak out on any issue as the National Governors Association, at least two-thirds of them need to be on the same page. On health reform, governors were divided into four camps: Democrats who rallied for reform regardless of the fiscal impact, more conservative Democrats with fiscal concerns, Republicans with concerns who wanted reform, and Republicans who wanted nothing to happen. Each party had sufficient numbers to block any statement or initiative from the NGA unfavorable to their national party; in particular, Valerie Jarrett, the White House senior advisor and assistant to the president for intergovernmental affairs, reached out to friendly Democratic governors—chiefly Pennsylvania governor Ed Rendell—to organize opposition to most NGA statements, resulting in only one letter to Congress from the NGA on health reform, a July 20 letter declaring it "steadfastly opposed to unfunded federal mandates and reforms that simply shift costs to states."[7] That was it. As a result, NGA had a low profile, though individual governors spoke out often as the debate progressed.

Governors wanted the federal government to pick up 100 percent of the cost of covering any expansion population—and then some. From their perspective, the reform effort would attract a substantial number of the millions of low-income Americans already eligible prior to the ACA though unenrolled in Medicaid, expanded enrollment that would cost states significant dollars to pay for them at the lower historic matching rate. Also, greatly expanding Medicaid would place extra pressure on states to increase payment rates to providers, and that would affect spending for the entire state's Medicaid population. However they looked at it, governors saw more financial obligations coming their way when they felt least able to afford it.

Complicating a complicated picture, some states had already expanded coverage to childless adults up to at least 100 percent of the federal poverty level, and some well beyond that—Arizona, Delaware, Hawaii, Maine, Massachusetts, New York, and Vermont. Paying these states more for something they had already done increased the already high cost of the legislation.

The House was more sympathetic than was the Senate to the states' viewpoint, proposing to pay 100 percent for the entire expansion population permanently in its initial plan released in June 2009, though budget pressures and Blue Dog demands compelled it to pull back, and the final bill approved in November 2009 paid states 100 percent for 2013 and 2014, and 91 percent thereafter. The Senate bill approved in December 2009 offered 100 percent for 2014, 2015, and 2016, and a bifurcated formula for 2017 and 2018 between expansion and nonexpansion states, with all states receiving a 32.3 percent FMAP increase—capped at 95 percent—in 2019 and beyond. Additionally, the Senate bill contained a special provision requiring permanent 100 percent reimbursement for Nebraska, a controversial provision nicknamed the "Cornhusker kickback," done to secure the reluctant vote of Senator Ben Nelson (D-NE) before the final Senate vote on Christmas Eve. Nelson had wanted to make the Medicaid expansions optional for all states, something Democratic leaders would not do. The kickback was the agreed-upon alternative.

The final ACA legislation approved in March 2010 jettisoned the Nebraska arrangement and gave all other states a boost as follows: 100 percent in 2014, 2015, and 2016; 95 percent in 2017; 94 percent in 2018; 93 percent in 2019; and 90 percent in 2020 and beyond. Expansion states (states that had already expanded eligibility prior to 2010) will phase into the higher rates paid to other states, reaching parity with them in 2019 and beyond. Also, all Medicaid programs will pay primary care providers at Medicare rates in 2013 and 2014 with 100 percent federal financing.

How will states fare under the final deal? The Kaiser Commission on Medicaid and the Uninsured released a report in May 2010 concluding that 15.9 million Americans will enroll in Medicaid through the expansion—11.2 million of them formerly uninsured, substantially lower than the CBO estimate of 16 million. Federal spending for the expansion will rise by $443.5 billion, and state spending will increase by $21.1 billion between 2014 and 2019, so 95 percent of new overall spending on this population will be federal.[8]

MEDICAID'S FUTURE

Prior to passage of the ACA, the unheralded stepchild of the U.S. health care system had already become the nation's biggest health program, and it will grow substantially larger over the coming decade. Because of its state-based administration, poor reputation, and lower rate of payment, it has not been able to act as a coherent and unified force for health system reform. The authors of Title II are hopeful Medicaid will become a much more national and consistent program in the days and years ahead and will assume a larger role in shaping the U.S. health system's future.

The new Center for Medicare and Medicaid Innovation established in Title III is one pathway for new directions that can bring together both enormous programs to act in a consistent and coherent way, as is the new Coordinated Health Care Office, which focuses on transforming care for the large population of dual eligibles. The quality-of-care initiatives in Subtitle I, including those affecting accountable care organizations, medical homes, bundled payments, and quality-of-care measures, have numerous champions. Medicaid advocates hope the new MACPAC—the Medicaid and CHIP Payment and Access Commission—will bring a new level of attention and accountability, a new day for Medicaid.

Other dramatic changes are in the works. If Title II is implemented as written, by 2014, there will be near-uniform Medicaid eligibility across the nation, a single method to calculate income to determine eligibility, and no more categorical distinctions. Officials involved in implementation believe the program will begin to look different in many basic ways. No longer a program of "last resort," Medicaid will be open to nearly everyone with family incomes below 133 percent of the federal poverty level. A substantial bump up in federal support means the program will be run differently.

CHIP—THE FAVORED CHILD

The Children's Health Insurance Program was created in 1997 as part of that year's Balanced Budget Act, the only significant federal program expansion in a law otherwise devoted to cutting the federal deficit. Its creation is due to the odd coupling of Senators Edward Kennedy (D-MA) and Orrin Hatch (R-UT), who teamed up on a plan to establish a new children's health insurance program funded by new taxes on tobacco products. It was seen as one of the principal bipartisan accomplishments in the late 1990s in a bitterly partisan Congress. Many members of Congress in both parties and branches took pride and ownership in preserving and strengthening it as it grew to cover more than five million lower- and lower-middle-income children in families not eligible for Medicaid.

The original ten-year CHIP authorization expired in September 2007, and the new Democratic majorities in the House and Senate, elected in November 2006, were committed to a full and robust reauthorization. Yet a veto threat by President George W. Bush compelled Democrats to make compromises to attract Republican support, including the continuation of a five-year exclusion from CHIP of newly arrived legal immigrant children. While the compromise was sufficient to achieve a veto-proof majority in the Senate, it did not succeed in the House, and only temporary reauthorizations passed in 2007, extending the program into 2009. In early 2009, a burgeoning Democratic majority pushed CHIP reauthorization as one of the earliest legislative wins for the new Obama administration. The blanket five-year exclusion on legal child immigrants was also changed to a state option in order to address concerns by members of the House Hispanic Caucus. Their mollification resulted in the alienation of Senator Charles Grassley (R-IA) and other Republicans who had bucked their party to support the compromise. The Children's Health Insurance Program Reauthorization Act (CHIPRA), extending the program through at least 2013, was signed by President Obama on February 4, 2009.

Some had urged folding the CHIP reauthorization into the slowly emerging health reform package or the faster-moving stimulus bill, but those voices were overruled by the new White House chief of staff Rahm Emanuel, who wanted CHIP as an early victory for the new president. Still, there were issues to be addressed in the context of health reform: How would CHIP align with coverage available through the new state exchanges? Would families have a choice between CHIP and an exchange? Why would states continue to participate in CHIP, which required them to pay part of the bill, when the exchange could cover the same children completely on the federal dime? Meanwhile, the children's advocacy community, which had worked for over a decade to build and improve CHIP, did not want its progress erased.

The House of Representatives dismayed children's advocates by including in its health reform legislation—released in the summer of 2009—a repeal of CHIP beginning in 2014, when the new exchanges would be up and running. Children in families with incomes over 150 percent FPL would enroll with their parents in the exchanges, and children in families below this level would be eligible for enrollment in Medicaid with their parents. Children in families over 150 percent of the federal poverty level already in CHIP plans could stay, and states would receive enhanced federal matches for those children, but no new children would be allowed to join them. In September, Senator Baucus brought to the Finance Committee a similar proposal to move CHIP children into the exchanges and to require states to provide additional "wraparound" benefits that would otherwise have been provided through CHIP. Senator Jay Rockefeller (D-WV), a passionate CHIP supporter, prevailed with the full committee for his amendment to maintain the existing CHIP structure through 2019 with a 23 percent increase in the state matching rate. In Senate Majority Leader Harry Reid's December "Manager's Amendment," included as Title X, two additional years of directly authorized funding were included for 2014 and 2015. The vision of some to "mainstream" CHIP enrollees into private coverage faltered, and with a valid reason: the cost sharing in the new exchange policies will be much steeper than what is permitted in CHIP; many enrollees will be much better staying where they are.

Rather than facing elimination, CHIP has been preserved and extended two years beyond CHIPRA's 2013 authorization. Many questions remain about the alignment of CHIP with the new exchanges and the ongoing role of states. For the time being, CHIP continues.

· · ·

The lengthy period between the ACA's enactment in March 2010 and the implementation of Medicaid reforms in January 2014 reminds some of a parched landscape. States have held their Medicaid programs together during difficult budgetary stresses only with significant supplemental financial support from the federal government—support that is a low priority and often opposed by Republicans in Congress. One of the most difficult challenges in implementing Title II may simply be getting to 2014 with minimal damage to the underlying program.

Beginning in 2014, the context will change. It is a truism that public programs, once established, are difficult to eliminate. That has proved true in the case of Medicaid and CHIP and further validated in the process leading to passage of the ACA. Advocates and program defenders, with years of experience and success in patching over gaps and deficiencies, are reluctant to embrace a hypothetically better future relative to what exists now, with its well-worn paths of accessibility, accountability, legal protections, culture, and more. Even CHIP, a "patch on a patch" of America's disjointed health care system, had a phalanx of supporters inside and outside the government to fight its absorption into the state exchanges. It is a new day dawning for CHIP and especially for Medicaid.

7. Title III—Medical Care, Medicare, and the Cost Curve

May 11, 2009—Leaders of six key health organizations representing the insurance industry, hospitals, physicians, medical-device makers, pharmaceutical makers, and health care workers stood with President Barack Obama at a White House press briefing to announce their commitment to help to achieve $2 trillion in health care system savings over a ten-year period, a large portion of which would help pay the bill for health care reform. The president lauded the leaders:

> Over the next 10 years—from 2010 to 2019—they are pledging to cut the rate of growth of national health care spending by 1.5 percentage points each year—an amount that's equal to over $2 trillion. Two trillion dollars.[1]

After the event, some industry leaders pointed to the precise language in their letter to the president:

> As restructuring takes hold and the population's health improves over the coming decade, we will *do our part* [emphasis added] to achieve your Administration's goal of decreasing by 1.5 percentage points the annual health care spending growth rate—saving $2 trillion or more.

TITLE III—IMPROVING THE QUALITY AND EFFICIENCY OF HEALTH CARE

For decades, health system thought leaders have declared the U.S. health care system to be fraught with waste and overtreatment. In recent years, many have grabbed on to the number $700 billion in annual health care waste as though it were a scientifically derived number.[2] Various analysts and research groups all point to the same $700 billion and yet produce different sets of waste configurations.[3] Whether the real number is $700 billion or more or less, broad consensus exists for the belief that there is a lot of waste in U.S. health care. In the spirit of "continuous improvement," the U.S. health system's quality paradigm, every defect is a treasure because it points the way toward greater efficiency and improved care. In 2009, $2 trillion worth of defects seemed a tantalizing treasure to address the hardest part of health reform, how to pay for it. Since about half of U.S. health spending comes from public sources, it was reasonable to estimate about $1 trillion in public savings from the industries' commitment. Extracting those savings while improving quality, increasing value, and expanding access—what could be better? It could be a health policy grand slam. And beginning in May 2009, it was time to get specific.

In the end, policy makers approved about $449 billion in system savings now embedded in Title III and, specifically, Medicare; most of the other $500 billion needed to pay for the ACA came from revenue increases included in Title IX (and smaller amounts of new revenue and savings in Titles I and II). While much of the $450 billion in system savings was accomplished with the agreement of the affected industries, much was not. And much more of the savings came from old-fashioned rate reductions than from cutting-edge system and quality improvements. Many, many innovative system improvements are in the act; they just got miserly savings projections from the estimating oracle, the Congressional Budget Office.

This chapter provides some essential background on Medicare, an overview of Title III's key sections, a detailed description of the process leading to $449 billion in ten-year savings, and an exploration of Title III's prospects to control health care spending and "bend the cost curve."

SOME ESSENTIAL BACKGROUND ON MEDICARE

Medicare covered about forty-six million Americans in 2010, about eight million of whom are under age sixty-five and permanently disabled. Medicare has four Parts—A, B, C, and D. Before diving into Title III, it will be helpful to define these parts.

Part A, called Hospital Insurance, is financed by a portion of the Social Security tax (2.9 percent of earnings split equally between employers and employees) and pays for inpatient hospital care, skilled nursing care, hospice care, and other services. Part A accounted for 35 percent of spending in 2010. A and B are the two original parts of Medicare set up in the 1965 law. When the suggestion is made that "Medicare is going broke," it is the Part A Hospital Trust Fund being referenced.

Part B, called Medical Insurance, is financed by monthly premiums of enrollees and by general funds from the U.S. Treasury. It pays for physicians' services, outpatient hospital visits, and medical services and supplies not covered by Part A; it accounted for 27 percent of benefit spending in 2010.

Part C, once called Medicare + Choice, has been known as Medicare Advantage (MA) since 2003. MA allows enrollees to receive all their medical services through a private insurer or provider organization, which is paid a lump sum (or "capitated" payment) by the U.S. Centers for Medicare and Medicaid Services (CMS). Part C accounted for 24 percent of benefit spending in 2010.

Part D covers prescription drugs offered through private plans under contract with Medicare and is financed through monthly enrollee premiums and the federal treasury. It accounted for 11 percent of spending in 2010.

The percentage share of costs under the four parts equals 97 percent; the other 3 percent involves the administrative costs to run the program.[4]

UNDERSTANDING TITLE III

Title III sets in motion changes to every part of Medicare, among the most significant and comprehensive set of changes since the program's establishment in 1965. Many changes will improve the benefits and operations of the program for beneficiaries, many will improve the efficiency and quality of the care provided to them, and many will generate savings that are a large part of the ACA's overall financing scheme—and some of these will have adverse impacts on some beneficiaries. Title III has ninety-eight sections, the most of any title in the law, included within its seven subtitles. Here is a brief overview of the subtitles, followed by an explanation of the most important and controversial sections.

Subtitle A: Transforming the Health Care Delivery System implements new strategies to improve the quality and efficiency of medical care and instigates changes in how Medicare pays providers to foster quality and better outcomes rather than promoting more services to Medicare patients.

Subtitle B: Improving Medicare for Patients and Providers implements other specific program changes to Medicare, including savings provisions such as those affecting the home health industry.

Subtitle C: Provisions Related to Part C alters the financing of Medicare Advantage, the private insurance option used by approximately 25 percent of Medicare enrollees.

Subtitle D: Medicare Part D Improvements for Prescription Drug Plans and MA Drug Plans eliminates the so-called Medicare Part D doughnut hole and makes other changes to Medicare prescription drug plans.

Subtitle E: Ensuring Medicare Sustainability changes Medicare market basket (payment) updates for hospitals, home health agencies, and other providers; increases Part B premiums for higher-income beneficiaries; and establishes the Independent Payment Advisory Board (IPAB).

Subtitle F: Health Care Quality Improvements implements provisions to improve the quality of medical care and treatment for the entire U.S. health care system.

Subtitle G: Protecting and Improving Guaranteed Medicare Benefits provides "a statement of intent by Congress on the impact of Title III provisions on Medicare benefits."

It is challenging to pick out the key Title III sections both because there are so many and because the real impact of these will not be known until they are implemented and in operation for at least several years. With that caveat, here is a brief overview of key sections within each subtitle, including CBO estimated costs and savings in brackets. A plus sign (+) means the provision costs billions (B) or millions (M), and a minus sign (–) means the provision will save federal dollars. If there is no bracketed item, the CBO estimates zero cost or savings.

SUBTITLE A: TRANSFORMING THE HEALTH CARE DELIVERY SYSTEM

- Quality reporting: Beginning in 2014, physicians who do not submit data to the Physician Quality Reporting Initiative to assess the quality of the care they deliver will have their Medicare payments reduced [–$100M] (section 3002, Subtitle A). A new national quality-reporting system is established for long-term care hospitals, inpatient rehabilitation hospitals, inpatient psychiatric hospitals, hospice programs, and certain cancer hospitals; nonparticipating providers will see payment reductions [–$100M] (sections 3004 and 3005, Subtitle A).

- CMS innovation: A new Center for Medicare and Medicaid Innovation is established within the federal Centers for Medicare and Medicaid Services (CMS) to research, develop, test, and expand innovative payment and delivery arrangements to improve quality and reduce the cost of care provided to patients [–$1.3B] (section 3021, Subtitle A).

- Shared savings: A program is established to share savings with Medicare providers to reward organizations that take responsibility for the cost and quality of care received by their patients; these organizations will be called accountable care organizations (ACOs) [–$4.9B] (section 3022, Subtitle A).

- Bundling: A national pilot program on payment bundling will be developed by 2013 to encourage hospitals, doctors, and post-acute-care providers to combine their current separate payments into "bundles" to improve patient care and achieve savings (section 3023, Subtitle A).

- Hospital readmissions: Hospitals that have high levels of preventable patient readmissions will face reduced payments based on the cost of each hospital's potentially preventable Medicare readmissions [–$7.1B] (section 3025, Subtitle A).

- Other noteworthy provisions: A hospital value-based purchasing program will start in 2013 to tie hospital payments to performance on quality measures (section 3001). Medicare's physician resource user feedback program will develop individualized reports by 2012 comparing physicians who see similar patients (section 3003). Starting in FY 2015, hospitals in the top 25th percentile of rates of hospital-acquired conditions for high-cost and common conditions will be penalized [–$1.4B] (section 3008). The HHS secretary will establish and update annually a national strategy to improve the delivery of health care services, patient outcomes, and population health (section 3011). The president will convene an Interagency Working Group on Health Care Quality to develop quality initiatives as part of the national strategy (section 3012). A community-based-care transitions program will fund hospitals and community-based entities that offer evidence-based transition services to Medicare beneficiaries at high risk for readmission [+$500M] (section 3026).

SUBTITLE B: IMPROVING MEDICARE FOR PATIENTS AND PROVIDERS

· Home Health Care: The HHS secretary will restructure payments for home health services starting in 2014, achieving nearly $40 billion in payment reductions through 2019 [–$39.7B] (section 3131).

· Disproportionate Share Hospital (DSH) payments: The secretary will update hospital payments in the Medicare DSH program to better account for hospitals' uncompensated care costs. Starting in FY 2014, Medicare DSH payments will be reduced to reflect lower hospital uncompensated care costs due to increases in the numbers of insured [–$25.1B] (section 3133, Subtitle B).

· Other noteworthy provisions: The secretary will change hospice payments to improve payment accuracy in FY 2013 and impose requirements on hospice providers to increase accountability in Medicare [–$100M] (section 3132). The equipment-utilization factor for advanced imaging services is modified [–$2.3B] (section 3135). The Medicare option to purchase power-driven wheelchairs with a lump-sum payment when the chair is supplied is eliminated. Medicare will make the same payments for power-driven chairs over a thirteen-month period [–$800M] (section 3136). The secretary will recommend to Congress ways to reform the Medicare wage-index system by December 31, 2011, and will restore the hospital reclassification thresholds to the percentages used in FY 2009 [+$300M] (section 3137).

SUBTITLE C: PROVISIONS RELATED TO PART C

· Medicare Advantage: MA payments are frozen in 2011. Beginning in 2012, MA payment benchmarks are reduced. New benchmarks will vary from 95 percent of Medicare fee-for-service spending in high-cost areas to 115 percent in low-cost areas, with all benchmarks increased by 5 percent for high-quality plans [–$135.6B] (section 3201, Subtitle C).

· Other noteworthy provisions: MA plans may not charge beneficiaries more for cost sharing for covered services than what is charged under the fee-for-service program. Plans providing extra benefits must give priority to cost-sharing reductions, wellness, and preventive care, before benefits not covered under Medicare (section 3202). MA beneficiaries may disenroll from an MA plan and return to the fee-for-service program from January 1 to March 15 of each year (section 3204).

SUBTITLE D: MEDICARE PART D IMPROVEMENTS FOR PRESCRIPTION
DRUG PLANS AND MEDICARE ADVANTAGE PART D PLANS

· Part D: Drug manufacturers will provide a 50 percent discount
to Part D enrollees for brand-name drugs and biologics purchased during the coverage ("doughnut hole") gap beginning
January 1, 2011 [+$42.6B] (section 3301, Subtitle D).

· Other noteworthy provisions: The Part D premium subsidy
is reduced for beneficiaries with incomes above Part B income
thresholds [−$10.7B] (section 3308). Cost sharing is eliminated
for beneficiaries receiving care under a home- and community-
based waiver program who would otherwise require institutional care [+$1.1B] (section 3309). Part D plans must develop
drug-dispensing techniques to reduce prescription drug waste
in long-term care facilities [−$5.7B] (section 3310).

SUBTITLE E: ENSURING MEDICARE SUSTAINABILITY

· Market basket updates: A productivity adjustment is added to
the market basket payment update for inpatient hospitals, home
health providers, nursing homes, hospice providers, inpatient
psychiatric facilities, long-term care hospitals, and inpatient
rehabilitation facilities [−$156.6B] (section 3401).

· Higher-income beneficiaries: For higher-income beneficiaries
who pay a higher Part B premium rate, income thresholds are
frozen at 2010 levels through 2019 [−$25B] (section 3402).

· Independent Payment Advisory Board: A new fifteen-member
IPAB will present Congress with proposals to reduce excess cost
growth and improve quality of care for Medicare beneficiaries.
In years when Medicare costs are projected to be unsustainable
(that is, exceeding the target growth rates), IPAB proposals
will take effect unless Congress passes an alternative measure
achieving the same level of savings. The board cannot make
proposals that ration care, raise taxes or Part B premiums, or
change Medicare benefit, eligibility, or cost-sharing standards.
Hospital spending is exempted from IPAB recommendations
until 2019. Beginning in 2020, the board's binding recommendations to Congress will occur every other year if the growth in
overall health spending exceeds spending growth in Medicare
[−$15.5B] (section 3403).

FOLLOWING THE MONEY

While a substantial portion of Title III deals with "Improving the Quality and Efficiency of Health Care," the title's official name, Title III has two overriding purposes: first, to make improvements to Medicare for the benefit of the program's forty-five million beneficiaries, and second, to make changes to lower the program's anticipated rate of growth to provide federal budget flexibility to help finance the access expansions in Titles I and II. Savings, reductions, and cuts in Title III, all affecting only Medicare, amount to $449 billion, or a little less than half the total cost of the whole ACA.

A word about these estimates: They are all embedded in the ACA analysis done by the Congressional Budget Office, the nonpartisan agency created in 1974 to advise Congress on the federal budget and the budgetary impact of pending federal legislation. The CBO consists of about 250 economists and public policy analysts. While many from all political persuasions regularly take issue with various aspects of CBO analyses and reports, both political parties accept its role as the official word on the expected financial impact of legislation. The final CBO estimate on the ACA was released on March 20, 2010, three days before the final House vote.[5] Less noticed, though also producing estimates on the ACA's impact, was the Office of the Actuary within the Centers for Medicare and Medicaid Services, another office of professional economists and public policy analysts, with an exclusive focus on health, Medicare, and Medicaid. Its final report on the ACA was released on April 22, 2010.[6]

At the big-picture level, the CBO and Actuary estimates are remarkably close: $938 and $948 billion, respectively, for a ten-year net cost of coverage expansions, and $455 and $457 billion, respectively, for a ten-year net savings in Medicare and Medicaid.[7] On specific sections, though, their estimates vary, often widely, in both directions. For example, section 3404 sets up an Independent Payment Advisory Board, a controversial panel that will devise ways to control future Medicare cost increases. The CBO estimates $15.5 billion in ten-year savings, which the actuary estimates at $23.6 billion. Unless otherwise indicated, the numbers in this chapter (and book) reflect the CBO estimates in deference to its role as Congress's official scorekeeper.

The question arises, who is right? In the IPAB example and others, the likely answer is—neither. And because there is a reasonable chance Congress will amend the IPAB in some way before it ever takes effect, there may never be an answer in real life. The differences in estimates highlight the uncertainty in making them. While estimates are essential in the legisla-

TABLE 4. Key savings provisions in Title III

Section	Purview	Ten-year savings estimates (in billions of dollars)
3401	Revision of provider market basket updates and incorporation of productivity improvements	156.6
3201	Medicare Advantage (Part C) payments	135.6
3131	Payment adjustments for home health	39.7
3402	Temporary adjustment to calculation of Medicare Part B premiums for high-income beneficiaries	25.0
3133	Medicare payments to disproportionate share hospitals	22.1
3112	Revision to Medicare Improvement Fund	20.7
3403	Independent Payment Advisory Board	15.5
3308	Reductions in Part D subsidy for higher-income beneficiaries	10.7
3025	Hospital readmissions-reduction program	7.1
3310	Dispensing of outpatient drugs in long-term care facilities	5.7

tive process, they are often a poor guide to how a law will fare once implemented. In the case of the three most significant Medicare reforms since the CBO was established in 1974—creation of the prospective payment system for hospital payments in 1983, adoption of the Balanced Budget Act of 1997, and creation of the Medicare Part D program in 2003—the CBO was off in its estimates by wide margins, and each time in the same direction, underestimating revenues or savings and overestimating costs.[8] Noting this is not to knock the CBO's integrity or skill; it recognizes the uncertainties involved in this task. If this pattern holds true with the ACA, it is good news for the law's financial stability and longer-term viability. Still, three prior examples, even big ones, provide no guarantees regarding future events.

Just ten out of the ninety-eight sections in Title III account for $439 billion of the $449 billion in anticipated Medicare savings. These are shown, in order of magnitude, in table 4.

Over the past decade leading up to the ACA's signing, many ideas have been advanced to save money in the U.S. health care system, and many of those ideas made their way into the final version of the ACA: medical homes, accountable care organizations, payment bundling, community health teams, a high-powered board with extraordinary powers, and lots more. Precious few of them, though, achieved estimates of significant savings from the CBO or the CMS actuary. So, when White House, Senate, and House officials had to devise ways to pay the $940 billion–plus ten-year price tag for the ACA, they found the money where they could, mostly the old-fashioned way, through adjustments in payment rates.

Congress has many sources of information when it comes to Medicare. In the realm of Medicare savings, one source stands out, the Medicare Payment Advisory Commission. MedPAC is an independent federal body set up in 1997 solely to advise Congress on Medicare. The commission consists of seventeen members appointed by the U.S. comptroller general for three-year terms, backed by a professional staff. MedPAC releases two reports with recommendations each year, in March and June. Its reports invariably include the best up-to-date and detailed information about most aspects of Medicare, including the financial state of health industry entities that serve Medicare enrollees, such as hospitals, physicians, home health agencies, hospices, skilled nursing homes, and more. When Congress looks to find savings in Medicare, MedPAC reports are often one of the first places it looks, and 2009–10 was no exception.

Hospitals

More than any other segment of the health care industry, acute care hospitals saw an upside in national health reform generally and universal coverage in particular. Along with community health centers, hospitals are the frontline resource for uninsured and underinsured Americans. Many observers believe hospitals are legally required to treat all Americans for free under a misunderstood 1986 federal law known as EMTALA (the Emergency Medical Treatment and Active Labor Act), which requires most hospitals to provide an examination and stabilizing treatment, if needed, without consideration of insurance coverage or ability to pay, when a patient comes to an emergency room with an emergency medical condition.[9] Yet hospitals are permitted under EMTALA to bill for all services provided and to take action to collect payment after providing the services. Often, patients are unable to pay and resentful of the collection activities by hospitals. More than any other segment of the health care industry, hospitals are on the hook for the failure of U.S. society to provide universal coverage, and they want to get off the hook.

Acute care hospitals are the largest recipient of Medicare payments, having received $109 billion for fee-for-service inpatient care and $30 billion for outpatient fee-for-service care in 2008. They obtain more from Medicare for other services they provide, including home health, skilled nursing, psychiatric, rehabilitation, and more. Inpatient spending per enrollee grew 3.2 percent annually between 2003 and 2008, and outpatient grew 8.8 percent during the same period. It is accepted wisdom among health care providers and many others that Medicare underpays hospitals and thus forces hospitals to shift costs by charging private payers more, leading to higher-than-justified increases in the cost of private health insurance. This is not accepted wisdom by MedPAC:

> If providers can negotiate higher prices with non-Medicare payers, it is because of their market power and not the level of Medicare payment. . . . Specifically, hospitals under high financial pressure (that is, hospitals with low non-Medicare profit margins) tended to control their costs, and thus have better financial performance under Medicare, whereas those under low financial pressure (those with relatively high non-Medicare profit margins) had higher costs and lower or negative Medicare margins. As revenue rises from non-Medicare payers, the financial pressure the hospital is under declines, costs increase, and Medicare margins fall, putting pressure on policymakers to increase Medicare rates. Rather than reflecting inadequate Medicare payments, these losses may reflect inadequate cost control.[10]

In other words, hospitals do not find a sympathetic ear in Washington DC to their financial pressures. As a result, industry leaders understood early on that any move to universal coverage would require a financial contribution from the hospital sector to help pay the bill—and a big one, in recognition of the financial gains hospitals would realize from the implementation of near-universal coverage. The hospital community, recalling its experience with the 1993 Clinton reform and subsequent deficit-reduction efforts in the mid-1990s, recognized that whether Democrats won or lost in their 2009–10 health reform efforts, pressures to reduce the federal budget deficit would follow. Better to agree to spending reductions in a health reform effort that provided new revenue from paying customers, the hospitals reasoned, than take another round of cuts with no compensating gains, as occurred in 1997 under the Balanced Budget Act.

The three key hospital organizations, the Federation of American Hospitals, the American Hospital Association, and the Catholic Health Association, had committed to achieving universal coverage, understood the realities, and were ready to negotiate right after the $2 trillion announcement on May 11, 2009. The negotiation involved the White House and high-level Senate Finance staffers. The agreement involved two numbers:

$155 billion in reductions over ten years, and health insurance coverage for 95 percent of all Americans. At these numbers, hospital leaders were convinced that the revenue from the added covered lives would more than make up for their losses on the Medicare side, and it was a deal they could embrace. That was the number announced on July 8, 2009, by Vice President Joe Biden, and that number stuck.

How the $155 billion was to be reached and what program changes were to be made were the subjects of constant negotiation, tweaking, and alteration between July 8, 2009, and March 2010. Different segments of the industry had unique preferences (regions, for-profits, publics, safety nets, rural, urban—each had its own), while Senate, House, and White House staffers had their own as well. Ultimately, $112 billion of the $155 billion came from pure rate reductions, $36 billion more from reducing Medicare and Medicaid Disproportionate Share Hospital (DSH) payments, $7 billion from reducing hospital readmissions, and $1.5 billion from penalizing hospitals with high rates of hospital-acquired infections. Hospital leaders negotiated hard and successfully to be kept out of any payment reductions triggered by the creation of the Independent Payment Advisory Board (IPAB) until 2019 because they were already on the hook for major reductions through 2018. Hospital officials also made clear they opposed any public plan option as part of the insurance exchanges.

Republicans in the Senate and House attempted to make hay from the hospital reductions, but the attacks did not stick because the hospitals had agreed to the deal. When other Democrats attempted to change the terms, Baucus and the hospital leaders stuck to their bargain. Industry leaders and Senate staffers hate the word *deal* to describe the agreement and the taint that word carries. Yet hospitals were at the table to construct an agreement on how to reduce their revenues by $155 billion in a way that would work for them. If it was a deal, it was a deal in the best sense of the word, not the worst sense.

Home Health

Nurses, physical, speech, and occupational therapists, home health aides, medical social workers, and others, all providing individual care to Medicare clients in their homes—who wants to take a knife to them? But there's more to the home health care story than that. Home health has been a highly profitable activity, with profit margins averaging 17.4 percent annually between 2001 and 2007. Says MedPAC: "This consistent pattern of high margins indicates that Medicare payments have been well in excess of costs, even in years when the annual payment update has been reduced or eliminated."[11] Standards for service to clients are often ambiguous, and the industry is regarded as a significant source of Medicare fraud and abuse, particularly in states that have been regarded as rife with illegal payments—California, Florida, and Texas. In 2007, 60 percent of all home health care outlier claims nationwide were made to providers in just one county, Miami-Dade in Florida.[12]

In Medicare, home health has been in a boom-or-bust cycle for more than twenty years. With the arrival of prospective payments for Medicare hospital services in the mid-1980s, home health growth surged as agencies provided care for Medicare patients facing shorter hospital stays. In the 1997 Balanced Budget Act, Congress slashed home health care payments, resulting in a drop in visits by about 65 percent, a 52 percent drop in Medicare home health spending, and a 31 percent agency closure rate by 2000. In the first decade of this century, the industry came back, and by 2010 the number of agencies was close to the 1997 peak.

Industry leaders realized they would not emerge unscathed from the health reform process. Also, the industry faced internal divisions, especially between for-profit and nonprofit agencies. The House of Representatives went first and put forward $54 billion in cuts over ten years. The Senate advanced a plan with about $40 billion in reductions over the same time frame. Senate Finance staffer Neleen Eisinger made a concerted effort to engage with industry leaders to address their detailed concerns, with all sides understanding that a significant reduction was in the works. Industry leaders decided they preferred the Senate's $40 billion to the House's $54 billion and publicly supported the Senate's plan. During the PPACA Senate floor debate, Republican senators spent floor time explicitly attacking the home health care reductions. Their good sound bites did not obscure the reality that a large part of the industry had decided to support the Senate version and was sticking with it. On the passage of the ACA, the president of the Visiting Nurse Associations of America issued this statement:

> While the healthcare package is not perfect, particularly as it relates
> to nonprofit providers and the patients they serve, we support it
> and look forward to opportunities to work with Congress and the
> Administration to build upon the foundation laid by this historic
> legislation.[13]

Private Insurers

Few parts of Medicare divide Republicans and Democrats as much as Part C, also called Medicare Advantage (MA). Few issues in Title III generated more contention than MA—in a title that generated lots of tension.

Medicare Advantage allows Medicare beneficiaries to join a private health insurance plan for their covered benefits instead of participating in the traditional fee-for-service structure of Parts A and B, by which medical providers are paid piecemeal for every service they provide. Republicans like MA because they prefer medical care organized and delivered by the private sector as opposed to the government; if they could do it, Republicans would prefer that all Medicare services be delivered through private plans with no fee-for-service option. By contrast, Democrats tend to dislike and mistrust private insurance companies and prefer health coverage provided by the government and not the private sector. By extension, they are far less supportive of MA, though more circumspect in states with a high market penetration for these plans (for example, Oregon with 41 percent, Pennsylvania with 36 percent, and California with 34 percent).[14]

It has been a roller coaster history for private plans in Medicare. First admitted through the 1976 HMO Act, Medicare enrollees in private health maintenance organizations would (it was thought) receive better, more coordinated care at less cost. So initially, private plans were paid 95 percent of the average Medicare fee-for-service cost in each county, theoretically saving the federal government 5 percent on each enrollee who would get better care to boot. Enough seniors liked it that by 1999 the program had enrolled about 6.9 million of them, fully 18 percent of all Medicare beneficiaries. But when the federal government lifted the hood on the HMO car to see what was underneath, it discovered many plans deliberately attracting younger, healthier seniors who cost on average only about 90 percent of the fee-for-service cost. In reality, the government was paying more for these enrollees rather than less.

Congress clamped down in the 1997 Balanced Budget Act, giving the program a fancy new name, Medicare + Choice, while lowering payments to urban plans and increasing them to rural ones. Many plans closed or withdrew from unprofitable urban counties, the expected rural increases did not happen, and enrollment plummeted to 5.3 million, 13 percent of enrollees, by 2003. That same year, in the Medicare Modernization Act, which created the Part D drug benefit, the Republican-controlled Congress rechristened the program as Medicare Advantage, created more types of plans, and boosted federal payments to plans to encourage enrollment, particularly in hard-to-engage rural areas. Once again, enrollment grew—to 10.9 million, or 24 percent of Medicare beneficiaries by November 2009, the highest level in the history of private plans in Medicare. Medicare Advantage, by 2010, no longer had any pretense of costing less than fee-for-service; in fact, overall, the program cost had reached as much as 117 percent of the average fee-for-service cost, a differential costing the federal government $14 billion each year. Also, because of the intricacies of Medicare financing, fee-for-service Part B enrollees had to pay a higher Part B premium, $3.35 per month, to finance the higher cost of enrollees in Medicare Advantage.[15] Time for another haircut.

In the 2008 presidential debates, when Democratic candidate Barack Obama was asked to identify one federal program he would cut, his response was "Medicare Advantage."[16] The Democratic Congress started taking whacks at the program in mid-2008, using Medicare Advantage reductions to pay for legislation to avert a Medicare Part B physician-payment cut. Senator Max Baucus showed his hand in his November 2008 health reform white paper: "Congress must act to level the playing field between traditional Medicare and Medicare Advantage payments and the Baucus plan would do so."[17]

Karen Ignagni, president of America's Health Insurance Plans (AHIP), knowing that Medicare Advantage could not emerge unscathed if health reform were to succeed, led her industry to offer about $80 billion in reductions to the program in negotiations with Senate Finance staffers Shawn Bishop, Tony Clapsis, Liz Fowler, and John Selib in the summer of 2009, along with some specific restructuring ideas. She put other system reform proposals on the table, including simplifying administrative tasks, improving health literacy, and expanding the use of personal health records—none of which the CBO scored high in real savings. Senate Finance staffers wanted the insurance industry to deliver savings at least equivalent to those from the hospital industry, $155 billion or more. Unlike the pharmaceutical and hospital negotiations, all these talks were held exclusively with Senate staffers and without participation of the White House, which was even less eager to be associated with an insurers' deal than it was with the drug industry. In June and July, the war of words between the insurance industry and health reformers in the House, White House, and Senate began to escalate sharply. Talks ceased without resolution, and AHIP began secretly funneling a total of $86.2 million to the U.S. Chamber of Commerce to bankroll most of the cost of its anti-health-reform advertising campaign. Insurers still hoped Republicans in Baucus's Gang of Six would help them avert deeper reductions, but the cessation of that group halted that hope. Baucus brought a package to the Senate Finance Committee in September with steeper MA reductions, a new excise tax on the insurance industry, and more. In October, AHIP released a report from the accounting firm PricewaterhouseCoopers projecting major premium increases as a result of the Senate Finance Committee's reform plan. From that point on, talks were more than over—the camps were at war.

House and Senate health reform teams were in complete agreement on reducing Medicare Advantage payments as a major funding source but had starkly different visions of how to achieve that goal. The House wanted to pay MA plans 100 percent of fee-for-service rates in each county: it was a simple and direct "administered pricing" approach. House Ways and Means leaders and staffers had done extensive education to convince House Democrats it was the way to go. Democratic senators, by contrast, found the 100 percent fee-for-service option unacceptable because lower payment rates in rural areas would chase all the MA plans away and make the program exclusively urban. Instead, the Senate opted for a "competitive bidding" scheme where payments to plans would be based on the average plan bid in each area, with bonus payments for quality and improved-quality plans. In the fall 2009 Senate negotiations leading to Majority Leader Harry Reid's December 2009 Manager's Amendment, changes were made to grandfather existing MA plans in Florida and New York in order to address concerns by Senator Bill Nelson (D-FL) and Chuck Schumer (D-NY)—triggering similar (though less vehement) criticism to that leveled against Senator Ben Nelson (D-NE) for the Nebraska Medicaid deal. The White House initially accepted and then criticized the arrangement, angering Florida's Nelson.

When House and Senate staffers sat down to negotiate differences in January 2010 before the special Massachusetts Senate election, neither side could accept the other's structure. The House had one big advantage—its plan saved an estimated $75 billion more than did the Senate version over ten years. Still, the only option was to devise a third way resembling neither branch's ideal and saving money in the neighborhood of the House's plan. That is what happened. The final agreement, hammered out in mid-January, was incorporated into the "reconciliation sidecar" legislation signed by President Obama one week after he signed the ACA. It was not competitive bidding and not 100 percent fee-for-service. It was, like the House's plan, administered pricing—a new set of benchmark payments for Medicare Advantage plans at different percentages of Medicare fee-for-service rates, by area, with bonuses for quality and enrollee satisfaction, and lower plan payments for "low-quality" plans. High-cost urban areas would be paid at 95 percent of fee-for-service and lower-cost rural plans would be paid at 115 percent. The final ten-year savings were estimated by the CBO at $135.6 billion, along with $53 billion in Medicare Part B savings because of interactions between Parts B and C—$188.6 billion in all.

There is one irony in the final result. Although the compromise structure did not resemble either the Senate or House version, it did resemble the proposal advanced by AHIP's Karen Ignagni in the summer of 2009, not in the actual dollar savings, but in the revised program structure. And so the roller coaster for private insurance plans in Medicare continues—up from 1976 until 1997, down between 1998 and 2003, up from 2004 until 2010, and down from here, at least until the next transformation.

Prescription Drugs

It was the first "deal" or "stakeholder agreement" of the ACA health reform process—a three-way understanding among the White House, Senator Max Baucus, and the pharmaceutical industry represented by its trade organization, the Pharmaceutical Research and Manufacturers of America (PhRMA). Announced by President Obama himself at the White House on June 20 with a representative of the seniors organization AARP at his side while PhRMA reps sat in the audience, the $80 billion agreement resulted from weeks of intense negotiations, and it generated animus toward all three parties from the House of Representatives, Republicans, the media, and progressive groups, as well drug-industry players who felt their trade group gave away too much.

The most featured aspect of the agreement was a strategy over ten years to close the Medicare Part D doughnut hole, the coverage gap that leaves enrollees paying 100 percent of drug costs between $2,831 and $6,440 in 2010, which expands each year. Medicare pays 75 percent of costs lower than the hole and 95 percent of costs higher; the hole was created by Part D's designers in 2003 to hold down the total cost of the law. The industry's 2009 agreement is to sell brand-name drugs to Medicare beneficiaries who enter the doughnut-hole payment zone at a 50 percent discount for seniors with incomes below 400 percent of the federal poverty level. Beginning in 2013, the federal government will add an additional subsidy that will grow yearly until it reaches 25 percent in 2020. At that point, the manufacturer and government subsidies will equal 75 percent, the same subsidy rate as for drugs below the doughnut-hole opening. Beneficiaries will still be liable for 25 percent of the costs. That is what officials mean by "closing the doughnut hole."

Closing that hole had been a Democratic priority for years, including a priority for Democratic presidential candidate Obama. As public support for national health reform plummeted among seniors in the spring of 2009, the White House and congressional leaders focused on addressing the doughnut hole as the best way to shore up political support among this crucial constituency. Addressing the hole was also a demand from the seniors lobbyist AARP, which was facing rising membership cancellations (about 400,000, or 1 percent of its membership) because of its members' growing antipathy toward the organization's supportive stance on health reform.

Creating the Part D benefit had been a stormy controversy in 2003 as Democrats favored a government-managed benefit resembling Parts A and B, and Republicans, with solid majorities in both branches, favored a private sector model with competition among plans. Some Democrats, notably Max Baucus, then the Senate Finance ranking member, joined Republicans while most were in solid opposition. Implementation of the new benefit in 2005 and 2006 was rocky, with beneficiaries bewildered by a dizzying array of drug plan choices, as Democrats promised an overhaul at their first opportunity. But confusion dissipated, and in the 2008 presidential campaign, Democrats talked only about closing the doughnut hole and allowing the federal government to negotiate prices, not about overhauling the private structure. Even under the Democrats, privately run Part D is here to stay.

Part D was the source of prescription drug coverage in 2010 for 40.5 million of Medicare's 45 million enrollees. About 27 million of them are enrolled in private Part D plans—one-third of those as part of their Medicare Advantage coverage. About 13 million obtain drug coverage through other sources such as employer-sponsored retiree benefit plans, the Department of Veterans Affairs, and other sources. About 10 million enrollees qualify for the low-income subsidy, enabling them to avoid premiums, most cost sharing, and the doughnut hole. In 2007, about 8.3 million Part D enrollees had prescription drug needs high enough to land inside the doughnut hole, though only 10 percent of those faced 100 percent of the doughnut-hole costs—most were wholly or partially subsidized by the low-income subsidy or other benefits. In 2009, the Part D program cost $53.3 billion—$19.9 billion was for the low-income subsidy, $18.8 billion for the cost of the direct subsidy for all enrollees, $10.9 billion for reinsurance for the highest-cost enrollees, and $3.7 billion for the subsidy to employers who maintain retiree drug coverage. Between 2010 and 2019, the expected federal cost for Part D will total nearly $1 trillion. The law was written so that these costs are financed through general revenues. Unlike those who drafted the ACA, Part D's Republican designers made no effort in the 2003 law to offset the cost.[18]

Baucus and his staffers who were working to close the doughnut hole saw the PhRMA agreement as the only viable path that could pass muster in the Senate, where a significant number of Democrats were friendly with the pharmaceutical industry, including Baucus and Edward Kennedy (D-MA). The House preferred to close the doughnut hole with direct federal financing and increases in mandatory drug-industry rebates, an approach politically unworkable in the Senate and more costly to the federal treasury. But the Senate plan did not go far enough to satisfy AARP and other advocates. It left enrollees facing 50 percent of brand-name costs inside the doughnut hole, an unacceptable exposure in light of the other reductions and changes being made to Medicare in Title III. The final Reconciliation Act added the 25 percent federal government subsidy starting in 2013, as well as a $250 check to each enrollee entering the doughnut hole zone in 2010 as an early deliverable.

Rather than undermining or transforming the underlying structure of Part D, the ACA and the reconciliation law strengthened and continued the basic structure, modifying it in a way that maintained industry support. Advocates from AARP and similar constituencies, as well as the House, did not get what they wanted (reimportation and price controls), though they did get what they needed (a closed doughnut hole).

Physicians

Of all provider constituencies, physicians got one of the best deals. And of all provider constituencies, physicians got one of the worst deals. The two statements are equally plausible. Physicians were the only provider stakeholder asked to give up nothing in terms of reimbursement cuts or savings to pay for the law—even the hospice industry came up with $7.5 billion over ten years. At the same time, the 570,000 physicians who bill Medicare were promised by House and Senate leaders fundamental reform of an obscure and financially threatening Medicare payment rule known as the sustainable growth rate (SGR), because of the formula's accepted flaws and in consideration for their public support of health reform—and they ended the process with no positive outcome on the SGR rule.

Many physician organizations are scattered across the U.S., including physician specialty societies, fifty state medical associations, and other groupings, though the largest, claiming approximately 20 percent of physicians and medical students as members, is the American Medical Association, begun in 1847, which now has a reported membership of 244,000 retired and active physicians, medical students, residents, and fellows. Though its proportionate representation of U.S. physicians has been shrinking for years, its brand recognition, the large number of rival physician organizations with widely varying positions and political perspectives, and its generous political action committee donations keep the AMA the preeminent voice on physician policy in Washington DC.

Historically, the AMA has been among the most ardent and vociferous opponents to all forms of national health insurance, having led both the successful opposition to FDR and Truman's proposals in the 1930s and 1940s as well as the unsuccessful opposition to LBJ's plan in 1965. After the enactment of Medicare, physicians openly discussed a national boycott of the new program, a threat deftly thwarted by President Johnson[19] and by the lure of reimbursement rules permitting them to charge the federal government their "usual, customary, and reasonable fees." The formula, also applicable to hospitals, triggered an early Medicare cost explosion abated only somewhat in 1975, when fees were first limited by a Medicare economic index. Starting in 1975, Congress set yearly annual limits on physicians' Medicare fees until 1992, when it established a fee schedule and a "volume performance standard," which resulted in volatile and unpredictable annual changes in physician reimbursement.

In the 1997 Balanced Budget Act, Congress tried a fresh start with a sustainable growth rate for Part B physician payments to begin in 1998. The SGR sets an overall physician spending target each year so that physician payments are adjusted upward if actual spending goes below the target and downward if spending moves above the target. The principal drivers of the increases in Part B spending are the volume and intensity of services provided by physicians. The major error in the SGR formula is the assumption that individual physicians will voluntarily reduce the volume and intensity of services they provide to Medicare enrollees to avoid payment cuts; if a physician does not believe that his or her colleagues will act the same way, then that doctor faces double jeopardy—a rate cut in addition to voluntary reductions in services delivered. More than a decade of experience has proven the model to be fatally flawed.

Since 2002, the SGR formula has required reductions in payment rates to doctors because actual increases have annually exceeded targets. In 2002, for the only time, Congress allowed the reduction, a 4.8 percent cut, to take effect. Since 2003, Congress has stepped in each time to stop the cut and to add a small increase in physician service payments.[20] Between 2003 and 2006, Republican Congresses halted the cuts with no effort to offset the federal cost with revenues or savings. In 2007, the new Democratic majorities in the House and Senate adopted "pay-go" rules requiring any unbudgeted expenditures to be financed in a deficit-neutral manner. For example, in July 2008, the House and Senate approved legislation to avert yet another looming Medicare physician-payment cut, financed by compensating payment reductions to the Medicare Advantage program. Even though physicians have averted the impact of direct SGR-triggered cuts, their 2010 reimbursement rate is 17 percent below the rate for 2001 when adjusted for medical inflation; so the SGR has had an indirect and substantial effect in depressing physician payments below what they might otherwise be, even with the congressional fixes.[21]

The greatest impediment to eliminating the SGR is the large and fast-growing cost to the federal treasury, which, for CBO scoring purposes, is viewed over a ten-year budget window and was estimated at $210 billion during the 2009–10 health reform process. The estimated cost of fixing the SGR keeps growing at an alarming rate—in an August 24, 2010, letter, the CBO estimated the ten-year cost of eliminating the SGR from 2011–20 had grown to $330 billion.[22] In his November 2008 white paper, Senator Max Baucus noted: "Moving toward a more value-driven physician-payment system in Medicare must start with reform of the current system used to update physician payments."[23] His paper, though, discussed options, not a single proposal. In the optimistic days of 2008 and early 2009, many hoped that systemic payment reform would provide a pathway to solve this expensive problem. But physician-payment reform as part of comprehensive reform proved too heavy a challenge and financial lift.

Democrats in the House of Representatives came up with a solution—pay for all of health reform except for the elimination of the SGR, something even the conservative Democrat Blue Dog caucus embraced. But President Obama's declaration in his September 2009 joint address to Congress that the total health reform legislation would not cost more than $900 billion put an insoluble obstacle in the middle of that path. The House's comprehensive health reform legislation, approved on November 7, 2009, did not include any resolution of the physician-payment issue, though House leaders assured AMA leaders they would address the matter quickly through separate legislation—which the Senate was then unable to muster sufficient support to pass. The AMA expressed qualified support for the House health reform bill and endured withering criticism from individual physicians and a number of its state affiliates. "As Congress considers new coverage commitments to the American people through health reform, it must ensure that commitments already made are fulfilled through passage of the Medicare Physician Payment Reform Act of 2009," said AMA president James Rohack following the House vote.[24]

The plan to address the SGR—without a pay-for—in the Senate was filed as legislation in October by Senator Debbie Stabenow (D-MI) and got only forty-six votes in a Senate roll call, with Democratic budget hawks led by Budget chair Kent Conrad (D-ND) in indignant opposition. The final Senate health reform legislation could have included a short-term SGR fix, but AMA leaders demanded a longer-term resolution as part of separate legislation if it could not be addressed in the health reform bill. The final Senate bill, approved on December 24, 2009, had no provisions relating to the SGR, nor did the final ACA; nor did the reconciliation side-car legislation include any fix.

The physician community had other issues of concern, some resolved (a Senate proposed tax on elective cosmetic surgery, opposed by dermatologists, was removed) and some not (physicians are included in the stakeholders potentially affected by decisions of the Independent Payment Advisory Board). The AMA supported universal coverage, including an individual mandate, as well as insurance-market reforms. It backed investments in prevention, wellness, and administrative simplification as well as some quality initiatives that did not impinge on its members' practices. It did not achieve significant progress regarding medical-liability issues. And most important for the AMA, it did not eliminate the SGR.

THE FUTURE: WILL THE ACA LOWER U.S. HEALTH CARE COSTS?

Among many contested arguments involving the ACA, one of the most consequential is the question of the law's impact on slowing the growth in overall health care spending over the next two decades. The ACA will undoubtedly slow the rate of growth in Medicare at least by the CBO-estimated $449 billion between 2010 and 2019. That those savings will help to pay for coverage expansions in Titles I and II does not diminish that fact. Reductions in Medicare payments may, however, create pressure for even higher private health spending. Alternatively, it is also possible that the ACA innovations in Medicare and Medicaid may have positive spillover effects that will improve efficiency and also lower costs in the private health sector. And with so many changes occurring simultaneously, it will be challenging to tease the impact of any single intervention from the others.

It is possible to examine the key ACA innovations and consider their potential impact on private health spending. Table 5 lists eleven specific cost-lowering interventions.

Five of the eleven innovations, if implemented as designed, should lower private sector health spending in addition to public sector spending. These include the "Cadillac" excise tax on high-premium plans, discussed in more

TABLE 5. Key ACA innovations to lower Medicare, Medicaid, and private health spending

Innovation and ACA section	CBO/JCT ten-year estimated federal savings or revenue (in billions of dollars)	Medicare impact	Medicaid impact	Private sector impact
High-premium "Cadillac" excise tax (9001)	32	No	No	Yes
Independent Payment Advisory Board (3403)	15.1	Yes	No	Yes
Administrative simplification (1104)	11.6	Yes	Yes	Yes
Preventable hospital readmissions (3025)	7.1	Yes	Spillover	Spillover
Pathway for generic biologic agents (Title VII)	7.0	Yes	Yes	Yes
Fraud- and abuse-prevention measures (Title VI, Subtitles E, F)	7.0	Yes	Yes	Spillover
Accountable care organizations, shared savings (3022)	4.9	Yes	Yes	Spillover
Hospital-acquired infections (3008)	1.4	Yes	Spillover	Spillover
Center for Medicare and Medicaid innovation (3021)	1.3	Yes	Yes	Spillover
Physician quality reporting (3002)	0.1	Yes	Spillover	Spillover
Patient Centered Outcomes Research Institute (6301–02)	2.2*	Yes	Yes	Yes

* Net increase 2010–19

detail in chapter 13; the creation of the Independent Payment Advisory Board, whose purview was expanded during the crafting of the reconciliation bill beyond Medicare to cover private spending; administrative simplification, which is aimed at the entire health sector and may see results far more extensive than the CBO estimate of $11.6 billion in federal savings, according to many industry leaders; a pathway for generic-like biopharmaceuticals, discussed in chapter 11; and the new public-private institute to conduct comparative effectiveness research. All of these initiatives, if implemented effectively, have the potential to save far more in spending in the second decade than in the first.

The other six may have a positive impact on private sector health spending because changes in medical care delivered at hospitals or in physician's offices should have a positive spillover on private spending. For example, Medicare payment policies will penalize hospitals that have higher-than-average rates of preventable readmissions and hospital-acquired infections (also known as health-care-associated infections). Hospitals will reengineer their medical care systems to avoid the penalties. It is unlikely that hospitals will change their care processes only for Medicare patients; rather, the changes will benefit privately insured patients and the private bill payers as well. A similar dynamic can be envisioned with the greatly expanded fraud- and abuse-prevention system in Title VI; according to health care fraud and abuse experts, fraudulent perpetrators are indifferent to the source of their funds; more effective control systems in the federal and state governments may hamper illegal operations that are stealing private health dollars as well.[25]

Are there other innovations that could have been included in the ACA? And could any of the innovations have been structured to have a more effective and significant impact? Yes and yes. An example of the former would have involved permitting Medicare to pay physicians to provide end-of-life counseling to beneficiaries—a proposal dropped because of political attacks charging that Democrats were creating "death panels." An example of the latter is the Patient Centered Outcomes Research Institute (PCORI), included in Title VI, which could have been structured to consider cost-effectiveness in addition to clinical effectiveness, which was not done for reasons similar to the end-of-life issue. The ACA took every idea on how to reduce health care spending, public and private, and pushed as far as the political system would tolerate in 2009 and 2010. Some of these innovations will fail, either completely or mostly. Some will succeed, far beyond the estimates calculated by the CBO. Some of these innovations will be altered by Congress in the coming years, and no one will know how they might have otherwise worked. Let's take a look at one of the more controversial innovations.

The Independent Payment Advisory Board and Triggers. The sustainable growth rate is triggered only if certain conditions are met. If Part B physician payments go above a certain level, then automatic rate cuts are triggered—unless Congress intervenes, which it has done every time the trigger point has been hit since 2003. In 2003, the Republican-controlled Congress created another trigger in that year's Medicare Modernization Act, requiring the president to submit legislation to reduce Medicare expenditures whenever two consecutive Medicare Trustee Reports indicate that general revenues are funding more than 45 percent of total Medicare outlays; the Democratic-controlled Congress suspended operation of this trigger in 2009.[26] Nonetheless, support for triggers or some new device or board with special powers continues, including triggers in the ACA.

In his 2008 book, *Critical*, former Senate majority leader Tom Daschle called for the formation of a Federal Health Board "charged with establishing the system's framework and filling in most of the details . . . insulated from political pressure and, at the same time, accountable to elected officials and the American people . . . making the complex decisions inherent in promoting health system performance."[27] In late 2008, Peter Orszag, then director of the CBO (and President Obama's first director of the Office of Management and Budget in 2009 and beyond), issued a set of "budget options" on ways to finance national health reform and limit federal health care spending. Option 113 was to "Devise an Enforcement Mechanism for the Medicare Funding Warning."[28] The CBO laid out an option to "apply an automatic 1.0 percent reduction in payments for services furnished in Medicare's fee-for-service sector" whenever the 45 percent trigger point was reached.

For a long time, it appeared the idea had lost any support. Baucus conspicuously left any board, trigger, or other limitation out of his November 2008 white paper. The January 2009 derailment of Daschle's nomination as health and human services secretary left the idea of a Federal Health Board by the wayside. When death panels, government takeovers, and health care rationing by bureaucrats became a refrain among Republicans and tea party activists, Democrats retreated from such discussions for much of 2009.

Senator Jay Rockefeller (D-WV), though, kept pushing in private meetings, roundtables, and public hearings the idea of a "MedPAC on steroids," whether expanded powers for the existing MedPAC or extraordinary powers for a new MedPAC-like entity composed of experts one or two steps removed from the political process. Over the summer and fall of 2009, business groups and others began to demand provisions to "bend the cost curve" in addition to expanding access to coverage. The White House, prodded by Orszag and their other economists, echoed these sentiments, which were viewed with suspicion by the House of Representatives and by progressive groups such as AARP.

Baucus's September 2009 proposal to the Senate Finance Committee included the establishment of an "Independent Medicare Commission . . . that would develop and submit proposals to Congress aimed at extending the solvency of Medicare, slowing Medicare cost-growth, and improving the quality of care delivery to Medicare beneficiaries" with expedited rules of consideration and automatic reductions in the event of congressional inaction. The final PPACA, approved in the Senate in December 2009, required the creation of a fifteen-member Independent Medicare Advisory Board (IMAB) along the lines of Baucus's proposal, with a prohibition on proposals that rationed care, raised taxes or beneficiary premiums, or changed Medicare benefit, eligibility, or cost-sharing standards. Through 2019, an exemption was included against further cuts to any provider group that had already taken a substantial level of cuts in the ACA, keeping hospitals, hospices, and other constituencies out of the initial impacts of the board's decisions.

The final reconciliation sidecar changed the entity's name to the Independent Payment Advisory Board, adding a mandate to examine the rate of cost growth in the private sector as well as Medicare, and clarifying that the board would make binding recommendations to change Medicare only in years when that program's spending was above the targeted growth rate—a new trigger. The IPAB is one of the key reforms trumpeted by the Obama administration and Democratic congressional leaders to address long-term health care spending.[29] Critics on the right point to it as evidence of rationing and a government takeover in the new law.[30] Even the hospital and pharmaceutical industries, supporters of the ACA, jumped on the bandwagon to repeal the IPAB within eight months of the law's enactment. Critics on the left worry it will lead to erosion in Medicare. And critics in the middle are concerned Congress will never allow the reforms to take effect. Because it is impossible to predict how the world will look in 2014 and beyond, it is impossible to refute any of these assertions with certainty.

.   .   .

Medicare started in the 1965 as one tree with two branches. More than thirty-five years later, it has four major trunks and a vast array of secondary and tertiary branches and shoots. Its roots now intertwine with Medicaid and private health insurance in ways not seen or understood by the American public. Like a living organism, these trunks and branches keep evolving, some growing, some shrinking and falling off, with new formations sprouting in ways the creators could never have imagined.

Changes brought by the ACA will alter some trajectories, though the tree will keep growing. It is now the mighty oak of U.S. health policy.

Republicans attempted to thwart passage of the ACA by decrying and opposing changes to Medicare. Their complaints ring hollow. In discussions about Medicare over many years, Republicans led the charge to cut the program, especially in 1995 and 1997. The ACA's savings and reductions to Medicare are balanced by gains that will help stabilize the health care industry. Such gains were never part of plans offered by Republicans, either in the past or in the current tight-budget environment. In truth, Republicans are less opposed to the ACA's Medicare changes than to the use of those savings. Democrats were determined to use Medicare savings to help finance coverage expansions for uninsured Americans; Republicans would use such savings for tax cuts or deficit reduction. That is a legitimate disagreement—one Republicans chose not to advance this time. Regardless of the purpose for which the savings were used, savings of the scope brought by the ACA are legitimate. And Medicare will survive them just fine.

8. Title IV—Money, Mammograms, and Menus

"Prevention is better than cure," is a widely accepted truism among the public, and among public officeholders, especially in matters relating to health and medical care. It is better to prevent or detect a cancer early than to treat it late. When money is added to the equation, things change. While prevention may be better, it is not always cheaper, and often it is more expensive, depending on the preventive measure, to whom it is applied, the rate at which the condition strikes, and other variables. Evidence for this has been known for decades, documented by Louise Russell in her 1986 book, *Is Prevention Better than Cure?*[1] Her work was updated in a 2008 article incorporating the latest evidence:

> The broad generalizations made by many presidential candidates can be misleading. These statements convey the message that substantial resources can be saved through prevention. Although some preventive measures do save money, the vast majority reviewed in the health economics literature do not.[2]

There is nothing wrong with prevention, even with preventive measures that do not save money if they save lives or improve the quality of life. It is just not the magic bullet it is often characterized to be. Congressional Budget Office director Douglas Elmendorf agrees:

> Expanded government support for preventive medical care would probably improve people's health, but would not generally reduce total spending on health care. The evidence suggests that for most preventive services, increased utilization leads to higher, not lower, medical spending.[3]

An alternative view is advanced by Dr. Ken Thorpe, an Emory University health economist who worked diligently to bring a prevention focus to the health reform debate. He notes that there are three classes of preventive measures: primary (eliminating risk factors like smoking and obesity before an individual gets sick); secondary (detecting an underlying disease before symptoms appear, such as with cancer or diabetes screening); and tertiary (working with ill individuals to manage and coordinate their care—for example, to reduce unnecessary hospitalizations). Thorpe argues that secondary prevention measures "are not fundamentally intended, and never have been, to save money. The other two forms of prevention do save money and it is here we need to invest."[4] Agreeing with Thorpe was the Trust for America's Health, a national nonprofit that drew up an influential report, "Blueprint for a Healthier America," in October 2008 with a focus on community preventive measures.[5]

TITLE IV—PREVENTION OF CHRONIC DISEASE AND IMPROVING PUBLIC HEALTH

In a victory for prevention advocates of all persuasions, a good number of breakthrough prevention provisions are embedded in the ACA, most notably in Title IV: Prevention of Chronic Disease and Improving Public Health, along with some significant and controversial prevention measures in Title I. After an overview of Title IV, we will explore four key prevention and wellness initiatives and controversies in the ACA, in both Titles IV and I: the Prevention and Public Health Trust Fund, coverage for services recommended by the U.S. Preventive Services Task Force, incentives for healthy behaviors and wellness, and menu labeling.

UNDERSTANDING TITLE IV

Title IV seeks to upgrade and expand the nation's efforts to prevent disease on all three levels described by Thorpe: first, to prevent disease from occurring; second, to treat illness before it becomes symptomatic through screening; and third, to reduce |disability and restore the functionality of those already affected by disease. Title IV has twenty-seven sections spread across five subtitles, including items added by the Manager's Amendment in Title X. Following is a brief overview of the subtitles, followed by an explanation of the most important and controversial sections.

Subtitle A seeks to better orient the U.S. health system to promote healthy policies and to establish for the first time a national disease prevention and health promotion strategy.

Subtitle B authorizes new clinically based preventive care service programs.

Subtitle C establishes new programs to promote individual and community health and to prevent chronic disease.

Subtitle D provides new funding for research in public health services and systems to identify best prevention practices.

Subtitle E directs the CBO to develop better tools to score the costs and benefits of prevention programs, and directs the Department of Health and Human Services to conduct evaluations of federal health and wellness initiatives.

Key Sections of Title IV

Following are some of the key and most controversial sections of each subtitle. In brackets is the ten-year savings score estimated by the CBO. A plus sign (+) means the section will cost the federal treasury billions (B) or millions (M) and a minus sign (−) means the provision will save federal dollars. If there is no bracketed item, the CBO estimates zero cost or savings.

Subtitle A: Modernizing Disease Prevention and Public Health Systems promotes healthy policies and establishes a national prevention and health promotion strategy.

- Prevention and Public Health Investment Fund: A new dedicated fund will make a national investment in prevention and public health to improve health and restrain the growth in health care costs, with a dedicated, stable funding stream [+$12.9B] (section 4002).

- A new interagency federal council will set national prevention and health promotion strategies (section 4001). Two existing federal task forces—the U.S. Preventive Services Task Force and the U.S. Task Force on Community Preventive Services—are expanded and coordinated (section 4003).

- The HHS secretary will convene a national public-private partnership to conduct a national prevention and health promotion outreach and education campaign. Each state will design a public awareness campaign to educate Medicaid enrollees regarding preventive services (section 4004).

Subtitle B: Increasing Access to Clinical Preventive Services authorizes new clinically based programs related to preventive care services.

- Medicare Preventive Services: Medicare will cover, without co-payments or deductibles, an annual wellness visit and personalized prevention services, including a health-risk assessment [+$3.6B] (section 4103). Medicare co-insurance will be waived for most preventive services, including any service given an A or B grade by the U.S. Preventive Services Task Force [+$800M] (section 4104). The secretary will conduct outreach regarding covered preventive services [−$700M] (section 4105).

- Medicaid Preventive Services: State Medicaid programs may provide diagnostic, screening, preventive, and rehabilitation services including: (1) any clinical preventive service given an A or B grade by the U.S. Preventive Services Task Force; and (2) adult immunizations recommended by the Advisory Committee on Immunization Practices [+$100M] (section 4106). State Medicaid programs must cover counseling and pharmacotherapy for pregnant women for tobacco cessation with no cost-sharing [−$100M] (4107). HHS will award grants to states to provide incentives for Medicaid beneficiaries to participate in healthy-lifestyle programs [+$100M] (section 4108).

- A grant program will promote school-based health clinics to provide preventive and primary services to medically under-served children and families, with $50 million in funding each year for fiscal years 2010 to 2013 [+$200M] (section 4101).

Subtitle C: Creating Healthier Communities establishes new programs to promote individual and community health and to prevent chronic disease.

- Calorie Labeling on Chain Restaurant Menus: Any chain restaurant with twenty or more locations must disclose in written form the calories of each item on menus and the menu board, as well as information on total calories and the calories from fat, and the amounts of fat, saturated fat, cholesterol, sodium, carbohydrates, sugars, dietary fiber, and protein. These rules also apply to drive-up menu boards and to vending machines (section 4205).

- The HHS secretary will establish a Healthy Aging, Living Well program to improve the health of the pre-Medicare-eligible population [+$100M] (section 4202).

- The U.S. Access Board will establish standards for the accessibility of medical diagnostic equipment for individuals with disabilities (section 4203).

- All employers with fifty or more employees must provide break time and a place for breastfeeding mothers to express milk (section 4207).

Subtitle D: Support for Prevention and Public Health Innovation provides funding for public health research to identify best prevention practices.

- The HHS secretary, through the Centers for Disease Control and Prevention (CDC), shall fund research relating to public health services and systems (section 4301).

- Any ongoing or new federal health program must collect and report data by race, ethnicity, primary language, and any other indicator of disparity [+$200M] (section 4302).

- A childhood obesity demonstration program will be appropriated up to $25 million through 2014 (section 4306).

The Prevention and Public Health Fund

Title IV includes many new programs and initiatives across the spectrum of public health, prevention, and wellness. Most of them received a zero score from the CBO, meaning they cost or save nothing according to the budget estimator's analysis. This is because the CBO never gives a score to legislative spending authorizations that must rely on the federal appropriations process for actual funding. Federal funding may happen or it may not, and there is no reliable way for the CBO to tell until each such item emerges from the fierce competition for scarce appropriated dollars. This is one reason many public health advocates express disappointment with Title IV.

There is one significant exception, and it is section 4002, a new Prevention and Public Health Fund, to be administered by the HHS secretary to provide for "expanded and sustained national investment in prevention and public health programs to improve health and help restrain the growth in private and public sector health care costs." Unlike the other sections, this fund receives a direct appropriation embedded in the statute at these levels:

fiscal year 2010	$500,000,000 ($500 million)
fiscal year 2011	$750,000,000 ($750 million)
fiscal year 2012	$1,000,000,000 ($1 billion)
fiscal year 2013	$1,250,000,000 ($1.25 billion)
fiscal year 2014	$1,500,000,000 ($1.5 billion)
fiscal year 2015 and each fiscal year thereafter	$2,000,000,000 ($2 billion)

In the Senate HELP Committee markup in June–July 2009, the final committee bill earmarked $80 billion for the fund, though that amount was subject entirely to the appropriations process, meaning none of that money was guaranteed. Some advocates were disappointed to see the funding level drop from $80 billion to $15 billion in the final ACA and missed the essential difference that the $15 billion is guaranteed while the $80 billion was soft and speculative. Committee Republicans, including ranking member Mike Enzi (R-WY), Judd Gregg (R-NH), and Tom Coburn (R-OK), criticized the $80 billion provision as a "slush fund" for jungle gyms and walking paths. The challenge moving forward is to ensure that the funding is used to generate meaningful results instead of scattering it in numerous directions with no impact in any focused area.

Senator Tom Harkin (D-IA), who managed the prevention issue for Senator Kennedy, spearheaded this win, as well as all the key provisions included in Title IV. He was named HELP Committee chair following Kennedy's death in August 2009 and continues to serve as chair in addition to maintaining his prior role as Appropriations Subcommittee chair for Labor, Health, Human Services and Education. The Senate's leading advocate for health promotion and disease prevention is now in an enviable position to implement and advance this agenda.

In June 2010, HHS secretary Kathleen Sebelius announced the first round of spending from the trust fund for federal fiscal year 2010, with $500 million in available funds. The Obama administration decided to spend half of the funding for public health investments in Title IV and half to address health care workforce priorities specified in Title V. Workforce advocates were pleased because very few workforce provisions received any direct funding, though prevention and public health advocates were concerned about siphoning half the new resources away from Title IV. Obama administration officials explained there was insufficient time in the four months remaining in federal fiscal year 2010 to spend all available funds on public health needs. The decision puts a spotlight on the tension that will surround the decision making on this new funding source in the coming years, though the bigger issue will be the attitude of the new Republican-controlled House of Representatives. Beginning in fiscal year 2011, decisions on how the annual funding allotment will be spent is to be made by congressional appropriators. Some Republicans have already proposed elimination of the fund to pay for other changes in the ACA. In spite of guaranteed funding, the future of the Prevention and Public Health Fund is far from certain.

Covering Preventive Services and the U.S. Preventive Services Task Force

Inside and outside Title IV are far-reaching initiatives to provide nearly every American with access to evidence-based preventive health services as part of their insurance coverage and without cost sharing.

For Medicare enrollees, these provisions are spelled out in Subtitle B of Title IV. Starting in 2011, beneficiaries will have access to all preventive services that receive an A or B recommendation from the U.S. Preventive Services Task Force. Families and individuals with private coverage will have access to the same services spelled out in Subtitle A of Title I, which took effect in September 2010 (though, importantly, not for enrollees in "grandfathered" plans that have been in operation without major changes since March 2010). For adults in state Medicaid programs, covering these services is a new option for states—and states that choose to provide them will receive a 1 percent payment increase in their Federal Medical Assistance Percentage for these services.

What are A and B services? The U.S. Preventive Services Task Force gives an A for any service with a "high certainty" that the net benefit is substantial and a B for a service with a "moderate certainty." The task force recommends against the routine provision of services graded C (judged to have "no net benefit") or D (whose "potential harm outweighs the gain"). The task force also gives an I grade when evidence is "insufficient." The grades may differ depending on an individual's age or gender. Table 6 provides some examples of A and B services, indicating whether they are recommended for adult men, adult women, pregnant women, or children.

What is the U.S. Preventive Services Task Force? It was started in 1984 during President Ronald Reagan's term by the U.S. Public Health Service

TABLE 6. Examples of A or B services recommended by the U.S. Preventive Services Task Force

Recommendation	Adult men	Adult women	Pregnant women	Children
Alcohol misuse, screening and behavioral counseling	X	X		
Cervical cancer, screening		X		
Colorectal cancer, screening	X	X		
Dental caries in preschool children, prevention				X
Depression, screening	X	X		
Hearing loss in newborns, screening				X
Hepatitis B virus infection, screening			X	
HIV, screening	X	X	X	X
Lipid disorder in adults, screening	X	X		
Obesity in adults, screening	X	X		
Sexually transmitted infections, counseling	X	X	X	
Syphilis infection, screening	X	X	X	
Tobacco use and tobacco-caused disease, counseling	X	X	X	
Type 2 diabetes mellitus in adults, screening	X	X		
Visual impairment in children <5, screening				X

SOURCE: U.S. Preventive Services Task Force, A and B Recommendations, August 2010, http://www.uspreventiveservicestaskforce.org/uspstf/uspsabrecs.htm.

to provide advice and recommendations to health professionals about clinical preventive services—what works and what doesn't work according to unbiased evidence. Its initial *Guide to Clinical Preventive Services*, published in 1989, was the first comprehensive effort to apply a systematic and explicit process to review evidence and link clinical practice recommendations directly to the quality of science. Since 1998 the task force has been sponsored by the Agency for Healthcare Research and Quality (AHRQ), which is part of the U.S. Department of Health and Human Services. In 2010, the task force had twelve members (eleven physicians and one PhD) who serve as volunteers without salary. The federal Public Health Service statute governing the task force—prior to changes made in the ACA—is succinct enough to reprint in full here:

SEC. 915. (A) PREVENTIVE SERVICES TASK FORCE

(1) Establishment and Purpose. The Director may periodically convene a Preventive Services Task Force to be composed of individuals with appropriate expertise. Such a task force shall review the scientific evidence related to the effectiveness, appropriateness, and cost-effectiveness of clinical preventive services for the purpose of developing recommendations for the health care community, and updating previous clinical preventive recommendations.

(2) Role of Agency. The Agency shall provide ongoing administrative, research and technical support for the operation of the Preventive Services Task Force, including coordinating and supporting the dissemination of the recommendations of the Task Force.

(3) Operation. In carrying out its responsibilities under paragraph (1), the Task Force is not subject to the provisions of Appendix 2 of title 5, United States Code.

In this case, the "agency" is AHRQ and the director runs it. Title 5, mentioned in paragraph 3, is the Federal Advisory Committee Act, and the task force is declared exempt from its numerous process requirements. Note that the AHRQ "may periodically convene" a task force and also that the task force "shall review the scientific evidence related to . . . cost-effectiveness." When the task force became embroiled in a public controversy over recommendations for mammography screening in late 2009, task force members indicated they took no account of cost considerations in their recommendations, and they seemed unaware that the term *cost-effectiveness* was included in their enabling law. Section 4003 of the ACA further clarifies and defines the responsibilities of the task force without undermining its role and purpose, as well as the related Community Preventive Services Task Force.

The reputation of the Preventive Services Task Force was so positive that no criticism or negative amendment surfaced on the issue at all during five committee markups in the House and Senate in the summer and fall of 2009. Even Senator Tom Coburn (R-OK), a physician on the Senate HELP Committee and a harsh critic of the Democratic package, publicly endorsed coverage of clinical preventive services without cost sharing. Coverage of preventive services with A or B task force recommendations had been agreed to by Democrat and Republican staffers in the spring of 2009 before negotiations ceased.

The era of good feeling ended abruptly in mid-November 2009, when the task force published recommendations for revised standards for mammography screening in the medical journal *Annals of Internal Medicine.*[6] After a review of clinical evidence, it advised against the routine screening of women in their forties with no known risk factors and recommended screening every other year (instead of every year) for women aged fifty to seventy-four. Though its recommendation was not mandatory, organizations such as the American Cancer Society and the American College of Radiology strongly contested the task force's conclusions.

The Preventive Services Task Force routinely promulgates new recommendations in journal articles prepared long before actual publication, as was true in this case. The task force members had no idea their recommendations would reach public view in the middle of the health reform debate. From the viewpoint of health reform proponents, the timing was disastrous; from the viewpoint of health reform opponents, fortuitous. After the 2009 summer of "death panel" accusations had subsided, here was prima facie evidence of Democratic designs for health care rationing, according to opponents. The task force members did not help themselves with their "deer in the headlights" response of surprise to the controversy, prompting HHS secretary Kathleen Sebelius to distance herself publicly from the recommendation and to note that "this panel was appointed by the prior administration, by former President George Bush."[7] Feisty and combative Senator Barbara Mikulski (D-MD) who was battling unsuccessfully for mandatory coverage of women's preventive services, warned a meeting of the Senate Democratic Caucus, "Women are vibrating everywhere."

To stem the political damage, Mikulski's language was added in Majority Leader Harry Reid's Manager's Amendment (Title X) to the ACA section on coverage of clinical preventive services in Title I, subsection A. The amended language reads:

(5) for the purposes of this Act, and for the purposes of any other provision of law, the current recommendations of the United States Preventive Service Task Force regarding breast cancer screening, mammography, and prevention, shall be considered the most current other than those issued in or around November 2009. Nothing in this subsection shall be construed to prohibit a plan or issuer from providing coverage for services in addition to those recommended by the United States Preventive Services Task Force or to deny coverage for services that are not recommended by such Task Force.

The provisions relating to coverage of preventive services for enrollees in Medicare, Medicaid, and private coverage emerged intact, more than did the pride of the task force members. Ironically, this episode highlights what the original provision was designed to avoid—elected officials making ad hoc decisions about coverage.

Incentives for Healthy Behaviors and Wellness

Among Capitol Hill staffers, the word was that Steve Burd had senators and House members nearly dancing on tables with joy. The president of the Safeway grocery store chain since 1992, Burd convinced Democrat and Republican members alike that he had found a personal-responsibility path to controlling health care costs, as he outlined in a June 2009 *Wall Street Journal* op-ed:

> At Safeway we believe that well-designed health-care reform, utilizing market-based solutions, can ultimately reduce our nation's health-care bill by 40 percent. The key to achieving these savings is health-care plans that reward healthy behavior. As a self-insured employer, Safeway designed just such a plan in 2005 and has made continuous improvements each year. The results have been remarkable. During this four-year period, we have kept our per capita health-care costs flat (that includes both the employee and the employer portion), while most American companies' costs have increased 38 percent over the same four years.[8]

Under Burd's plan, Safeway employees receive substantial discounts on their health insurance premiums if they meet benchmark goals on four tests: tobacco use, weight, blood pressure, and cholesterol levels—$780 for individuals and $1,560 for families. The "problem," noted Burd, is that "we are constrained from increasing these incentives" by existing federal law. Health reform, he said, should relax the federal limits.

In this case, the law is the 1996 Health Insurance Portability and Accountability Act (HIPAA), which prohibits discrimination in eligibility and costs for similarly situated employees when they enroll in their employer's health plan. However, HIPAA also says that nothing in the act should "prevent a group health plan from establishing premium discounts or rebates or modifying otherwise applicable copayments or deductibles in return for adherence to programs of health promotion and disease prevention." It took until 2006 for federal regulations to be issued defining this exception. The final rules define two types of health-plan-linked wellness programs: those requiring participation only and those requiring an individual to meet a standard or result. No additional constraints apply to the former, but the latter must pass five tests to conform with the rules: (1) the incentive cannot exceed 20 percent of the employee's premium share; (2) the program must be capable of improving health or preventing disease among participants; (3) every individual must have an annual opportunity to participate; (4) the incentive must be offered to every similarly situated individual; and (5) there must be alternative standards and waiver opportunities.

Burd wanted to vary his employee premiums by more than 20 percent and undertook strenuous advocacy to spread his good news and his agenda for change. He founded the Coalition to Advance Healthcare Reform to promote his ideas nationally, meeting with senators and representatives, Democrats and Republicans, and even President Obama. Here are statements from Senator Ben Cardin (D-MD) and John Barrasso (R-WY):

> Safeway, one of the largest food and drug retailers in North America, is an example of how wellness and preventive care can make a difference. Safeway has devised an innovative approach called Healthy Measures that recognizes the role of personal responsibility. . . . Safeway has built a culture of health and fitness, and it has made a difference. Obesity and smoking rates among Safeway employees are 30 percent lower than the national average, and the company has been able to keep health costs constant over a four-year period. That's a real achievement, and one that should be emulated nationally. (Cardin)[9]

> They individualize the incentives so if you get your weight down and your blood pressure under control, and your cholesterol and blood sugar, if you don't use tobacco products, they know that will help save the company money, and they share that with you. So it's money in your pocket to stay healthy. And the company saves money too. (Barrasso)[10]

At a closed-door HELP Committee meeting with Democrats and Republicans, just prior to the start of the committee markup in June 2009, Senator Orrin Hatch (R-UT) pressed CBO director Doug Elmendorf on his agency's failure to show positive scores for preventive health measures such as the Safeway approach. Elmendorf's staffer, Phil Ellis, provided an answer that caught the senator short: "Safeway is largely a myth."[11]

The *Washington Post's* David Hilzenrath put numbers behind Ellis's comment in a January 2010 report. Safeway's health insurance costs did drop in 2006, by 12.5 percent, not in connection with the wellness program—which did not start until 2009—but because Safeway switched its insurance to high-deductible policies that increased the financial exposure for workers who used more medical services. After 2006, the cost increases resumed. The wellness discount applies only to the company's 28,000 nonunion management and office workers, not its full workforce of about 200,000.[12] Beyond Safeway, there is disagreement within the health services research community on the effectiveness of such incentives—with some concluding they work and others reaching the opposite finding.[13] Disease advocacy organizations such as the American Cancer Society, the American Heart Association, and the American Diabetes Association pushed back, charging that the incentives would raise insurance costs for sicker people.[14]

Nonetheless, Burd achieved his goal. Subtitle C of Title I allows employers to motivate workers to participate in approved wellness programs by varying premiums up to 30 percent, up from the 20 percent level permitted under HIPAA, and allows the HHS, labor, and treasury secretaries in the future to agree to raise the premium variance threshold to 50 percent. Also, the secretaries of HHS, labor, and the treasury will establish by 2014 a demonstration of a similar approach in individual insurance markets in ten states.

Most influential for members from both parties was the belief that individuals should be required to pay more for their unhealthy behaviors. In its bill markup, Senate Finance voted eighteen to four in favor of an amendment by Tom Carper (D-DE) and John Ensign (R-NV) to expand employer wellness incentives along the lines of the HELP Committee proposal. The final law enshrined that principle for tobacco use—under Title I, smokers can be required to pay 50 percent higher premiums than nonsmokers. Under the wellness provisions, there will be more to come. This is one argument that is not over.

Menu Labeling

Section 4205 of the ACA includes a new mandate on all restaurant chains with at least twenty outlets to disclose the calories for each item on menus, the menu board, drive-thru displays, and vending machines, as well as additional information in written form, available to consumers on request, regarding calories from fat and amounts of fat, saturated fat, cholesterol, sodium, carbohydrates, sugars, fiber, and protein. This requirement for more government regulation was included in the ACA with the public support of the National Restaurant Association and leading national chains. How did this happen, and why did the industry support new regulations on their business?

In a word, it was federalism, the curious and always dynamic relationship and interaction between federal and state or local policies.

In 2003, Margo Wootan, a researcher at the Center for Science in the

Public Interest, and Kelly Brownell, a researcher at the Rudd Center for Food Policy and Obesity at Yale University, began talking about calorie labeling on menus as a strategy to change food consumption among Americans toward healthier and lower-calorie choices. Senator Harkin picked up on the idea and filed the first version of the Menu Education and Labeling (MEAL) Act in 2003, teaming up with Congresswoman Rosa DeLauro (D-CT), who filed companion legislation in the House. They talked with restaurant-industry leaders, who said they already were doing enough by putting this information on their websites and in pamphlets available in their outlets. The federal legislation did not move.

Soon thereafter, cities, counties, and state governments—most prominently New York City—began considering and approving legislative proposals to require various forms of nutritional and calorie labeling on restaurant selections, creating a patchwork of regulations and requirements the restaurant industry could not thwart or avert. Suddenly, the industry was facing a new wave of rules differing in every jurisdiction, and it was unable to slow the wave. The industry backed alternative federal legislation—the Labeling Education and Nutrition (LEAN) Act sponsored by Senators Tom Carper (D-DE) and Lisa Murkowski (R-AK), which would have established weaker national standards, combined with strong preemption of all state and local laws.

Section 4205 of the ACA gives the industry what it most wanted, preemption of any new state or local laws, though existing nonfederal statutes may stay in place at the discretion of that governmental entity. In exchange, the new standards require the prominent display of calorie information on all menus, menu boards, drive-through menu boards, and vending machines for all affected restaurant chains. The agreement was announced on June 10, 2009, with the endorsement of many organizations, including the American Academy of Pediatrics, American Diabetes Association, American Dietetic Association, the Center for Science in the Public Interest, the Coalition for Responsible Nutrition Information, Dunkin Donuts, the National Restaurant Association, and the Rudd Center for Food Policy and Obesity at Yale University.

Without pressure in the form of new laws enacted by states, cities, and counties, this would not have happened.

. . .

How effective will Title IV be in creating a new "culture of prevention" in the United States and in the nation's health care system? The question cannot be answered before several years of implementation activity as well as research on the policy outcomes. The new Prevention Trust Fund has the capacity to finance important and strategic investments, but its resources may be siphoned off in less effective directions or eliminated in the future appropriations processes. The cost of some preventive services will be covered, and research will provide evidence to inform conclusions on their impact. Wellness incentives and menu labeling will also require time to be judged. What can be said with certainty is that prevention was an important part of the conversation leading to passage of the ACA. The results can be seen in Title IV and beyond. Prevention's time in the spotlight has arrived, and it is not likely to fade fast.

9. Title V—Who Will Provide the Care?

Of the ACA's ten titles, Title V stands out in a peculiar way. It was the only title that generated no public conflict and no attacks in the legislative process leading to enactment. The need to address health care workforce issues is viewed by both parties as urgent regardless of health reform. Two key factors motivated policy makers to act: an aging and growing population with expanding rates of chronic illness combined with an aging and dispirited health care workforce. A frequent criticism of the 2006 Massachusetts health reform law was the law's failure to address health care workforce shortages, which exacerbate access problems, especially in some geographic areas and within primary care and some specialties. Title V signals a desire by the Congress to avoid this part of the Massachusetts experience and to address the long-term interests of many individual senators in various aspects of the workforce issues. One important question in evaluating Title V is whether its potpourri of member-generated initiatives leads to a coherent workforce policy in the face of pressures already in existence as well as those that will be brought on by the ACA.

Avoiding the Massachusetts experience, though, may be harder than it seems. Even prior to reform, Massachusetts had a much lower proportion of uninsured individuals than most other states—8–10 percent versus 16–17 percent nationally. Massachusetts had a more robust system to provide care to lower-income persons, insured or uninsured, than exists nationally or in most other states. Also, Massachusetts has among the highest professional-to-population ratios among a host of categories including physicians, primary care physicians, physician assistants, registered nurses, nurse practitioners, nurse midwives, dentists, psychiatrists, psychologists, social workers, and many others.[1] Indeed, one explanation for Massachusetts having the nation's highest per capita health costs is the higher proportion of teaching hospitals and medical professionals of nearly all stripes. Given that context, it is difficult to see how the nation avoids even more daunting workforce challenges regardless of the ACA.

TITLE V—HEALTH CARE WORKFORCE

Title V is the Senate's best answer to addressing the nation's workforce challenges; the House of Representatives wrote its own workforce title, which included a number of significant initiatives, including more guaranteed funding, not included in the Senate version. These House provisions would have been included in the merged House-Senate bill that was thwarted by the Massachusetts Senate election on January 19, 2010. Nonetheless, Title V still has a lot in it and, standing alone, is the broadest health workforce law ever passed by any Congress. Still, of the fifty-three sections, only eight have direct funding. The rest must compete for scarce dollars in the appropriations process. Many promising initiatives may never take root due to lack of money. More promising, the prime mover of Title V, Senator Patty Murray (D-WA), is a senior member of the Senate Appropriations Committee and in a strategic position to advance funding for these provisions.

The Obama administration, shortly after passage of the ACA in spring 2010, opened the door for long-term funding by designating $250 million from the Prevention and Public Health Fund established in Title IV—half of the first-year funding allotment—to address workforce needs. This is on top of $500 million directed to the federal Health Resources and Services Administration in the American Recovery and Reinvestment Act of 2009 to address the nation's healthcare workforce needs. After the first year, allocation of the Prevention and Public Health Fund moves to congressional appropriators, and Congress will decide whether to continue the Obama administration's path. It may be the most feasible way to realize the promise and possibilities of Title V, though at a cost to the promise of Title IV. More new funding has been targeted for health workforce investments since 2009 than ever before. The problem is recognized, and steps are being taken to address it.

UNDERSTANDING TITLE V

Title V's purpose is to expand and upgrade the U.S. health care workforce to better meet the needs of the U.S. population, and to meet an increasing demand for services with the implementation of coverage expansions in Titles I and II. Title V has fifty-three sections included among eight subtitles.

Subtitle A: Purpose and Definitions sets out the purposes of Title V as gathering data about, increasing the supply of, enhancing the education and training of, and providing support for health care workers.

Subtitle B: Innovations in the Health Care Workforce establishes a national health care workforce commission to advise Congress. It is the major innovation in this subtitle and perhaps in the entire title.

Subtitle C: Increasing the Supply of the Health Care Workforce expands the numbers of physicians, nurses, and other professionals.

Subtitle D: Enhancing Health Care Workforce Education and Training provides training for physicians, dentists, nurses, direct care workers, and others.

Subtitle E: Supporting the Existing Health Care Workforce reauthorizes Centers of Excellence for minority applicants and expands scholarships for disadvantaged students.

Subtitle F: Strengthening Primary Care and Other Workforce Improvements focuses resources on needs of the primary care workforce.

Subtitle G: Improving Access to Health Care Services directs new resources to Federally Qualified Health Centers (FQHCs), the National Health Service Corps, and others.

Subtitle H: General Provisions requires evaluations of the programs' effectiveness to be submitted to Congress.

Following is a brief overview of key sections in Title V, including the CBO's estimated costs in brackets. A plus sign (+) means the provision costs billions (B) or millions (M), and a minus sign (−) means the provision will save federal dollars. If there is no bracketed item, the CBO estimates zero cost or savings. Also, each section includes the names of the senators (where identified) who instigated its inclusion—unlike most other title sections, nearly all the sections in Title V were generated by members.

Key Sections of Title V

Because most of the sections in Title V do not have dedicated funding attached to them, it is difficult to predict which sections will have the most impact. As a result, the number of key sections is lower than that of other titles. They include:

- National Health Care Workforce Commission: A permanent commission is established to review projected health care workforce needs and to provide comprehensive, unbiased information to Congress and the administration about how to align federal resources with national needs (Patty Murray, D-WA, and Jeff Bingaman, D-NM) (section 5101).

- Medicare Payment for Primary Care: Beginning in 2011, all primary care practitioners and general surgeons who practice in health professional shortage areas will receive a 10 percent Medicare payment bonus for five years [+$3.5B] (section 5501).

- Community Health Center Medicare Payments: The HHS secretary will implement a prospective payment system for Medicare-covered services furnished by Federally Qualified Health Centers (Blanche Lincoln, D-AR; Olympia Snowe, R-ME; and Bingaman) [+$400M] (section 5502).

- Community Health Centers and National Health Service Corps Fund: A fund is established to create an expanded and sustained national investment in community health centers and the National Health Service Corps. As amended by section 2303 of the Reconciliation Act, mandatory funding is increased for community health centers to $11 billion over five years. (Bernie Sanders, I-VT) [+$11B] (section 10503). Table 7 shows the funding schedule.

- Primary Care: Beginning in 2011, the HHS secretary will redistribute residency positions that have been unfilled for primary care physician training [+$1.1B] (sections 5503 and 5504–6). Hospitals may receive indirect medical education and direct graduate medical education funding for residents who train in nonprovider settings so that time spent in a nonprovider setting may count (section 5504). A grant program will help low-income individuals obtain education and training for health care occupations projected to experience labor shortages or high demand (Max Baucus, D-MT, and Herb Kohl, D-WI) [+$400M] (section 5507). A grant program will support primary care residency programs at teaching health centers (Jeff Bingaman) [+$200M] (section 5508). A program will increase graduate nurse education training under Medicare (Debbie Stabenow, D-MI) [+$200M] (section 5509).

TABLE 7. Funding increases for community health centers
and the National Health Service Corps, 2011–2015

Fiscal Year	Community health centers (in billions of dollars)	National Health Service Corps (in millions of dollars)
2011	1.0	290
2012	1.2	295
2013	1.5	300
2014	2.2	305
2015	3.6	310

The National Health Care Workforce Commission

In late 2008, realizing that his illness would prevent him from engaging fully in the health reform process, HELP Committee chair Edward Kennedy named other senior HELP Committee Democrats to assume coordinating roles on key health reform priorities: Barbara Mikulski on quality, Jeff Bingaman on access, Tom Harkin on prevention and public health, and Chris Dodd in an overall coordinating role. In the weeks leading up to the start of the HELP Committee's health reform markup, members huddled in Kennedy's Capitol Hill hideaway to review the proposed bill. Mikulski and other members complained that the workforce proposals lacked focus and clout. With weeks to spare, Dodd asked Washington senator Patty Murray, the Senate's fourth-ranking Democrat and a subcommittee chair on workforce issues, to take ownership of a workforce title. Murray had worked on workforce issues generally and health care workforce issues specifically; she had a global perspective on the policy terrain, including education, training, and certification issues as well as establishing pipelines to keep young people coming into the various professions.

In constructing Title V, members and staff reviewed more than a hundred health care workforce bills filed in recent years by senators from both parties, culling through each to find compelling themes and ideas. Because the HELP Committee lacks jurisdiction over Medicare—the nation's biggest funder of graduate medical education—Finance Committee staff developed Subtitle F to cover physician training, especially for primary care and general surgery, and other changes affecting residents and teaching capacity.

The centerpiece idea for Title V—establishing a National Health Care

Workforce Commission (section 5101)—was Senator Jeff Bingaman's. The model on which it is based is MedPAC, the highly respected and influential Medicare Payment Advisory Commission.[2] The purpose is to create a body to provide thorough and regular reports and recommendations to the Congress (also to the president, states, and localities) on priority needs and issues affecting the health care workforce. As with MedPAC, the U.S. comptroller general—considered an independent and nonpartisan appointing authority—names the commission members. The notion of a "vacuum" in workforce policy had confirmation beyond Senate and House members. In 2008, an Association of Academic Health Centers report concluded:

> The dysfunction in public and private health workforce policy and infrastructure is an outgrowth of decentralized decision-making in health workforce education, planning, development and policy-making; the costs and consequences of our collective failure to act effectively are accelerating due to looming socioeconomic forces that leave no time for further delay.

The association urged the creation of

> a national health workforce planning body that engages diverse federal, state, public and private stakeholders with a mission to: Articulate a national workforce agenda; Promote harmonization in public and private standards, requirements, and prevailing practices across jurisdictions; Address access to the health professions and the ability of educational institutions to respond to economic, social, and environmental factors that impact the workforce; and Identify and address unintended adverse interactions among public and private policies, standards, and requirements.[3]

With creation of the commission, whose first members were appointed in the fall of 2010, the stage is set for a new level of attention to ongoing policy development and planning for the nation's workforce needs. The commission got almost no attention in the legislative process leading to ACA, and it has the potential, assuming it receives sufficient resources to meet its mandate, to be a breakthrough panel. Unfortunately, in spite of the enthusiasm for the commission, senators left its funding subject to the vagaries of the appropriations process, jeopardizing the ability of the commission to undertake its work.

Primary Care, Community Health Centers, and the National Health Service Corps

The health care workforce shortage involves more than primary care. The Association of American Medical Colleges, for example, tracked twenty-nine studies commissioned by individual states since 2002 on physician workforce needs, finding shortages beyond primary care, particularly in allergy and immunology, cardiology, child psychiatry, dermatology, endocrinology, neurosurgery, and psychiatry, and recommends increasing U.S. medical school enrollments by 30 percent to address these needs.[4] The AAMC estimates a shortage of forty-six thousand primary care physicians by 2025, and as many as twenty-one thousand by 2015.[5] The Council on Graduate Medical Education has predicted that by 2020 the nation will have a 10 percent shortage of physicians.[6]

Though the estimates vary, it often appears to be a consensus opinion that the nation faces a serious physician shortage. It is important, then, to note dissenting voices. Dr. Fitzhugh Mullan, a professor of pediatrics at George Washington University and the former head of the Bureau of Health Professions in the U.S. Health Resources and Services Administration, concludes that the current number of U.S. physicians is not far off the right mark, but that the distribution and specialization are way off target.[7] David Goodman and Elliott Fisher, of the Dartmouth Center for Health Policy Research, argue that physician shortages reflect a broader health system dysfunction that would not be improved, and might be worsened, by increasing the numbers of physician training slots.[8] It is also noteworthy that in the ACA, Congress chose not to heed the call of the medical profession to increase the number of Medicare-funded graduate medical education positions by 15 percent, choosing instead to redistribute nine hundred unused slots for primary care and general surgery (section 5503).

All informed voices agree on the legitimacy of one part of the workforce crisis: primary care involving physicians, nurse practitioners, physician assistants, and nurses, among others. Problems training and retaining primary care physicians were not created by national health reform, and a crisis would exist with or without the ACA. Incentives embedded in medical education and future earnings, along with the growing appeal of specialization, are more at fault for this crisis than efforts to improve health insurance coverage.

Members of Congress, determined to get national health reform as right as possible, chose to pay particular attention to the primary care crisis side of the workforce issue. Title V includes primary care, community health centers, and the National Health Service Corps initiatives to address the primary care needs of the entire U.S. population—and not just those newly covered because of the health insurance expansions. Subtitle F of Title V was assembled by the Senate Finance Committee and provides direct funding of $5.6 billion over ten years to provide bonuses for primary care practitioners as well as general surgeons who practice in health professional shortage areas, to redistribute unfilled residency positions for primary care, to permit flexibility in residency training programs, and to increase teaching capacity in primary care residency programs. These steps are considered a start, not the full solution.

Of special significance is the ACA's financial commitment to community health centers and the National Health Service Corps. CHCs have a long history in the U.S. health care system, and federal support for them dates back to 1965 and the Office of Economic Opportunity, part of President Lyndon Johnson's Great Society. The medical home for an estimated twenty million Americans, or more than 5 percent of the U.S. population, they focus on the delivery of "primary medical, dental, behavioral and social services to medically underserved populations in medically underserved areas."[9] By 2010, CHCs were operating in more than eight thousand sites in every state.

Investing in CHCs has been a bipartisan project for over a decade, and they were a favorite of President George W. Bush, who agreed to a doubling of the annual appropriations in 2008 to $2.1 billion. The American Recovery and Reinvestment Act of 2009—also known as the stimulus law—directed an additional one-time $2 billion investment into CHCs. The ACA will continue this doubled investment through 2015 at least, allowing CHCs to serve as many as twenty million additional clients, with an additional $1.5 billion set aside for the construction of new centers. The ACA also doubles funding for the National Health Services Corps, "a brilliant but underfunded asset available to redistribute health professionals" to underserved areas.[10]

The new funding for CHCs and the NHSC was not easily obtained, and it occurred because of the determined advocacy of House Majority Whip James Clyburn (D-SC) and Senator Bernie Sanders (I-VT). Clyburn had obtained a $14 billion commitment in the House. Sanders had obtained a commitment in the HELP legislation, though only for a funding authorization, which would have needed to weather the uncertain appropriations process. Sanders, an avid advocate for a Medicare for All/single-payer system, had pulled back from his more expansive ambitions and agreed to support the final health reform law as long as it contained a robust public-plan option. When Majority Leader Harry Reid (D-NV) abandoned a public option in December 2009 in order to obtain the sixty Senate votes needed for final passage of the ACA, Sanders threatened to vote against the final package. At the eleventh hour, just before the release of Reid's Manager's Amendment, Senate leaders agreed to $10 billion in direct funding for

CHCs and the NHSC. In the final negotiations in March on the reconciliation bill to accompany the ACA, at Clyburn's urging, negotiators agreed to up the final CHC-NHSC number to $12.5 billion.

State governments have historically been an important part of the health care workforce puzzle, especially those with their own state medical and nursing schools. Their support has diminished over the years because of growing financial constraints. Most do not have the fiscal capacity to make major new investments in workforce development, at least not to match the capacity and potential of the federal government. Because of Title V's workforce investments, including the funding drawn from the Prevention and Public Health Trust Fund, the federal government has made a real and meaningful start to meet the workforce challenges associated with national health reform.

10. Title VI—The Stew

Most public policy experts believe that smaller bills and smaller measures can win approval more easily than larger bills and larger programs. This hypothesis fits reality much of the time, and sometimes it does not. The ACA was one of those other times. Embedded in the health reform law are many smaller initiatives that had been clamoring for attention for years, in some cases a decade or longer. No one denied the legitimacy of these issues; they just could not generate sufficient attention or controversy to get high enough in the queue, and so always got left behind.

An example is the Elder Justice Act. It will create, for the first time, a national framework to address financial, physical, and other forms of abuse against older Americans. It is a breakthrough that senators and representatives from both parties sought to advance for over a decade. The measure even passed one chamber in some years and failed to get through the other. The Elder Justice Act finally made it to the president's desk, not by itself, but as part of the ACA. Were it not for the opportunity provided by the health reform process, the Elder Justice Act—and similar measures embedded in the ACA—would still be waiting for their moment, many for a long, long time.

TITLE VI—TRANSPARENCY AND PROGRAM INTEGRITY

Title VI is a little-noticed ACA title with a lot in it, and nearly all of it was distinctly bipartisan. Two subtitles launch an aggressive effort to deter fraud and abuse in federal health programs. Elsewhere, there is a far-reaching transparency provision to discourage inappropriate marketing influence on physicians and hospitals. There is a new national program to compare the clinical effectiveness of medical treatments—a controversial provision parked in Title VI to avoid attention. There are new protections and disclosure standards for nursing home residents. There is an initiative to address medical-liability reform. It's a stew, a potpourri of provisions that fit together loosely if at all. Their importance should not be underestimated. After reviewing the structure and key sections of Title VI, we will explore in detail five significant components: fraud and abuse, the Physician Payments Sunshine Act, comparative effectiveness research, the Elder Justice Act, and medical-liability reform.

UNDERSTANDING TITLE VI

These are the major elements of Title VI. It has fifty sections included within nine subtitles. The first two sections include the names of the senators who instigated its inclusion.

Subtitle A limits participation in Medicare by physician-owned hospitals; requires manufacturers of drugs, medical devices, biologics, and medical supplies to report publicly nearly all gifts and other transfers of value to physicians and hospitals (Herb Kohl, D-WI, and Charles Grassley, R-IA).

Subtitle B requires new forms of public reporting by skilled nursing facilities, establishes new compliance and ethics programs, and makes new quality information available on the Internet (Grassley-Kohl).

Subtitle C establishes a nationwide program of background checks on direct care workers.

Subtitle D creates a public-private Patient-Centered Outcomes Research Institute to generate comparative clinical outcomes research.

Subtitle E sets new requirements on providers and suppliers in federal health programs to deter fraud and abuse.

Subtitle F places new responsibilities on states to police their Medicaid programs to deter fraud and abuse.

Subtitle G sets new powers for the U.S. Department of Labor and state governments to deter fraudulent multiple employer welfare arrangements.

Subtitle H seeks to prevent and eliminate elder abuse, neglect, and exploitation.

Subtitle I expresses the view of the Senate regarding medical malpractice and medical-liability insurance reform and establishes state demonstrations to evaluate alternatives to tort litigation.

Key Sections of Title VI

Unlike the previous titles, Title VI makes it difficult to pull out discrete sections as most important or significant. In Title VI, the subtitles themselves are more coherent, thematic, and distinct than in other ACA titles. Following is a brief overview of key sections, including CBO estimated costs in brackets. A plus sign (+) means the provision costs billions (B) or millions (M), and a minus sign (–) means the provision will save federal dollars. If there is no bracketed item, the CBO estimates zero cost or savings.

Subtitle A: Physician Ownership and Other Transparency addresses physician-owned hospitals and requires public disclosure of financial arrangements involving health providers.

- Physician-owned hospitals without a provider agreement prior to December 31, 2010, may not participate in Medicare. Hospitals with a prior agreement may participate under new rules regarding conflicts, investments, patient safety, and expansions [–$500M] (section 6001).

- The Physician Payments Sunshine Act. Drug, device, and biological and medical supply manufacturers must report transfers of value to physicians, medical practices, physician group practices, and teaching hospitals. Duplicative state and local laws are preempted, though not in the case of state or local laws beyond the section's scope (section 6002).

Subtitle B: Nursing Home Transparency and Improvement makes available to the public new information on ownership and quality indicators.

- Nursing home transparency: Skilled nursing facilities (SNFs) under Medicare and nursing facilities (NFs) under Medicaid must provide information on ownership upon request by the secretary, the HHS inspector general, states, and state long-term care ombudsmen (section 6101). SNFs and NFs must implement a compliance and ethics program for the facility's employees and its agents within thirty-six months (section 6102). The HHS secretary will publish standardized staffing data, links to state websites regarding survey and certification programs, a model complaint form, a summary of substantiated complaints, and the number of instances of criminal violations by a facility or its employees (section 6103). The HHS secretary will require facilities to report staffing information uniformly, taking into account services provided by agency or contract staff (section 6106).

- Nursing home enforcement and improvement: The HHS secretary will establish a national independent monitoring program to oversee interstate and large intrastate chains (section 6112). The administrator of a facility preparing to close must provide written notice to residents, their legal representatives, the state, the secretary, and the Long-Term Care Ombudsman program at least sixty days in advance. Facilities must prepare a closing plan for the state, which must approve it and ensure the safe transfer of residents (section 6113). Facilities must include dementia management and abuse prevention training in pre-employment training for staff, and if the secretary determines, for ongoing in-service training (section 6121).

Subtitle C: Nationwide Program for National and State Background Checks on Direct Patient Access Employees of Long Term Care Facilities and Providers establishes a national program for federal and state background checks on direct patient access employees of long-term supports and services facilities and providers [+$100 M] (section 6201).

Subtitle D: Patient-Centered Outcomes Research sets up a public-private Patient-Centered Outcomes Research Institute to generate comparative clinical outcomes research. The institute will be governed by a public-private sector board appointed by the comptroller general to identify priorities and provide for the conduct of comparative outcomes research. The institute will ensure that patient subpopulations are accounted for in research designs. Findings that may be construed as mandates on practice guidelines or coverage decisions are prohibited, and patient safeguards will protect against discriminatory coverage decisions based on age, disability, terminal illness, or an individual's quality-of-life preference. Funding is authorized [Medicare: −$300 M; Non-Medicare: +$2.5 B] (section 6301).

Subtitle E: Medicare, Medicaid, and CHIP Program Integrity Provisions sets new measures to combat fraud, waste, and abuse in federal health programs.

- The secretary will establish procedures to screen providers and suppliers participating in Medicare, Medicaid, and CHIP prioritized according to the risk of fraud, waste, and abuse for each provider or supplier category. All providers and suppliers will be subject to licensure checks. The secretary may impose additional screening. Providers and suppliers enrolling or reenrolling in Medicare, Medicaid, or CHIP will be subject to new disclosure requirements [−$100 M] (section 6401).

· Enhanced Medicare and Medicaid program integrity provisions [−$2.9 B] (section 6402).

> Data banks at the Centers for Medicare and Medicaid Services will include claims and payment data from Medicare, Medicaid, CHIP, health programs of the Social Security Administration, Departments of Veterans Affairs and Defense, and the Indian Health Service. The HHS secretary will create data-sharing agreements with the commissioner of Social Security, the secretaries of the VA and DOD, and the director of the IHS to identity fraud, waste, and abuse.

> The HHS secretary will require that all Medicare, Medicaid, and CHIP providers include their National Provider Identifier numbers on enrollment applications. The secretary will withhold federal matching payments from states when the state does not report enrollee encounter data promptly.

> Providers and suppliers will be excluded for providing false information on any application to enroll or participate in a federal health care program. The use of civil monetary penalties is expanded to individuals who make false statements on applications or contracts to participate in a federal health care program, or who know of an overpayment and do not return the overpayment.

> The HHS secretary may issue subpoenas and require the attendance and testimony of witnesses and the production of evidence in matters under investigation or in question by the secretary. The HHS secretary shall consider the volume of billing for a durable medical equipment supplier or home health agency when determining the size of the surety bond. The HHS secretary may suspend payments to a provider or supplier pending a fraud investigation.

> Funding for the Health Care Fraud and Abuse Control is increased by $350 million over the next decade.

· The HHS secretary will maintain a national health care fraud and abuse data collection program to report adverse actions against providers, suppliers, and practitioners and submit information to the National Practitioner Data Bank (section 6403).

· Durable medical equipment or home health services must be ordered by a Medicare-eligible professional or physician enrolled in Medicare [–$400 M] (section 6405).

· The HHS secretary may disenroll, for no more than one year, a Medicare-enrolled physician or supplier failing to maintain and provide access to written orders or requests for payment for DME, certification for home health services, or other referrals (section 6406).

· Physicians must have a face-to-face encounter with an individual prior to issuing a certification for home health services or DME [–$1 B] (section 6407).

· Persons who fail to grant HHS timely access to documents for audits, investigations, or evaluations may be subject to penalties of $15,000 for each day. Persons who knowingly make, use, or cause to be made or used any false statement to a federal health care program will be subject to a penalty of $50,000 for each violation (section 6408).

· HHS will expand the number of areas in the DME competitive bidding program from seventy-nine to one hundred of the largest metropolitan statistical areas, and to use competitively bid prices in all areas by 2016 [–$1.4 B] (section 6410).

Subtitle F: Additional Medicaid Program Integrity Provisions addresses fraud, waste, and abuse issues involving the federal government and state Medicaid programs.

· States must terminate individuals or entities from their Medicaid programs if they were terminated from Medicare or another state's Medicaid program (section 6501). Medicaid agencies must exclude individuals or entities from participation for a period of time if the entity or individual owns, controls, or manages an entity that (1) has failed to repay overpayments; (2) is suspended, excluded, or terminated from participation in any state Medicaid program; or (3) is affiliated with an individual or entity that has been suspended, excluded, or terminated from Medicaid participation (section 6502).

· Any agents, clearinghouses, or other payees that submit claims on behalf of providers must register with the state and the HHS secretary (section 6503). States may not pay for items or services provided under a Medicaid State plan or waiver to any financial institution or entity located outside of the U.S. (section 6505).

· States will have up to one year to repay overpayments when a final determination of the amount of the overpayment has not been determined due to an ongoing judicial or administrative process [+$100 M] (section 6506). States must make their Medicaid Management Information System methodologies compatible with Medicare's national correct coding initiative [-$300 M] (6507). States must implement new fraud, waste, and abuse programs before January 1, 2011 (section 6508).

Subtitle G: Additional Program Integrity Provisions addresses fraud and abuse issues in private health plans known as multiple employer welfare arrangements. MEWA employees and agents will be subject to criminal penalties if they provide false statements in marketing materials regarding a plan's financial solvency, benefits, or regulatory status (section 6601). A model uniform reporting form will be developed by the National Association of Insurance Commissioners (section 6603). The Department of Labor may issue summary cease-and-desist orders and summary seizure orders against plans in financially hazardous condition (section 6605).

Subtitle H: Elder Justice Act creates a national initiative to prevent and eliminate elder abuse, neglect, and exploitation. The HHS secretary will establish an Elder Justice Coordinating Council and Advisory Board to combat elder abuse, neglect, and exploitation. The secretary will make grants to operate mobile and stationary forensic centers regarding elder abuse, neglect, and exploitation. The secretary will award grants to protect individuals seeking care in long-term care facilities and provide incentives for individuals to seek employment at such facilities; owners, operators, and some employees will be required to report suspected crimes committed at the facility. The HHS secretary will establish an adult protective services grant program to enhance services by state and local governments. The secretary will make grants to improve and provide training for Long-Term Care Ombudsman programs. The secretary will help to establish a national training institute for federal and state surveyors of long-term care facilities (section 6703).

Subtitle I: Medical Malpractice conveys the sense of the Senate that health reform presents an opportunity to address issues related to medical malpractice and medical-liability insurance. States should be encouraged to develop and test alternative models to the existing civil litigation system, and Congress should consider state demonstration projects to evaluate such alternatives (section 6801). A State Demonstration Program to Evaluate Alternatives to Current Medical Tort Litigation is established. Grants will be available for up to five years to states to test alternatives to civil tort litigation. These models must emphasize patient safety, disclosure of health care errors, and early dispute resolution. Patients must be able to opt out of these alternatives (section 10607, added in Manager's Amendment, Title X).

FRAUD AND ABUSE

No one knows the true dollar cost of fraud and abuse in the U.S. health care system. The National Health Care Anti-Fraud Association estimates that at least 3 percent of all health care spending—public and private—is lost to fraud.[1] In the 1990s, the FBI made a back-of-the-envelope estimate that 10 percent of all federal health spending is lost to fraud and abuse—and that number has assumed biblical-truth status over the years. No one knows for sure, and the actual number could be higher or lower. What is known is that there is a large amount of fraud and abuse in public and private health care, and that "wherever we look, we find more," according to Peter Budetti, the chief fraud control officer at the HHS Centers for Medicare and Medicaid Services.[2] Common types of fraud include billing for services never rendered, billing for more expensive services than those provided, performing unnecessary services to obtain insurance payments, falsifying a patient's diagnosis to justify tests and procedures, billing each step of a procedure as if it were separate, accepting kickbacks for patient referrals, and more.

As Malcolm Sparrow, a health care fraud expert at Harvard University, documents, health care fraud is big business. In 1997, the *New York Times* reported that local mafia families were dropping traditional criminal enterprises to participate in the less risky business of health insurance fraud. In 2003, America's largest hospital chain, Columbia-HCA, paid $1.7 billion to settle fraud and abuse charges by the U.S. Department of Justice. In 2008, a Miami couple, Abner and Mabel Diaz, pleaded guilty to submitting $420 million in false medical equipment claims to Medicare.[3] In 2009, drug giant Eli Lilly pleaded guilty and paid $1.4 billion for illegally promoting the use of its drug, Zyprexa, for uses not approved by the Food and Drug Administration.[4] While some larger urban areas—for example, Detroit, Houston, Los Angeles, Miami, and New York City—appear to have disproportionate levels of fraud, there is evidence of the problem across the nation. In 2008, the federal government opened 1,750 new health care fraud investigations.[5]

It's not that no one is paying attention. In the 1996 Health Insurance Portability and Accountability Act (HIPAA), Congress established the Health Care Fraud and Abuse Control (HCFAC) program to address Medicare fraud and abuse. In 2005, Congress set up the Medicaid Integrity Program to match HCFAC's focus on Medicare. These efforts have results to brag about. According to data from the Office of Inspector General, savings from Medicare and Medicaid oversight averaged $2.04 billion and $1.22 billion each year between 2006 and 2008, for a return on investment of $17 for each dollar spent.[6] To Sparrow, a seventeen-to-one return is a bad sign, indicating that existing fraud efforts are only skimming the surface of the total amount of fraud being committed: "picking off the simple stuff with almost no effort."[7]

An entire bureaucracy is devoted to combating fraud and abuse in federal health programs and includes the Department of Justice and the Office of Inspector General within the Department of Health and Human Services. Efforts to combat fraud and abuse expanded significantly during the Clinton administration as a result of HIPAA, provoking a backlash from physicians, hospitals, and others who complained of overly aggressive antifraud activities aimed at Medicare providers. During the eight years of the Bush administration, attention waned, and requests for additional antifraud funding were not heeded by Congress. The Obama administration has again raised the profile of antifraud activities with the creation in May 2009 of a Health Care Fraud Prevention and Enforcement Action Team (HEAT), committed to making Medicare fraud a cabinet-level priority for both the DOJ and HHS.[8]

Revamping and stepping up antifraud activities as part of health reform legislation got its first public nod in Senate Finance chair Max Baucus's white paper released in November 2008: "The Baucus plan, which includes ideas articulated by HHS OIG, would focus on preventing fraud, waste, and abuse before they happen, and aggressively detecting them when prevention fails."[9] Baucus's ranking member, Charles Grassley of Iowa, has a reputation as one of the most committed and aggressive fraud fighters in the Congress. President Obama, on numerous occasions, cited stepped-up antifraud activities as a priority for health reform legislation. Indeed, it is difficult to find anyone in Washington DC who is not a cheerleader—at least rhetorically—for attacking fraud and abuse in Medicare and Medicaid . . .

. . . Except, perhaps, the nonpartisan scorekeepers at the Congressional Budget Office. In its "Budget Options" volume released in December 2008,

it concluded: "Boosting funding for program integrity under HCFAC probably offers diminishing returns, and increased investment in combating
waste, fraud, and abuse is unlikely to significantly slow overall growth in
spending for Medicare and Medicaid."[10] In its final ACA score for Title VI,
the CBO estimates that the key fraud and abuse Subtitles E and F will
generate a less-than-impressive net savings of $6.5 billion over ten years.
Part of this modest projection can be tied to the CBO's congressionally
mandated "scorekeeping guidelines" that prevent it from counting changes
from "administrative or program management activities," which include
fraud and abuse.

If any place in the ACA presents an opportunity to outperform CBO
estimates, the twenty new fraud and abuse sections may be leading candidates. Most of the reforms in Subtitles E and F were recommended by
the professional fraud fighters at the Centers for Medicare and Medicaid
Services, the HHS Office of Inspector General, and the Department of
Justice. Of particular promise to them is section 6401, which gives the
executive branch significant new powers to keep fraudulent parties out
of the Medicare program and to keep them from renewing their participation. Creating better alignment between Medicare and Medicaid is
another approach required in several sections. Also, the final reconciliation
law provided $250 million in new funding for antifraud activities between
2011 and 2016. In a June 2010 House hearing, Kimberly Brandt, director of
the CMS program integrity group, told lawmakers that the new authority
will help the agency to move away from its current "pay and chase" model
to one based on fraud prevention.[11]

Also, there is an assumption by many in Washington DC that most
fraud and abuse is perpetrated against public health programs, not against
private insurers, and that the private health insurance sector is effective in
guarding against fraud. It is true that all private insurers have their own
antifraud programs. Yet national antifraud groups such as the Coalition
against Insurance Fraud and the National Insurance Crime Bureau dispute
this view, suggesting that fraudulent actors target and steal from any and
all sources, including the private sector. One private sector source of fraud
involves corrupt multiple employer welfare arrangements, which provide
insurance to networks of small employers and which have been poorly
policed by the U.S. Department of Labor. In response to documented fraud,
Subtitle G provides new tools for DOL and state insurance departments to
protect consumers.

All experts concur that fraudulent operators are resourceful and adap-
tive. The tools that work today will be less effective in future years as

criminal enterprises change their operations to thwart new methods of discovery and to exploit newly discovered vulnerabilities. Fraud and abuse will always, it seems, be a part of health coverage programs. The ACA presents a new opportunity to do a much better job of resistance and in the process to support the cost of health reform implementation.

THE PHYSICIAN PAYMENTS SUNSHINE ACT

A sly definition of the word *culture* calls it "the way we do things around here," adding, "wherever *here* may be." The definition fits like a glove, whatever one might place before the word—Capitol Hill culture, New Orleans culture, South African culture, Red Sox Nation culture, gay and lesbian culture, on and on. The definition suggests why one of the hardest things to do in life is to change culture because it's the way people are used to doing things around there, wherever "there" may be.

In the American health care system are innumerable cultures, in each hospital or clinic (and part thereof), in each specialty, in each regulatory arena, and on and on. One significant part of the U.S. medical culture for many years has been the provision of gifts and financial benefits, often substantial, to more than 90 percent of U.S. physicians by pharmaceutical companies, medical-device makers, and other well-resourced interests in the form of speaking fees, honoraria, consulting fees, dinners, lunches, trips, tchotchkes (trinkets such as pens, squeeze balls, key rings), and much more, large and small.

Even the small transactions create worries because of the documented influence of such gifts in influencing physician-prescribing behavior toward the products of the benefactor, often in ways unnoticed by the recipient. Large transactions have drawn the attention of some senators and representatives who see a corrupting influence on scientific research leading to false or misleading information about the benefits of various drugs, devices, and more. Senator Charles Grassley (R-IA), the Congress's most dogged critic on this matter, lists by name on his U.S. Senate website one dozen physician researchers whose industry ties have raised concerns and criticism—with multiple news links for each.[12] Grassley and Senator Herb Kohl (D-WI), chair of the Senate Aging Committee, teamed up in 2007 to sponsor the Physician Payments Sunshine Act to require the public disclosure of payments by industry groups to physicians and hospitals. They were preceded in their interest by Representative Peter DeFazio (D-OR), who filed the first Sunshine Act in 2002 in the House, as well as Representative Pete Stark (D-CA), chair of the Ways and Means Subcommittee on Health, a longtime critic of financial conflicts involving physicians, and Commerce and Energy chair Henry Waxman (D-CA). Members in both chambers saw health reform as an opportunity to make progress in advancing the Sunshine Act.

Outside Congress, the Pew Charitable Trusts launched a national Prescription Project in 2006 to clamp down on medical-industry practices of questionable ethics and potential harm to consumers. Their national coalition eventually included nearly fifty national patient and consumer groups, hospital organizations, and professional medical associations. Their strategy focused not only on Washington DC but also on states that might move on their own absent federal action. Minnesota and Vermont had passed laws earlier in the decade, but beginning in 2008, a new set of states joined in, including Massachusetts, which passed extensive disclosure requirements that year; Maine, West Virginia, and the District of Columbia were among the other governments lining up to follow suit, with similar legislation filed in more than a dozen states.

In a dynamic similar to the Title IV requirement that chain restaurants must post the calorie content of food on their menu boards, the new transparency requirements passed by states presented the industry groups with the specter of a plethora of reporting requirements and compelled them to weigh the challenges of a growing state-by-state patchwork versus a consistent federal standard that would preempt state laws. Uniformity won out, and in 2008 leading health industry groups, including the Pharmaceutical Research and Manufacturers of America, AdvaMed (representing the medical-device industry), and leading drug companies such as Eli Lilly, endorsed the Physician Payments Sunshine Act. Preemption of state laws was included, but only for requirements that mirrored the federal standard—states could still adopt requirements in areas not addressed in the Sunshine Act. More than uniformity and preemption drove industry support, however—over the course of five years, numerous journalists had exposed unsavory and exorbitant financial relationships between leading physician researchers and industry. The drumbeat of exposés required an industry response, and several companies began their own disclosure initiatives before any legislation was enacted as a result of legal settlements.

The new law, included in Subtitle A of Title VI, requires all U.S. manufacturers of drugs, medical devices, biologics, and medical supplies covered under Medicare, Medicaid, or CHIP to report payments annually to the Department of Health and Human Services, which will post the information on a public website. The law requires the disclosure of payments to physicians and teaching hospitals, whether cash or in-kind, including compensation, food, entertainment, gifts, consulting fees, honoraria, research funding or grants, education or conference funding, stocks or stock options, ownership or investment interest, royalties or licenses, charitable contributions, and any other transfer of value. Payments of less than $10 are exempt unless the aggregate amount per company and per recipient reaches $100, at which point all must be disclosed. Exempted are educational materials for the benefit of patients, rebates and discounts, loans of covered devices, items provided under warranty, dividend or interest payments in a publicly traded security, and payments to a physician who is a patient or an employee of the reporting company.

Companies must start recording transactions on January 1, 2012, and begin reporting to HHS by March 31, 2013, for information that will first be available on the Web no later than September 30, 2013. Each failure to report can bring a fine of up to $10,000, not to exceed $150,000 annually. An organization or manufacturer that knowingly fails to submit the required information can draw a penalty as high as $1 million.

How will these requirements change American medicine and health care? The culture of physician-industry relationships was already changing before the passage of ACA and the Physician Payments Sunshine Act. Vermont, with one of the oldest reporting laws in the nation, reports substantial drops in the aggregate number of financial dealings with each new annual report. Across the nation, medical schools and academic medical centers are taking the initiative themselves to discourage the culture of gifts. The ACA takes this trend to a new level, accelerating the pace and scope of change.

PATIENT-CENTERED OUTCOMES RESEARCH

Around 2004, medical-device makers such as General Electric, Philips Electronics, Siemens, and Toshiba introduced a new generation of CT scanners for hospitals and physician's offices. These offered a faster and clearer way to look inside patients' arteries, enabling physicians to identify blocked arteries in need of stents or other treatments. The machines sell for about $1 million apiece and can be financed easily with billings between $500 and $1,500 per patient. The device, according to experts, also exposes patients to potentially dangerous levels of radiation and can be used to justify unnecessary medical treatments that also enhance physician pay (imaging fees now account for half or more of the average U.S. cardiologist's $400,000 annual income). In 2007, when the HHS Centers for Medicare and Medicaid Services demanded scientific evaluation of the technology before continuing to pay for it, the Society of Cardiovascular Computed Tomography went to work. Its lobbying of Congress persuaded CMS to back down and to continue paying for the procedure without evidence of safety or effectiveness. "Once the train leaves the station, once the technology gets on the marketplace, we don't get the evidence," concludes Dr. Rita Redberg, a cardiologist and researcher at the University of California, San Francisco. "We're spending a lot of money on technology of unclear benefit and risk."[13]

Making clinical decisions without clear evidence of benefits and risks has always been a reality of medicine worldwide. Some refer to 1912 as the "great divide" in the history of medicine. Harvard professor Lawrence Henderson commented, "For the first time in human history, a random patient with a random disease consulting a doctor chosen at random stands a better than 50/50 chance of benefitting from the encounter."[14]

Over the course of the twentieth century and around the globe, a slow though growing number of physicians, other researchers, and organizations began to apply scientific rigor to the study of health care delivery and services to improve the odds further and to develop a field known as health services research. Beginning in the 1970s, a branch of this field began to focus on comparing the effectiveness of services, treatments, and therapies beyond the traditional one-at-a-time approach. The most celebrated pioneer of this approach was a British epidemiologist, Archie Cochrane. The Cochrane Collaboration,[15] established and named after his death, encompasses twenty-seven thousand volunteer researchers from more than ninety nations. It is now the world's leading organization in preparing, maintaining, and ensuring the accessibility of systematic reviews of the effects of health care interventions.[16] Comparative effectiveness research (CER), the most common name for the field, is now a worldwide and burgeoning collaborative enterprise.

Other nations, notably Australia, Canada, Germany, and Great Britain, have established centralized structures and processes of their own to perform comparative clinical and economic assessments of health services. Interest in this endeavor has also grown in the United States, spurred in the late 1990s by exploding prices for pharmaceutical products and by state governments interested in using systematic reviews to compare the quality and price of competing prescription drugs. The Drug Effectiveness Review Project (DERP) at the Oregon Health and Sciences University spearheaded a rigorous and respected comparative effectiveness research program to inform policy makers; even consumers got access through the *Consumer Reports Best Buy* drug program, informed by DERP evidence.[17]

U.S. interest in a new, federally led CER effort grew in the first decade of the new century as burgeoning health costs reemerged as a national concern and as reports of the politicization of difficult and expensive coverage decisions grabbed media attention. For example, a controversy in 2003 about whether Medicare should cover an aggressive and expensive lung operation for patients with emphysema grabbed the attention of U.S. Senate Finance Committee staffer Shawn Bishop, who perceived weaknesses in the government's ability to make sound judgments on these difficult controversies.[18] A former high-level federal health official in the George H.W. Bush administration, Gail Wilensky, began writing about how an effective CER program could be developed:

> There is widespread agreement on the attributes that need to be associated with a comparative effectiveness center: objectivity in the selection of what is studied, credibility in the findings, and independence—from political pressures generated either by government or by private-sector stakeholders. How best to achieve this set of outcomes, not surprisingly, differs in the eyes of different beholders.[19]

Support for a U.S. CER enterprise was broad, including business, labor, consumer, and insurance interests. Even Republican thought-leader Newt Gingrich, former U.S. House Speaker, was a fan, cowriting an October 24, 2008, *New York Times* op-ed with Senator John Kerry to endorse the effort:

> Working closely with doctors, the federal government and the private sector should create a new institute for evidence-based medicine. This institute would conduct new studies and systematically review the existing medical literature to help inform our nation's over-stretched medical providers.[20]

Support was not unanimous. Pharmaceutical and medical-device interests wanted CER to focus solely on clinical issues and not at all on cost-effectiveness, and resisted any use of so-called quality-adjusted life year (QALY) indices that measure the value of therapies and devices according to expected life years. Right to Life and other conservative groups shared an antipathy to QALYs and feared a backdoor approach to health care rationing. Some patient and disease advocacy groups worried that the CER approach might discourage the development of therapies for "orphan" diseases affecting smaller populations.

The House of Representatives made the first move in 2007 during the reauthorization debate over the Children's Health Insurance Program (CHIP), proposing the creation of a Center for Comparative Effectiveness

Research to be based within the existing Agency for Healthcare Research and Quality within DHHS.[21] In 2008, Senate Finance chair Max Baucus (D-MT) teamed up with Budget Committee chair and Finance Committee member Kent Conrad (D-ND) to introduce legislation to establish a national CER program, after several years of preparation. Their approach aimed to assuage critics by setting up a CER institute outside the federal government with public financial support. The Senate HELP Committee also supported a robust CER program and favored the House approach, which relied on an existing federal entity to protect against inappropriate stakeholder influence on research.

The first big break for CER came in February 2009 with passage of the American Recovery and Reinvestment Act. Otherwise known as the stimulus bill, ARRA appropriated $1.1 billion for immediate investments in CER, allocating $300 million to the Agency for Healthcare Research and Quality (AHRQ), $400 million to the National Institutes of Health (NIH), and $400 million to the HHS secretary, and further established a Federal Coordinating Council for Comparative Effectiveness Research.[22] The work was not finished, though, because ARRA included only short-term measures; the broader health reform legislation would be needed as a vehicle to establish a permanent federal CER initiative.

The ARRA provisions jump-started not just a new federal CER process but also the first round of open public criticism. During the 2008 presidential campaign, candidates Obama and McCain publicly supported establishing some capacity for CER within the federal government. Around the time of Obama's inauguration and the passage of ARRA, the tone of the discussion began to change. Drug, medical-device, and biotechnology companies financed and formed the Partnership to Improve Patient Care, along with medical-professional societies and industry-supported patient advocacy groups to lobby to fashion the CER initiative according to industry preferences.[23] Betsy McCaughey, a fellow at the conservative Hudson Institute, former New York lieutenant governor, and the author of a flawed and widely criticized critique of the Clinton health plan in 1994,[24] falsely charged in a widely disseminated Bloomberg commentary: "Medicare now pays for treatments deemed safe and effective. The stimulus bill would change that and apply a cost-effectiveness standard set by the Federal Council (464)."[25] The CER attacks became contagious, and the Federal Coordinating Council became exhibit A for charges that health reform would impose systemwide health care rationing with the power to decide whether patients would live or die.

The CER attacks merged with assaults on provisions in the Senate HELP and House health reform bills that would reimburse physicians through Medicare to counsel patients on end-of-life issues such as living wills, powers of attorney, and end-of-life treatment preferences. Advanced in the Senate by Johnny Isakson (R-GA) and in the House by Earl Blumenauer (D-OR), the provisions provoked charges of euthanasia, rationing, and death panels among Republicans and the new conservative populist tea party movement, which had begun focusing its anger on health reform. The House measure, it was suggested by Republicans, would "put seniors in a position of being put to death by their government."[26]

Within the Senate Finance Committee's Gang of Six, attempting to negotiate a bipartisan deal during the heated summer of 2009, Democrats Baucus, Conrad, and Bingaman were joined by Olympia Snowe (R-ME) in support of CER, while Mike Enzi (R-WY) expressed reservations. Baucus had hopes that his Republican ranking member and frequent policy partner, Charles Grassley, would support CER. But in one CER discussion that summer, Grassley turned to his staffer to say: "This is going to pull the plug on grandma." In August, he repeated the charge in a town meeting in his home state of Iowa: "We should not have a government program that determines if you're going to pull the plug on grandma," he noted, combining thoughts on CER and end-of-life counseling.[27]

Despite the uproar, CER provisions remained in the legislation approved in the House of Representatives in November 2009, setting up the program within AHRQ. CER provisions also stayed in the HELP and Senate Finance legislation approved by both committees, and Senate Majority Leader Harry Reid (D-NV) kept the provision in the merged legislation he released in November, though Reid chose the Senate Finance formulation of a new, quasi-government entity to do the work. Publicly aired charges that the Senate version would cede "substantial influence to the medical products industries"[28] helped persuade Senate staffers to rewrite the legislation to lessen industry influence in setting the agenda. The term *comparative effectiveness research* was abandoned in favor of *patient-centered outcomes research*. Even the location of the provision within the ACA showed the sensitivity. Rather than locating the provision in Title III, which deals with delivery-system reform, staffers relocated it to Subtitle D of Title VI, where, they hoped, it would draw less attention.

Section 6301 refers to "comparative clinical effectiveness research" and, significantly, is silent on including cost-effectiveness within the scope of study. While the language states that "nothing in this Act shall be construed to permit the Institute to mandate coverage, reimbursement, or other policies for any public or private payer," it also does not bar CMS or any other public or private payer from using CER research to inform its own coverage decisions.[29] The program will be funded by $1 or $2 assessments on covered lives in most public and private health insurance plans, including Medicare.

CER is coming to town.

ELDER JUSTICE AND NURSING HOME TRANSPARENCY AND IMPROVEMENT

Three subtitles in Title VI address non-Medicare issues affecting older Americans. Each was a product of years of effort by members, staff, and interest and advocacy groups across the nation. Each is regarded by knowledgeable participants as landmark reform. None has received any particular attention in the torrent of publicity surrounding the ACA beyond their immediate communities of interest. Subtitle H, the most significant of the three, is called the Elder Justice Act; Subtitle B addresses nursing home transparency and improvement; and Subtitle C establishes a nationwide program for background checks on employees of nursing homes and other long-term care facilities who have direct access to patients.

Elder Justice

Between one and two million Americans over age sixty-five are estimated to have been injured, exploited, or otherwise mistreated each year by someone on whom they depend for care or protection, according to the National Center on Elder Abuse.[30] Between five and six hundred thousand cases of elder abuse are reported annually through state and local Long-Term Care Ombudsman programs, and experts estimate four times as many cases go unreported. A 2009 study estimates the annual financial loss to elderly victims of financial abuse at $2.6 billion per year.[31]

Advocates assert that media attention to elder abuse is erratic compared with coverage of abuse to children and women, though some cases have drawn a public spotlight. In October 2009, as the House and Senate were gearing up for floor action on their respective health reform laws, the son of Brooke Astor, philanthropist and matriarch of New York society who died in 2007 at age 105, was convicted on charges of defrauding his mother and stealing tens of millions of dollars from her as she suffered from Alzheimer's disease.[32] Another public case emerged in the spring of 2009 in Harry Reid's home state of Nevada, where a husband and wife were charged with duping and bilking elderly men out of tens of thousands of dollars.[33]

The Elder Justice Act, included in the ACA as Subtitle H of Title VI, is the result of more than ten years of work by a bipartisan group including former Democratic senators John Breaux of Louisiana, Bob Graham of Florida, and Blanche Lincoln of Arkansas, and current senators Orrin Hatch (R-UT), Herb Kohl (D-WI), and Charles Grassley (R-IA). In the House, the key supporter in recent years was Rahm Emanuel, who resigned his congressional seat in December 2008 to become Obama's first chief of staff; Emanuel helped keep the Obama administration involved in the provision, in contrast with the prior Bush administration, which called the act unnecessary. After his departure, key House voices were Peter King (R-NY), Tammy Baldwin (D-WI), and Jan Schakowsky (D-IL).

Outside Congress, a national network known as the Elder Justice Coalition provided public support. To the coalition, the act represents the largest federal commitment ever to fighting elder abuse. The funding commitment is $777 million over four years with more than $400 million of that directed to Adult Protective Services. Funding for new forensic investigation centers, ombudsman training, complaint-investigation systems, and a National Training Institute for Surveyors for the first time holds the prospect for a genuinely national system. Though all funding is subject to the uncertainties of the appropriations process, advocates believe they have finally emerged from the policy wilderness, and the act sets a valuable foundation upon which they can build in years to come.

Nursing Home Transparency and Background Checks

Subtitles B and C are also viewed as welcome signs of progress by the nursing home advocacy community. The last major nursing home reform law was passed in 1987 as part of that year's Omnibus Budget Reconciliation Act (OBRA 87). The Senate Aging Committee held public hearings in 2007 to consider the accomplishments and limitations of OBRA 87 twenty years later. Aging Committee chair Herb Kohl and Senator Grassley worked collaboratively to move the reform discussion. The progress made by the Subtitle B amendments may appear mundane to laypersons, but they do not appear so to those close to the field.

- On the enforcement of standards, civil monetary penalties have proven ineffective because nursing home owners appeal and delay payments for lengthy periods, often getting fines reduced by administrative law judges. Subtitle B allows the Centers for Medicare and Medicaid Services to collect fines up front, placing them in escrow, with an expedited appeals process. Homes cited for quality violations will have to pay, and for the first time, pay right away.

- Some radical new ideas and models are being introduced in nursing homes and nursing home care. These include homes that have downsized and reconfigured themselves to resemble real homes where the administrators actually know residents by name, in a process called culture change. Subtitle B will support more of these demonstrations.

- Most nursing homes these days are owned by for-profit chains that have split themselves into numerous suboperations, separating the real estate from the overall business and carving the operations into various limited liability corporations where accountability and responsibility are split in many directions, often leaving regulators, residents, and relatives at a loss to know who is in charge. As a result of changes in Subtitle B, all contractual relationships must be disclosed to federal and state regulators, and to nursing home ombudsmen.

- Since 1987 nursing homes have been required to report their staff-to-resident ratios but were required to show data only for the two weeks before inspectors show up. Under Subtitle B, they will have to report staffing data quarterly, based on payroll data, and the data will be made available to the public on the federal Nursing Home Compare website.

Subtitle C establishes a new nationwide program for national and state background checks on employees of long-term care facilities and providers who have direct patient access. In the 2003 Medicare Modernization Act, Congress set up a pilot program giving grants to seven states to clean up their background-check systems. State systems have been plagued by lack of consistency and coordination, with different registries for sex offenders, child care workers, and others that were not connected with each other, even within the same state, or with the Federal Bureau of Investigation. The seven pilot states demonstrated the feasibility of cleaning up and connecting the systems, and Subtitle C provides funding for all states to implement this new system.

Congressional staffers involved with these issues all agree that these issues might never have achieved sufficient attention to move forward as stand-alone legislation. The ACA provided the opportunity to advance these reforms and trigger meaningful systemic improvements.

MEDICAL-LIABILITY REFORM

In 2006, before they were president and secretary of state, and before they were Democratic presidential nomination rivals, Barack Obama and Hillary Clinton were the coauthors of an article in the *New England Journal of Medicine* on medical-liability reform. It was a joint effort to carve an alternative path on yet another sharply divisive and long-standing health policy controversy:

> Instead of focusing on the few areas of intense disagreement, such as the possibility of mandating caps on the financial damages awarded to patients, we believe that the discussion should center on a more fundamental issue: the need to improve patient safety.[34]

Senate Finance chair Max Baucus sounded a similar theme in his November 2008 white paper, looking for new alternatives. Earlier in 2005, Baucus had signed on as the sole cosponsor with then HELP Committee chair Mike Enzi (R-WY) of legislation, the Fair and Reliable Medical Justice Act, to authorize ten demonstration grants to states to develop, implement, and evaluate alternatives to tort litigation to resolve disputes over health care injuries.[35] Beyond Obama, Clinton, Baucus, and Enzi, the conversation on medical-liability reform (physicians strongly dislike the term *medical malpractice*) assumed familiar outlines.

Republicans presented liability reform as a centerpiece of their health reform agenda under the banner of eliminating "frivolous lawsuits" and reducing the practice of "defensive medicine," medical treatments done solely for the purpose of averting potential lawsuits. Their major reform proposal was to set strict limits on noneconomic damages such as pain and suffering arising from successful malpractice lawsuits. Though twenty-six states have some form of cap already in place, the $250,000 caps in California and Texas are considered the most restrictive. Also, there is nothing in the California and Texas mechanisms to distinguish frivolous from nonfrivolous actions. In advancing this cause, Republicans are viewed as champions by physicians and medical-liability insurers. Democrats generally oppose Texas- and California-style caps—suggesting they reduce the ability of injured patients to obtain damages for legitimate and serious claims. In this they are the heroes of the medical-liability trial bar—at least the plaintiff's side. In general, consumer organizations have sided with Democrats against strict limits, though they have not been a significant voice in the process, and public opinion polls show consistent support for the Republicans' stance. The most widely accepted estimate of patient deaths in hospitals due to preventable medical errors is between forty-four thousand and ninety-eight thousand, provided by the Institute of Medicine in 1999.[36] Although the IOM estimate is now more than a decade old, there is no credible alternative estimate, nor is there disagreement that a significant burden is placed on patients by poor care and medical errors.

For many years, the Congressional Budget Office has looked at the evidence and found it negligible regarding potential federal and overall health system savings from Texas- or California-style liability reform. In its late 2008 *Budget Options* report, it estimated only $5.6 billion in ten-year federal savings.[37] In October 2009, in the midst of the congressional health reform debate, the CBO announced a change of mind based on new evidence, declaring that as much as $54 billion could be saved in the federal budget from a package of reforms, including the tight caps.[38] Republican members did their best to trumpet the CBO change of heart, but it was too late to influence the course of the health reform debate. No Republican except Maine's Olympia Snowe was open to supporting the final version of Senate reform, and Democrats had both policy and political justification to oppose onerous Texas- and California-style caps. Senator Sheldon Whitehouse (D-RI) led the opposition to caps on policy grounds, while Majority Leader Harry Reid made clear to the White House—which was hoping to find middle ground on the issue—that anything strong on malpractice would gain Democrats nothing and lose a lot in political contributions from the trial bar.

When Reid unveiled his proposed health reform legislation in mid-November 2009, the only reference to liability reform was a token Sense of the Senate resolution included at the tail end of Title VI. That was not enough for some moderate Democrats who agreed on the need for some liability reform and did not want to vote for a package without any. Senator Tom Carper (D-DE) insisted on adding more in Reid's December Manager's Amendment and won the inclusion of section 10607, State Demonstration Programs to Evaluate Alternatives to Current Medical Tort Litigation under the direction of the HHS secretary. The section authorizes up to $50 million in funding between 2011 and 2015, though the funding is not directly allocated. In the final push to produce the reconciliation sidecar legislation, efforts were advanced to make the funding mandatory, but the Senate parliamentarian would not agree. So the final version of ACA has medical-liability reform demonstration projects without guaranteed funding.

In this case, President Obama got the last word. In his September 2009 address to Congress, he indicated his intention to press ahead in the direction he and Hillary Clinton had first laid out in 2006:

> I don't believe malpractice reform is a silver bullet, but I've talked to enough doctors to know that defensive medicine may be contributing to unnecessary costs. So I'm proposing that we move forward on a range of ideas about how to put patient safety first and let doctors focus on practicing medicine. I know that the Bush Administration considered authorizing demonstration projects in individual states to test these ideas. I think it's a good idea, and I'm directing my Secretary of Health and Human Services to move forward on this initiative today.[39]

In October 2009, HHS secretary Kathleen Sebelius launched a Patient Safety and Medical Liability Initiative with $25 million to reduce preventable injuries, foster communication between doctors and patients, ensure that patients are compensated fairly and timely, and reduce liability premiums. In June 2010, the Obama administration announced the awarding of twenty projects to plan, implement, and evaluate reforms that address limitations of the current medical-liability system, such as costs, patient safety, and administrative burden.[40]

The American Medical Association's position on liability reform is that Texas- and California-style caps on noneconomic damages are the proven, effective path to stabilize medical-liability premiums, and it will continue to seek their adoption at the federal and state levels. Still, the Obama administration initiative was a result of direct discussions with the AMA, which officially praised the effort and worked with a number of state medical societies to initiate state proposals. Between 2001 and 2006, while Republicans controlled the White House, the Senate for all but eighteen months—with a physician majority leader in Senator Bill Frist (R-TN)—and the House of Representatives, no medical-liability initiative was enacted or implemented. To the AMA, the Obama initiative is not enough, and it also the first meaningful federal physician-liability reform measure to be implemented. It is noteworthy the extent to which the resolution of this issue—to this limited point—resembles the policy positions taken in 2005 and 2006 by Senators Obama, Clinton, Baucus, and Enzi.

11. Title VII—Biosimilar Biological Products

The scene was Senator Edward Kennedy's Capitol Hill hideaway, steps away from the Senate chamber on a late afternoon in June 2009. Of the thirteen Democratic members of the Senate Health, Education, Labor and Pensions (HELP) Committee, Kennedy was the only one not seated around the chain of tables pulled together for a high-stakes meeting on a contentious health reform issue—how to structure legislation to permit the manufacture and sale of generic-like biopharmaceutical drugs.

The key decision was how many years to permit makers of original biopharmaceutical products to avoid competition from new "biosimilars" beyond the life of their patents. The drug and biotechnology industries wanted at least twelve years of exclusivity, and their opponents—representing generic-drug manufacturers, consumers, insurers, business, and others—were pushing for no more than five years to keep potential competitors at bay. The conversation pivoted on an exchange between Barbara Mikulski (D-MD), the feisty lioness of the Senate, who preferred twelve years, and Sherrod Brown (D-OH), a hard-nosed progressive who wanted five.

Brown opened by stating his preference for five years, though he added a willingness to go up to six.

Mikulski explained her rationale for twelve years and said she perhaps could be persuaded to go down to eleven.

Brown expressed a desire to be reasonable and said he might be able to live with seven.

Mikulski, reciprocating Brown's reasonableness, said she could tolerate ten.

Brown thanked her for her flexibility and responded, "Eight."

Mikulski paused, reflected, and said, "Nine and no less."

Brown, smiling, offered, "Eight and a half?"

Mikulski didn't wait: "Nine and no less."

Brown paused. "I can't go to nine."

Game over, no deal. The matter was settled by the full committee on July 13 at a tense evening session where members voted sixteen to seven in favor of Orrin Hatch's (R-UT) amendment granting twelve years of exclusivity.

TITLE VII—IMPROVING ACCESS TO INNOVATIVE MEDICAL THERAPIES

How did a bare-knuckle stakeholder brawl about drug manufacturing get into the health reform debate? Except for the disagreement on the length of exclusivity, all sides agreed the issue was ready to go; and whichever version was adopted, the Congressional Budget Office had made clear it would score about $7 billion in favorable federal budget consequences to help pay for health reform; this was one of the few items HELP could bring to the table with a positive revenue score. So the table was set, if only both sides could reconcile their disagreements and agree on a number.

UNDERSTANDING TITLE VII

With the exceptions of Titles VII and VIII, the titles in the ACA are lengthy, multifaceted, and complicated. Title VII has just six sections in two subtitles.

> Subtitle A establishes a process under which the Food and Drug Administration may license a biological product shown to be biosimilar or interchangeable with a licensed biological product.
>
> Subtitle B extends drug discounts through the federal 340B program.

Following is a brief overview of both subtitles, including the CBO's estimated costs in brackets. A plus sign (+) means the provision costs billions (B) or millions (M), and a minus sign (−) means the provision will save federal dollars. If there is no bracketed item, the CBO estimates zero cost or savings.

Subtitle A: Biologics Price Competition and Innovation directs the Food and Drug Administration to establish a process to license a biological product shown to be biosimilar to, or interchangeable with, a licensed biological product, called a reference product. The approval of an application for a biosimilar or interchangeable product is prohibited until twelve years from the date on which the reference product is first approved by the FDA. If the FDA approves a biological product on the grounds that it is interchangeable with a reference product, the agency may not make a determination that a subsequent biological product is interchangeable with that same reference product until at least one year after the first commercial marketing of the first interchangeable product. The FDA may issue guidance with respect to the licensure of biological products under this new pathway, including patent-infringement concerns such as the exchange of information, good-faith negotiations, and initiation-infringement actions. Certain provisions of the Food, Drug, and Cosmetic Act will apply to pediatric studies of biological products [−$7.0 B] (section 7002). The treasury secretary, in consultation with the DHHS, will annually determine the amount of savings to the federal government as a result of this subtitle. The federal government savings will be used for deficit reduction (section 7003).

Subtitle B: More Affordable Medicines for Children and Underserved Communities extends participation in the 340B program—which limits the price of outpatient drugs for designated entities such as community health centers—to certain children's hospitals, cancer hospitals, critical access and sole community hospitals, and rural referral centers. It also exempts orphan drugs from required discounts for new 340B entities (section 7101).

BIOSIMILAR BASICS

Biopharmaceuticals, also called *biologics,* are drugs derived from living cells and other natural sources to treat conditions such as cancer, heart disease, rheumatoid arthritis, anemia, multiple sclerosis, and more. The terms *follow-on biologics, biosimilars,* and *biogenerics* all refer to the same thing (though drug and biologics industry partisans reject the terms *follow-on biologics* and *biogeneric*): biopharmaceutical products sold after the expiration of patents and marketed as having properties similar to other biopharmaceutical products. Most people are familiar with the concept because of their familiarity with generic medications. The purpose of Subtitle A is to create a generic-like pathway that—until passage of the ACA—did not exist for most biopharmaceutical products in the United States.

Standard generic drugs and biosimilars differ in important ways. Standard generic drugs are products proven to be exactly the same as the original medication, but biological products are unique and cannot be duplicated by another manufacturer—so a follow-on biologic or biosimilar is similar to, but not the same as, the original product. Biopharmaceutical products at the molecular level are larger and more complex than standard chemical drugs (and are therefore called large-molecule drugs); they are manufactured inside living systems such as yeast or plant and animal cells, and they are more complicated to produce, making the process of determining "equivalence" much more challenging for their manufacturers and regulators than it is for small-molecule drugs.

Biopharmaceutical products have "improved medical treatments, reduced suffering, and saved the lives of many Americans," notes the Federal Trade Commission in its June 2009 report on the controversy.[1] Interest in biosimilars has grown as the size of the biologic drug market has mushroomed, and the cost of these drugs has far outstripped the cost of traditional pharmaceuticals. As the pipeline for traditional small-molecule drugs has slowed, biologic drug sales reached $75 billion in 2007, with spending increasing rapidly each year; in 2008, 28 percent of sales from the drug industry's top one hundred products came from biologics, a figure projected to increase to 50 percent by 2014.[2] Avastin, a biologic drug for patients with advanced colon, lung, or breast cancer, can cost up to $100,000 per patient per year.[3] Cerezyme, used to treat Gaucher's disease (a genetic condition), is priced at an average of $170,000 per patient per year. As of early 2009, there were more than 250 FDA-approved biological medicines and more than 300 in development.[4] Many of the leading biologic drugs have exhausted their patents or will do so by 2012, yet would likely face no competition without a federal pathway for the approval of biosimilar products. The cost of biopharmaceuticals has been noticed by private payers, including insurers, businesses, and consumers, as well as public payers, especially Medicare for Parts B and D and state Medicaid programs. The Medicare Payment Advisory Committee (MedPAC) found that by 2009, the top six biologics made up 43 percent of the drug budget for Medicare Part B, with costs increasing rapidly.

Other parts of the advanced world—including Australia, India, South America, and the European Union—are ahead of the United States in enabling their citizens to have access to biosimilars. The European Medicines Agency (EMEA), the EU's equivalent of the U.S. Food and Drug Administration, has implemented an approval scheme that recognizes differences between standard generic drugs and biosimilars. The EU provides ten years of exclusivity for biopharmaceuticals against biosimilars—and that can be extended to eleven or twelve years.

The regulatory regime for small-molecule drugs and generics in the

United States was established in a 1984 law called the Drug Price Competition and Patent Term Restoration Act of 1984, more familiarly the Hatch-Waxman Act, named after its two principal sponsors, Senator Orrin Hatch and Representative Henry Waxman (D-CA). Credited with creating the robust generic-drug industry in the United States, the law opened a pathway for the approval and production of generic drugs without manufacturers having to go through the lengthy review and approval process required for new nongeneric drugs. Running concurrently with the standard patent protection of twenty years, Hatch-Waxman allows brand-name drug makers five years of exclusivity before generics can receive FDA approval to come to market. The result of Hatch-Waxman has been a boon in generic medicines—by 2009, generics accounted for more than 70 percent of all prescriptions written in the United States though for only 20 percent of the total spending on medications.[5]

The hope in 2009–10 was that the establishment of a similar process for the manufacture and sale of biosimilars would create competition within this market and trigger the same dramatic price drops—in the neighborhood of 70 percent—that occur when a standard generic competitor enters the market of a traditional brand-name drug. The FTC, among others, suggests that because the challenges of making and using biosimilars are so different from those for traditional small-molecule drugs, the likely impact will be price drops of 10–30 percent at best, with far fewer market entrants, and the competition will more closely resemble that between two brand-name drugs than between a brand name and a generic.[6] Specifically, the costs to produce biosimilars will be much higher than for standard generics, the development time much longer in years; and most biosimilars will need to be administered as part of medical treatments and not by patients on their own, requiring different marketing strategies to win adoption.

In the federal legislative process, a host of contentious issues had to be resolved regarding the patent process and FDA authority; with one exception, all these issues were settled before the health reform process got fully engaged. In creating a pathway for biosimilars in the health reform legislation, the unresolved critical question was, how many years of exclusivity should biopharmaceutical makers enjoy so they can keep the data on their clinical trials confidential? The boundaries of this dispute boiled down to five versus twelve years. That was the fight.

On the twelve-year side were the key industry players: the pharmaceutical industry represented by PhRMA; the biopharmaceutical industry represented by a newer player, BIO (the Biotechnology Industry Organization); academic medical centers and biotech labs; and patient advocacy organizations with ties to the drug industry. On the five-year side was a coalition of players including the Generic Pharmaceutical Association, consumer groups including the Consumers Union and AARP, leading business organizations, and health insurers. Two worthy sets of adversaries.

CONGRESS DECIDES

The path to a legislative solution began well before the health reform process. A key event occurred among the HELP Committee and other members in 2007, including Senators Kennedy, Hatch, Mike Enzi (R-WY), Hillary Clinton (D-NY), and Chuck Schumer (D-NY). In the Senate, FDA matters are in the HELP Committee's jurisdiction, and key members decided to meet to see whether they could hammer out an agreement. When they met, the options ranged from zero to sixteen years of exclusivity. Senator Schumer had filed legislation on the subject proposing zero years, which he viewed as a starting point for negotiations. In the meeting, discussion began to focus on the European model, which allows ten years of exclusivity, with an additional year for product innovation and a further additional year for pediatric research. At one point, Senator Schumer said, "Let's do twelve." Everyone in the room nodded in agreement and the deal was done. Soon thereafter, the HELP Committee unanimously reported legislation incorporating the twelve-year deal. The bill did not make it through the Senate, in part because key House leader and Energy and Commerce Committee chair Henry Waxman (D-CA) made clear he would not support twelve years. The issue was held for inclusion in the larger health reform measure.

In a two-hour HELP Committee debate on the evening of July 13, 2009, in the Russell Senate Caucus room, members went back and forth on Sherrod Brown's amendment for seven years, Orrin Hatch's for twelve, and John McCain (R-AZ) and Barbara Mikulski's (D-MD) for ten. Hatch, Enzi, and North Carolina's Kay Hagan (D-NC) argued to uphold the 2007 agreement and warned of stifled drug innovation for any period less than twelve years. Brown, Bernie Sanders (I-VT), and Tom Harkin (D-IA) argued for a shorter period, citing the Federal Trade Commission report's conclusion that twelve years would be more stifling for innovation than five or seven. Brown's amendment was voted down five to seventeen, and Hatch's was approved fifteen to seven. The Senate laid down the first marker. Among the fifteen were Democrats such as Barbara Mikulski and Patty Murray (D-WA) who had thriving and developing biotechnology industries in their home states.

At the same time the HELP Committee was doing its markup, the White House and Senate Finance staff were negotiating with the pharmaceutical industry on an overall agreement to place the industry on the side of reform and to win specific financing commitments from it to help pay for the legislation. The deal included $80 billion in industry financing and, in return, commitments by the White House and Senate Finance staffers to keep negotiated pricing in Medicare and allowances for the reimportation of drugs from other nations out of the bill; also included was support for a pathway for FDA approval of biosimilars, though with no specific agreement on either side to a number of years for exclusivity beyond patent protection. The Senate Finance staffers had a jurisdictional issue—it was HELP's domain—preventing them from making a deal. The Obama administration, which supported five to seven years of exclusivity, decided to allow Henry Waxman to "work his magic," in the words of one close observer. In retrospect, the summer negotiation was the sole opportunity the White House had to move the industry toward a compromise and a different place—and it was forfeited.

The House Energy and Commerce Committee followed HELP in a matter of weeks. Its chair, Henry Waxman, had an interest and history in the issue every bit as compelling as did Orrin Hatch—the other half of the Hatch-Waxman duo who wrote the generic drug law in 1984. Waxman had gone back and forth between zero and five years of exclusivity and adamantly opposed the twelve-year option, preferring to take no action and wait for another day than to approve that long a period. His committee had been heavily and effectively lobbied by pharmaceutical and biotechnology companies, who had a champion in Representative Anna Eshoo (D-CA) from Silicon Valley. Making clear her intention to push the issue, she fashioned an amendment even more favorable toward biotechnology interests than the HELP bill was, incorporating the Senate deal for twelve years of exclusivity. Waxman's staffers believed she would not demand a recorded vote, but she did. Uncharacteristically, Waxman lost to Eshoo in his own committee by a vote of forty-seven to eleven. Waxman's team had a lot more going on in those hectic days of July 2009 than just biosimilars—and his staffers are certain there would have been a different outcome had they not been so distracted by the Blue Dog rebellion, abortion, and much more.

The die was cast on both sides of Capitol Hill, and the industry had won hands down—the biosimilar provisions were more bipartisan than perhaps any other element of reform; the key committees of jurisdiction had overwhelmingly voted for a biosimilar pathway with twelve years of exclusivity. Speaker Nancy Pelosi and Majority Leader Harry Reid both included the issue in the bills they advanced, honoring the respective committee votes. Many assumed the matter was settled as long as health reform got to the president's desk.

Barack Obama, though, had other ideas. The president believed twelve years were too many and preferred seven. When the negotiations on a final bill moved to the White House in January 2010, Obama personally pushed leaders from both chambers in meetings in the White House Roosevelt Room to reopen and reconfigure the deal for less than twelve years. Sitting around the table were Waxman, Chris Dodd (D-CT), and Harkin—all of whom had voted against the twelve-year exclusivity arrangement in their respective committees. The senators pushed back, saying Obama would have to personally engage in the negotiation if they were to have any chance to change the number of years, given prior actions in both chambers. This was one issue where the president's words were not matched by follow-up—in the HELP and Energy and Commerce Committees, as well as with the members themselves, the White House lacked a clear focus on an issue this contentious.

In a closed-door meeting with House Democrats on January 14, 2010, Obama openly suggested to them that a shorter period would be in order. Representative Eshoo stood up to remind the president that Congress had overwhelmingly backed twelve years, and that it would not be fair to eliminate that measure when other pharmaceutical elements of the bill seemed to be sacrosanct. Obama replied: "Nothing is sacrosanct."[7]

In the frenzied weekend of January 16–17, biotechnology interests began a frantic lobbying campaign to halt any change. Some biotech industry representatives in Massachusetts threatened to withdraw support for health reform if the terms were changed, while others indicated they were prepared to publicly endorse Scott Brown, the Republican candidate for the seat held by Senator Kennedy until his passing in August 2009. It was Brown's victory on the following Tuesday, January 19, that ended conclusively any possibility of altering the deal—though the real possibility of a change was remote in spite of the president's advocacy. Too many Democrats had put themselves firmly on the twelve-year side to back down, and leaders in both chambers had little room to spare in corralling the votes to complete the health reform process.

What can be expected now? The ACA defines a biosimilar as "highly similar" to its reference product and leaves it to the FDA to define that term, not only what it means, but also how much testing, potentially including randomized clinical trials, will be needed before the product can be marketed and sold. Some expect a rush once the FDA approves a regulatory structure, though nothing like what developed with standard generics. Industry lawyers advise their clients to devise broad patent protections around their existing products, covering the sequencing of molecules, formulation methods, dosing, delivery methods, and more. "You need to create a picket fence around the product," counseled one life sciences attorney.[8] The European Union created its approval process in 2004 and thirteen biosimilars had been approved by late 2010.[9] Others suggest Congress missed the mark by providing twelve years of exclusivity with opportunities for further extensions and that "U.S. patients and insurers will continue to pay unnecessarily high prices for these products for decades to come."[10]

· · ·

An esteemed political scientist, the late E. E. Schattschneider, described the three fundamental elements of political conflict: site, scope, and intensity.[11] *Site* refers to the location of the conflict—legislative chamber, executive department, bureaucracy, courtroom, boardroom, and living room. *Scope* refers to the number of contestants on the playing field—their relative power and the numbers on all sides. *Intensity* refers to the passion and determination of the combatants. In this case, many players joined on the biosimilars playing field—pharmaceutical companies, consumer and patient groups, generic-drug manufacturers, academic medical centers, labor unions, insurers, business groups, and the biotechnology industry. Except for the last constituency, everyone else had numerous issues of concern related to national health reform. For the biotechnology sector, the biosimilars fight was the whole shooting match—and its support or opposition to reform rested solely on the resolution of this one concern. Rightly or wrongly, it fought as though the outcome meant the difference between life or death for its growing sector. It threw everything it had into the fight—and the intensity it brought to the conflict made the difference.

12. Title VIII—CLASS Act

JULY 7, 2009. SENATE HELP COMMITTEE MARKUP—
OFFICIAL TRANSCRIPT

SENATOR JUDD GREGG (R-NH): So I'm offering amendment—
in fact—offer an amendment at this time. I would offer an
Amendment Number 6, my Amendment Number 6. Could
we pass that out?

SENATOR CHRISTOPHER DODD (D-CT—PRESIDING):
Amendment Number 6?

SENATOR GREGG: Which essentially says that, takes out the
number that's in here, the $65 premium, and just simply
directs that the Secretary shall set a premium that causes
the program to be solvent over seventy-five years. Why
seventy-five years? Because that's what we score Social
Security, Medicare, and Medicaid on. And when you start
reducing below seventy-five years, you're basically playing
games with the number. . . . So that's all this language
does, is it says, "Let's strike the number and let's tell the
Secretary make the program solvent." There seems to be
a consistency of thought around here that we should have
a solvent program. I'm not opposing the program. I'm just
saying let's have a solvent program. . . .

SENATOR DODD: Well, am I to understand my colleague, then,
that if we were—let's say for the purpose of discussion
here, to talk about working out a number here that would
at least project that kind of solvency, that my colleague
from New Hampshire would then support this plan?

SENATOR GREGG: Yeah. That's what I do here. . . . If you'll
accept my amendment, I'll support the language. That's
basically—

SENATOR DODD: So I'm prepared to accept this amendment
because it still is—as Senator Enzi said, it's a bargain. . . .
But let's accept the amendment. I want to—let me
hear from my colleagues, too. I'm prepared to accept it.
Any objection to that? All those in favor of the Gregg
amendment, say aye.

[*Chorus of ayes*]

SENATOR DODD: Those opposed, no.

[*No audible response*]

SENATOR DODD: The ayes appear to have it, and the ayes have it. Congratulations, Senator.

SENATOR GREGG: Thank you, Mr. Chairman, and I appreciate your willingness to be flexible. . . . But I want to second your comments on the concept. I mean, it's a voluntary program. If it is solvently structured, it could have a very positive impact.

SENATOR DODD: Yeah.

SENATOR GREGG: And to get people to buy long-term insurance is really helpful.

DECEMBER 2, 2009. CONGRESSIONAL RECORD

SENATOR JUDD GREGG: The CLASS Act is another classic gimmick of budgetary shenanigans . . . a classic Ponzi scheme.

DECEMBER 4, 2009. CONGRESSIONAL RECORD. Recorded Roll Call No. 360—Amendment by Senator John Thune (R-SD) to delete the CLASS Act from the pending health reform legislation.

SENATOR JUDD GREGG: Yea.

TITLE VIII—COMMUNITY LIVING ASSISTANCE SERVICES AND SUPPORTS

Many Democrats and progressives were disheartened to see the absence of a so-called public-plan option in Title I of the final health reform law. While it is true there is no public-plan option to be offered through the health insurance exchanges, there is a "public-plan option" in the ACA. It is in Title VIII and is known as CLASS, which stands for Community Living Assistance Services and Supports. It's public—it will be run by the Department of Health and Human Services (DHHS). It's a plan—it will provide specific benefits to enrollees who will pay premiums. And it's an option—when launched in 2013 or thereabouts, it will be available to all working Americans, and no one will be required to participate.

To its leading proponents, CLASS is a breakthrough, the most important innovation in helping Americans with disability and long-term care needs since the creation of Medicaid in 1965, an innovation that may open the long-closed door to more fundamental long-term care reform. To less enthusiastic advocates, CLASS is only a sliver of a solution and not the most important sliver at that, and it may preempt chances for more comprehensive reform in the future. To its opponents, CLASS is a ticking fiscal time bomb, a Ponzi scheme of the highest order, a Trojan horse, and that's just for starters. To those involved in CLASS implementation, it may just be the most challenging single part of the entire ACA to implement—with huge statutory, financial, and structural obstacles to overcome before anyone will be able to enroll. In this chapter we dive into the language and details of Title VIII. Then we examine the viewpoints of proponents and opponents as well as explore the process leading to its enactment as part of the ACA.

UNDERSTANDING TITLE VIII

These are only two sections in Title VIII (no subtitles). Section 8002 is estimated by the Congressional Budget Office to reduce the federal deficit by $70.2 billion from 2010 to 2019.

> Short Title merely says that the title may be called the CLASS Act (section 8001).

> Establishment of National Voluntary Insurance Program for Purchasing Community Living Services and Supports outlines the purposes and operations of the program [–$70.2B] (section 8002).

Here is the Senate's official description of section 8002:

> Establishes a new, voluntary, self-funded public long-term care insurance program, to be known as the CLASS Independence Benefit Plan, for the purchase of community living assistance services and supports by individuals with functional limitations. Requires the Secretary to develop an actuarially sound benefit plan that ensures solvency for seventy-five years; allows for a five-year vesting period for eligibility of benefits; creates benefit triggers that allow for the determination of functional limitation; and provides cash benefit that is not less than an average of $50 per day. No taxpayer funds will be used to pay benefits under this provision. Section 10801 made technical corrections to Title VIII.[1]

The CLASS Act, within the ACA, is Title VIII. The language in Title VIII locates the CLASS Act in a broad federal law known as the Public Health Service Act (PHSA), not in the Social Security Act, where this sort of program normally would be located. By placing CLASS in PHSA, the Senate Health, Education, Labor and Pensions Committee (HELP) obtains joint jurisdiction with the Senate Finance Committee. As we will see later in the chapter, that was a politically consequential choice. Within the PHSA, CLASS is now established as Title XXXII. Within this new Title XXXII are ten sections, and here they are, including brief descriptions of each:

Section 3201: Purpose. The purpose of this title is to establish a national voluntary insurance program for purchasing community living assistance services and supports in order to—

(1) provide individuals with functional limitations with tools that will allow them to maintain their personal and financial independence and live in the community through a new financing strategy for community living assistance services and supports; (2) establish an infrastructure that will help address the Nation's community living assistance services and supports needs; (3) alleviate burdens on family caregivers; and (4) address institutional bias by providing a financing mechanism that supports personal choice and independence to live in the community.

Section 3202: Definitions. There are thirteen, and several are particularly important. Eligibility for benefits is restricted to those with at least two or three deficits in "activities of daily living," and the six ADLs are eating, toileting, transferring, bathing, dressing, and continence. The HHS secretary will decide whether two or three ADL deficiencies will determine eligibility (it was left vague to give the secretary discretion to ensure fiscal solvency). An "eligible beneficiary" must have paid CLASS premiums for at least sixty months, and at least three of those five years must be spent working and earning enough to pay Social Security taxes, or at least $1,200 per year.

Section 3203: CLASS Independence Benefit Plan. Premiums will be set by the HHS secretary so that the program will be actuarially sound for seventy-five years; premiums for individuals with incomes under 100 percent of the federal poverty level and for full-time working students under age twenty-two cannot exceed $5 per month. Benefit payments are triggered for a period when an eligible individual has at least two or three ADL deficits for at least ninety days. The minimum cash benefit is $50 per day and can be higher for individuals with more ADL limitations. As long as an individual stays enrolled, premiums for that person will not increase— unless the HHS secretary has to revise the plan for solvency purposes. Premiums will vary only for age and not for health status.

Section 3204: Enrollment and Disenrollment Requirements. Employers, at their own option, may enroll their employees in CLASS automatically, and those employees will have the option to waive out. Participating employers may deduct CLASS premiums from the participants' payroll checks. An alternative premium payment method will be set up for other enrollees.

Section 3205: Benefits. The HHS secretary will establish an eligibility-assessment system to make disability determinations and benefit-eligibility calculations. Beneficiaries will receive a cash benefit, advocacy services, and assistance counseling. Each beneficiary will have a Life Independence Account established to pay for "nonmedical services and supports that the beneficiary needs to maintain his or her independence at home or in another residential setting of their choice in the community, including (but not limited to) home modifications, assistive technology, accessible transportation, homemaker services, respite care, personal assistance services, home care aides, and nursing support."

Section 3206: CLASS Independence Fund. The treasury secretary will maintain the CLASS Independence Fund that holds premium payments from CLASS enrollees. A board of trustees will include the secretaries of treasury, labor and health and human services, plus two public members, nominated by the president and confirmed by the Senate.

Section 3207: CLASS Independence Advisory Council. A fifteen-member council will advise the HHS secretary with regard to CLASS. A majority of members must be individuals who participate or are likely to participate in CLASS.

Section 3208: Solvency and Fiscal Independence Regulations; Annual Report. No taxpayer funds may be used to pay for CLASS benefits— the only source of payment for benefits will be premiums and associated interest.

Section 3209: Inspector General Report. The HHS inspector general will produce an annual report on CLASS, including "overall progress of the CLASS program and of the existence of waste, fraud, and abuse in the CLASS program."

Section 3210: Tax Treatment of Program. For IRS tax purposes, CLASS will be treated "in the same manner as a qualified long-term care insurance contract for qualified long-term care services." The HHS secretary will establish a Personal Care Attendants Workforce Advisory Panel. Finally, "nothing in this title or the amendments made by this title is intended to replace or displace public or private disability insurance benefits, including such benefits that are for income replacement."

CLASS BEGINNINGS

For Senator Edward Kennedy, CLASS was personal. In 1984 his mother, Rose Fitzgerald Kennedy, suffered a severe stroke and used a wheelchair until her death in 1995 at the age of 104. While the family could afford private duty nursing and other supports to enable her to stay at home, Senator Kennedy saw firsthand how complicated and difficult it was. He realized that this kind of care was completely unaffordable and inaccessible for the vast majority of Americans whose only real option was to exhaust nearly all their assets to qualify for widely varying services under a state Medicaid program.

In 1994, he hired for his HELP Committee staff a Philadelphia-bred pediatric and neonatal intensive care nurse practitioner with the determination of a pit bull by the name of Connie Garner. Kennedy and Garner observed a "failure paradigm" in U.S. disability policy—there was no way to qualify for services and supports unless the disabled individual was poor—a "wait to fail" model that consigned disabled persons to poverty and nonemployment before they could enroll in a state Medicaid program. As Garner would tell parents, it was common for young adults who experienced a serious life-altering accident to find themselves nonqualified for Social Security disability benefits because they had yet to pay payroll taxes for the requisite number of quarters. Long-term care insurance had not worked for the vast majority of Americans, financing only $4 billion out of the nation's $200 billion long-term care bill in 2008. Disability insurance, provided by employers on a voluntary basis, is not a solution because once a person resumes work, disability payments stop.

The vast majority of Americans with disabilities live in their homes in communities, not in nursing homes or other institutional settings, and many need extra support to keep doing so, even those able to work. For a disabled person needing nursing-home-level care, the $50 to $75 daily CLASS benefit is not a solution. For a disabled person attempting to live independently in a noninstitutionalized situation, the daily payment can make an enormous difference in being able to survive and thrive. The $50–$75 payment can be used to help retrofit a home with wheelchair ramps or to pay for transportation services to medical appointments, personal care attendant services, or other approved purposes.

After lengthy engagement and consultation, Kennedy unveiled his first CLASS proposal in 2005, drawing endorsements from more than 260 disability, elderly, health, labor, and religious organizations, including AARP, Easter Seals, Paralyzed Veterans of America, the Special Olympics, the Alzheimer's Association, and many more. For a number of these organizations, CLASS was their principal motivation to support national health reform, and to them, health reform that did not address the need for long-term services and supports for persons with disabilities was not worthy of the name health reform. There were also opponents—most prominently from the life insurance industry, especially two companies with large footprints in the long-term care insurance market, Genworth and John Hancock, as well as their trade organization, the American Council of Life Insurers. Health insurers did not see CLASS as competition and did not engage.

It was Kennedy's practice always to seek a Republican partner, and on this issue he found one in Senator Mike DeWine (R-OH). They jointly introduced the first version of CLASS in 2005, and both were taken aback at their first press conference on the bill when they saw firsthand the variety of individuals and families who expressed a need for the kind of support that would be available through CLASS, adults of all ages who had become disabled by accidents or illness, and family members struggling to keep them at home and in the community. DeWine lost his 2006 bid for reelection and Kennedy, uncharacteristically, was unable to find a Republican to replace him. He made the decision to run with CLASS as a Democratic initiative, teaming up with House members John Dingell (D-MI), then chair of the House Energy and Commerce Committee, and Frank Pallone (D-NJ), chair of the Energy and Commerce Subcommittee on Health.

As the health reform process got under way, the HELP Committee had to resolve many issues regarding CLASS and the overall legislation. One issue never in question, as far as Kennedy was concerned, was whether the committee's bill would include CLASS. When draft legislation was distributed to HELP members in early June 2009, CLASS was in it. Even though Kennedy was unable to participate in the markup because of his illness, his close friend Christopher Dodd carried the CLASS portfolio against expected opposition from Republicans, especially New Hampshire's Judd Gregg. There also were HELP Committee Democrats, notably Kay Hagan (D-NC), who were openly skeptical. Dodd was unsure he could hold together enough Democrats to keep CLASS in the bill. When Gregg moved his amendment to delete an explicit premium and replace it with an actuarially sound premium to be determined by the HHS secretary, Dodd peered at Garner for her call: "How about accepting it?" he asked in a whispered conversation. They decided on the spot to agree, surprising and disarming Gregg, and infuriating some Republican staffers who saw the move coming even before Dodd and Garner made the call. CLASS survived; arguably and ironically, Gregg's amendment did more to secure that survival than anything else in the lengthy process.

CLASS QUESTIONS

Senate Finance chair Max Baucus was a CLASS skeptic, and his chief health reform ally, Budget chair Kent Conrad, was a CLASS opponent. To them, the risks of adverse selection and the budgetary uncertainties, even with the lack of federal subsidies, were too great. The legislation Baucus brought to the Finance Committee in September contained no CLASS benefit, and no committee member attempted to insert one during the committee's monthlong markup. Majority Leader Harry Reid was a CLASS agnostic, with no stated position. As he combined the Finance and HELP bills into one merged bill in October and November, he faced strong pressures from both sides. Before his death in August, Senator Kennedy had personally pleaded with Reid for inclusion of CLASS, and his determination was backed up by Dodd, Kennedy's successor as HELP chair; Tom Harkin (D-IA); and Kennedy's temporary successor to his Senate seat, Paul Kirk (D-MA). At the same time, seven moderate Democratic Caucus members— Kent Conrad (ND), Joe Lieberman (I-CT), Mary Landrieu (LA), Evan Bayh (IN), Blanche Lincoln (AR), Ben Nelson (NE), and Mark Warner (VA)— wrote Reid to urge him "not to include these provisions (CLASS) in the Senate's merged bill."[2]

What was their concern?

Much involved the Congressional Budget Office estimates relating to CLASS. All sides agreed on one point—the CBO estimated that between 2010 and 2019, the CLASS program would generate far more premium revenue than would be paid out in benefits, $70.2 billion more. The reason for the surplus is that CLASS enrollees have to pay premiums for five years before they ever qualify for benefits—and then benefits only flow when an enrollee has a qualifying disability. That $70.2 billion, incidentally, amounts to slightly more than half the entire CBO estimated budget savings of the ACA in the first ten years—even though the revenues are all dedicated to CLASS and not available for other governmental purposes. In the second decade, the CBO projects CLASS "would reduce the federal budget deficit . . . but by smaller amounts than in the initial decade. By the third decade, the sum of benefit payments and administrative costs would probably exceed premium income and savings to the Medicaid program. Therefore, the programs would add to budget deficits in the third decade—and in succeeding decades—by amounts on the order of tens of billions of dollars."[3]

One reason the CBO counts CLASS as adding to the deficit in future decades is that its scorekeeping conventions do not permit it to count interest from accumulated premiums in the trust fund as counting toward the cost of the program. If those interest revenues were counted, they would change the budget picture in favor of CLASS. In truth, both sides can be accused of not fully representing CBO's CLASS analysis. Democrats take credit for $70.2 billion in deficit reduction, which will not really occur because those dollars are dedicated to paying CLASS obligations in future years. CLASS critics can be criticized for ignoring a CBO scoring convention—not counting interest—to mischaracterize the budget impact of CLASS in later decades.

Critics had more ammunition at their disposal. In December, the chief actuary for the Centers for Medicare and Medicaid Services (CMS), Richard Foster, provided his own estimate of the costs of the ACA, including CLASS, with a final estimate issued in April.[4] Foster's analysis projected budget savings from CLASS in the first ten years at $35.6 billion as opposed to the CBO's $70.2 billion calculation. Foster also estimated 2.8 million participants, or roughly 2 percent of eligible individuals, enrolled by the third year, as well as relatively high premiums that would trigger adverse selection into the program, while the CBO estimated about 3.5 percent of adults would enroll. While the CBO estimated average monthly premiums at $123 per month at the start, Foster predicted average monthly premiums around $240. His conclusion:

> In general, voluntary, unsubsidized, and non-underwritten insurance programs such as CLASS face a significant risk of failure as a result of adverse selection by participants. Individuals with health problems or who anticipate a greater risk of functional limitations would be more likely to participate than those in better-than-average health. Setting the premium at a rate sufficient to cover the costs for such a group further discourages persons in better health from participating, thereby leading to additional premium increases. This effect has been

termed the "classic assessment spiral" or "insurance death spiral."
The problem of adverse selection would be intensified by requiring
participants to subsidize the $5 premiums for students and low-income
enrollees. Although Title VIII includes modest work requirements in
lieu of underwriting, and specifies that the program is to be "actuarially
sound" and based on "an actuarial analysis of the 75-year costs of the
program that ensures solvency throughout such 75-year period," there
is a very serious risk that the problem of adverse selection would make
the CLASS program unsustainable.[5]

Foster's gloomy estimates were distinct outliers relative to other professional estimates. Even the American Council of Life Insurers, an ardent
CLASS opponent, projected premiums in the $140 range, while other
estimates varied between $65 and $125 in monthly enrollee premiums.
Beyond the hard estimates lurked the concern that if and when CLASS got
into financial difficulty, political pressure would compel Congress to fill
the financial hole with general revenues, much as Medicare Part B (physician and outpatient services) has moved from its original financing by
enrollees to one increasingly financed by general revenues.

Those wanting to make the countercase had their ammunition.

CLASS MAKES THE CUT

Majority Leader Harry Reid decided to include CLASS in the merged
health reform bill he unveiled on November 18. The Dodd-Harkin-Kirk
trio had worked the issue hard, and Reid was attracted by the $70.2 bil-
lion CBO-estimated deficit reduction, real or not. A number of moderate Democratic Caucus members, including Senators Ben Nelson and Joe
Lieberman, stated publicly they would not vote for a health reform bill
that included CLASS. When they got down to their final items in their
late negotiations with Reid, though, CLASS turned out not to be a deal
breaker. It was not eliminated in the Manager's Amendment, though it
was clarified so that all premium dollars were restricted to use for the
CLASS program.

The Senate floor showdown on CLASS happened on December 4, 2009.
Senator John Thune (R-SD) offered an amendment to strike CLASS from
the bill and asked for a recorded vote. Twelve Democrats joined thirty-nine
Republicans to strike CLASS, for a vote of fifty-one yes to forty-seven no
to strike Title VIII. So CLASS survived. How? The Senate rules of debate—
including the need for sixty affirmative votes to invoke cloture—required

that any and all amendments also needed at least sixty votes to prevail. The amendment failed and CLASS survived. Among Democrats joining the Republicans were the seven signatories to the October 23 letter to Reid, plus Baucus, McCaskill (D-MO), Udall (D-CO), and Webb (D-VA). Had Harry Reid not put CLASS into the underlying bill, there would not have been sixty votes or even a majority to support adding it. On the morning of the Thune amendment vote, Connie Garner started her day by visiting Senator Kennedy's gravesite at Arlington National Cemetery to chat with the boss. She, Dodd, and Harkin had an army of advocates behind them and faced daunting resources from the American Council of Life Insurers focused on killing CLASS. Once CLASS survived the Senate debate, its future in the bill was secure as long as the larger health reform vehicle prevailed. House negotiators mostly deferred to the Senate on CLASS. More difficult were January negotiations with the Office of Management and Budget, which wanted to raise the employment-income threshold needed to qualify for the three-year work requirement from about $1,200 up to $9,000. Senate and House leaders refused to budge.

Had Republicans in Max Baucus's Gang of Six and elsewhere stayed at the table and negotiated health reform to an agreement, CLASS likely would have been traded away to garner minority party support. Senator Gregg, who voted against CLASS on the Senate floor, may have done more than anyone else to save it, courtesy of his amendment in the HELP markup because it protected CLASS from attacks on its financing. CLASS, more than likely, would never have prevailed as a stand-alone piece of legislation—illustrating that it's easier sometimes to get something big through than something small.

As the Obama administration—not a fan of CLASS during the legislative process—moves toward implementation, CLASS has a challenging future ahead of it on many levels—financially, programmatically, and politically. Among a host of challenges is the $5 guaranteed premium for low-income and student enrollees; generally, when Congress creates a subsidized program, federal or other governmental dollars support all or some of the subsidy. In the case of CLASS, paying for benefits with any dollars beyond premium revenue and accumulated interest is explicitly prohibited, meaning that the premiums for all nonsubsidized enrollees— whose participation is essential for solvency and success—must be higher to finance the low-income and working-student option, a structural feature that will raise full premiums and discourage some number of potential full-premium payers from signing up—a potentially fatal adverse selection obstacle. Another issue: while the cash benefit is required to increase annually by inflation, the premiums are not, which will again trigger higher initial premiums that will discourage nonsubsidized enrollment. These are just two of the many challenges facing the Obama administration as it attempts to devise a feasible program. These obstacles may be fixable—the ACA gives the HHS secretary discretion regarding the setting of premiums when solvency is threatened—though there is disagreement on just how much flexibility the ACA language provides, for example:

> The Secretary shall establish all premiums to be paid by enrollees for the year based on an actuarial analysis of the 75-year costs of the program that ensures solvency throughout such 75-year period. . . . If the Secretary determines . . . that the monthly premiums and income to the CLASS Independence Fund for a year are projected to be insufficient . . . the Secretary shall adjust the monthly premiums for individuals enrolled in the CLASS program as necessary (but maintaining a nominal premium for enrollees whose income is below the poverty line).[6]

Ironically, CLASS was kept in the ACA in large measure because of its $70.2 billion contribution to deficit reduction, but the fixes needed to make it work may well lower that deficit projection.

Despite the obstacles, CLASS is also being celebrated by individuals with disabilities and their loved ones across the nation as a paradigm-shifting move in federal policy because for the first time, it provides coverage for custodial care. As elder law attorney Daniel Fish notes:

> Until now, health insurance has only reimbursed care that for the patient's safety had to be provided by medical personnel such as doctors, nurses, physical therapists, speech therapists, and occupational therapists. It ignored the demographic imperative of the aging population that increasingly needs important but less sophisticated care, such as assistance with eating and bathing.[7]

The challenge now is to make the structure work. While the regulatory, financial, and marketing challenges are imposing, the need for a more effective national policy for persons with disabilities only grows. If CLASS can overcome its intimidating obstacles and succeed, it will be yet another noteworthy ACA breakthrough in U.S. social policy.

13. Title IX—Paying for the ACA (or about Half of It)

When it came to paying for the ACA, the first question was, how much of it needs to be paid for? There was no agreement up front. Many health reform supporters saw that Republican congressional leaders made no effort to pay for the Medicare Part D program, the wars in Afghanistan and Iraq, or the 2001–3 Bush tax cuts. Some of the price tag could and should be paid for, but not all. Why was health insurance coverage for all Americans less important than those other priorities? Some stakeholders involved in the HELP Committee's negotiation process wrote a joint letter to key Democrats in the late winter of 2009 to press this point. In response, budget hawks led by Senator Kent Conrad (D-ND) made clear they would support health reform only if it was fully self-financed. When the Obama administration made clear their agreement with Conrad during the budget process in the winter and spring of 2009, the question appeared to be settled, even though some Senate and House staffers continued to believe that a fully financed health reform package was not achievable politically.

The next question was, how would Congress agree to pay for it? There were two schools of thought. Leaders in the House of Representatives thought the large bulk of the money should be raised from new taxes on the wealthy as well as penalties on employers not providing health insurance. Key Senate leaders, though, believed the law should be financed by capturing savings from within the health care system itself. The respective bills approved in each chamber in late 2009 reflected these divergent orientations—and the final ACA, approved in late March 2010, split the difference.

To understand the money flows in and out of the Affordable Care Act, think about the law in exaggerated terms—though not by much. First, of the total net price tag of approximately $940 billion over ten years, about half is intended to be spent on the private coverage expansions in Title I and about half is spent on public coverage expansions in Title II—not precisely, but close enough. Second, of that $940 billion, about half is financed by the Medicare changes in Title III, and about half is raised by the revenue provisions of Title IX—not precisely, but close enough. This chapter explores the Title IX revenue provisions—what the big ones are and how they got to be a part of the final law.

TITLE IX—REVENUE PROVISIONS

As with the presentations of previous titles, specific financial estimates for each section are included to understand which elements are most significant. There is one difference in this chapter's estimates. The official ones are not provided by the Congressional Budget Office. These estimates are produced by an entity known as the Joint Committee on Taxation.[1] The JCT is a nonpartisan committee of the Congress established in 1926 to advise both parties in the House and the Senate on every aspect of the legislative process involving tax policy. Readers of the CBO's final estimates on the Affordable Care Act, issued on March 20, 2010, will find a hole when they come to Title IX.[2] This is because estimating the tax provisions of legislation is the JCT's turf—the JCT also provided its final estimates on March 20, 2010.[3] Like the CBO, the JCT employs a respected professional staff of economists, attorneys, and accountants (about sixty in number), and the official committee itself consists of five members of the Senate Finance Committee and five members of the House Committee on Ways and Means (three majority and two minority from each committee). The committee is located on the House side of Capitol Hill in the Longworth House Office Building.

UNDERSTANDING TITLE IX

Welcome to Title IX. It has twenty sections divided between two subtitles:

Subtitle A: Revenue Offset Provisions

Subtitle B: Other Provisions

Following this key-section overview is a fuller discussion of the most important sections in this title, ranked by their respective revenue impact. All items listed in this summary include the JCT's ten-year revenue estimate in brackets. *Important Note:* Unlike the summaries in other chapters, in this summary, a plus sign (+) means the section will raise revenues for the federal treasury in billions (B) or millions (M) and a minus sign (–) means the provision will cost federal dollars. If there is no bracketed item, the JCT estimates zero cost or savings.

SUBTITLE A: REVENUE OFFSET PROVISIONS

- A new excise tax of 40 percent (the so-called "Cadillac" tax) is levied on insurance companies and plan administrators for any health coverage plan that is above a premium threshold of $10,200 for single coverage and $27,500 for family coverage beginning in 2018. The tax applies to self-insured plans and plans sold in the group market, but not to individual market plans (except when coverage is eligible for the self-employed deduction). The tax does not apply to stand-alone dental and vision coverage. It applies to the amount of the premium in excess of the threshold and is indexed to increase at the consumer price index plus 1 percent in 2019 and at the CPI in years thereafter. A threshold increase of $1,650 for singles and $3,450 for families is available for retired individuals aged fifty-five and older and for plans that cover family members in high-risk professions. An adjustment is made for firms whose health costs are higher due to the age or gender of their workers, and the initial threshold is adjusted if there is an unexpectedly high growth in premiums before 2018 [+$32B] (section 9001).

- Employers must disclose the value of employer-provided health benefits for each employee's health insurance coverage on the worker's annual W-2 form (section 9002).

- The definition of qualified medical expenses for health savings accounts (HSAs), flexible spending arrangements (FSAs), and health reimbursement arrangements (HRAs) will conform to the definition used for the medical-expense itemized deduction. Over-the-counter medicines obtained with a prescription will still be a qualified medical expense [+$5B] (section 9003).

- The additional tax for HSA withdrawals prior to age sixty-five that are used for purposes other than qualified medical expenses is increased from 10 percent to 20 percent. The additional tax for Archer medical savings account (MSA) withdrawals not used for qualified medical expenses increases from 15 percent to 20 percent [+$1.4B] (section 9004).

- The amount of contributions to health FSAs is limited to $2,500 per year beginning in 2013. The cap is indexed at CPI-U, the consumer price index—urban, in subsequent years [+$13B] (section 9005).

- Businesses that pay any amount greater than $600 during the year to corporate and noncorporate providers of property and services must file an information report with each provider and with the IRS (this is the so-called 1099 provision). Information reporting is already required on payments for services to noncorporate providers [+$17.1B] (section 9006).

- A new annual fee is imposed on the pharmaceutical manufacturing sector: $2.5 billion in 2011, $2.8 billion in years 2012–13, $3.0 billion in 2014–16, $4.0 billion in 2017, $4.1 billion in 2018, and $2.8 billion in 2019 and years thereafter [+$27B] (section 9008).

- A new excise tax is imposed on the sale of medical devices by the manufacturer or importer equal to 2.3 percent of the sales price. The excise tax does not apply to sales of eyeglasses, contact lenses, hearing aids, or any other medical device of a type generally purchased by the public at retail [+$20B] (section 9009).

- An annual fee is assessed on the health insurance sector: $8.0 billion in 2014, $11.3 billion in years 2015–16, $13.9 billion in 2017, and $14.3 billion in 2018. This nondeductible fee is allocated across the industry according to market share and does not apply to companies whose net premiums are $50 million or less. The fee does not apply to any employer or governmental entity. Nonprofit insurers that receive more than 80 percent of their gross revenues from government programs that target low-income, elderly, or disabled populations are exempt [+$60.1B] (section 9010).

- The deduction for the subsidy paid by the federal government to employers who maintain prescription drug plans for their Medicare Part D–eligible retirees is eliminated effective for taxable years beginning after December 31, 2012 [+$4.5B] (section 9012).

- The adjusted gross income threshold for claiming the itemized deduction for medical expenses is increased from 7.5 to 10 percent. Individuals aged sixty-five and older may claim the itemized deduction for medical expenses at 7.5 percent of their adjusted gross income through 2016 [+$15.2B] (section 9013).

- The deductibility of executive compensation under section 162(m) for insurance providers is limited if at least 25 percent of the insurance provider's gross premium income from health business is derived from health insurance plans that meet minimum essential coverage requirements. The deduction is limited to $500,000 per taxable year and applies to all officers, employees, directors, and other workers or service providers performing services for or on behalf of a covered health insurance provider [+$600M] (section 9014).

- The hospital insurance tax rate is increased by 0.9 percentage points on an individual taxpayer earning more than $200,000 ($250,000 for married couples filing jointly). Revenues will be credited to the Health Insurance Trust fund. The hospital insurance tax will also include a 3.8 percent tax on income from interest, dividends, annuities, royalties, and rents on taxpayers with income above $200,000 for singles ($250,000 for married couples filing jointly) [+$210.2B] (section 9015).

- Nonprofit Blue Cross Blue Shield organizations must have a medical loss ratio of 85 percent or higher to take advantage of tax benefits provided to them under Internal Revenue Code section 833 [+$400M] (section 9016).

- A 10 percent tax is imposed on amounts paid for indoor tanning services. The tax is effective for services rendered on or after July 1, 2010 [+$2.7B] (section 9017).

KEY SECTIONS OF SUBTITLE B

- Simple cafeteria-style plans are established so that small businesses can provide tax-free benefits to their employees. Self-employed individuals may be counted as qualified employees (section 9022).

- A two-year temporary tax credit subject to a $1 billion cap is established to encourage investments in new therapies to prevent, diagnose, and treat acute and chronic diseases [less than −$900M] (section 9023).

- The adoption tax credit and adoption-assistance exclusion ($12,170 for 2009) is increased by $1,000, and the credit is made refundable [−$1.2B] (section 9025).

- The $1.01 per gallon cellulosic biofuel producer credit is modified to exclude fuels with significant water, sediment, or ash content, such as black liquor. The provision is effective for fuel sold or used after January 1, 2010 [+$23.6B] (section 1408).

- The "economic substance doctrine" that has been used by courts to deny tax benefits for transactions lacking economic substance is clarified. The provision imposes a 40 percent strict liability penalty on underpayments attributable to a transaction lacking economic substance (unless the transaction was disclosed, in which case the penalty is 20 percent) [+$4.5B] (section 1409).

· · ·

A helpful way to understand Title IX is to rank the sections according to each item's share of the $452 billion in anticipated revenue (table 8). Here, we get a different view.

Item 1 in table 8 by itself accounts for close to half of the $452 billion in new revenue in Title IX, and the top five items account for about 80 percent. Each section, like every section of the ACA has a story behind it, and there are stories relating to the title as a whole. Several of these items were altered substantially in the final reconciliation bill approved in late March 2010—especially items 1 and 3. Two items—numbers 5 and 12—were newly added in the reconciliation process.

The most significant political fight in Title IX involved the proposed tax on high-cost health insurance plans (item 3), known as the Cadillac tax. In the December 24, 2009 PPACA approved by the Senate, this section was estimated by the JCT to generate $148.9 billion over ten years, and by March 2010, it had been whittled down to $32 billion. By contrast, the change in the Medicare Hospital Insurance Tax Base (item 1), generated $86.8 billion in December's ACA, and ballooned to $210.2 billion by the final March version. The cost of trimming the Cadillac tax was addressed by substantially increasing the hit on higher-income taxpayers. And the need for more revenue in Title IX was further addressed by adding items 5 and 12—both of which had been part of the House health reform bill approved in November 2009. In December, the total revenue generated by Title IX was estimated at $398.1 billion, and by the March final version, that revenue had been increased to $452 billion. Throughout the health reform process, the House Democratic leaders had wanted a financing package with a substantial share paid by affluent Americans, and they wanted

TABLE 8. Key revenue-raising sections in Title IX

Rank	ACA section	Purpose	JCT ten-year revenue estimate (in billions of dollars)
1	9015	Broaden Medicare hospital insurance tax base for high-income taxpayers	210.2
2	9010	Impose annual fee on health insurance providers	60.1
3	9001	Impose 40% excise tax on high-cost health coverage (a.k.a. the Cadillac tax)	32.0
4	9008	Impose annual fee on manufacturers and importers of branded drugs	27.0
5	1408	Exclude unprocessed fuels ("black liquor") from the cellulosic biofuel producer credit	23.6
6	9009/ 1405	Impose excise tax on manufacturers and importers of certain medical devices	20.0
7	9006	Require information reporting on payments to corporations	17.1
8	9013	Raise the 7.5% floor on medical-expenses deduction to 10%	15.2
9	9005	Limit health flexible spending arrangements to $2,500	13.0
10	9003	Conform the definition of medical expenses for health savings accounts	5.0
11	9012	Eliminate deduction for expenses allocable to Medicare Part D subsidy	4.5
12	1409	Codify economic substance doctrine and impose penalties for underpayment	4.5
13	9017	Impose 10% excise tax on indoor tanning services	2.7

nothing to do with the Cadillac tax or the earlier effort by Senate Finance chair Max Baucus (D-MT) to change the tax treatment of private health insurance. The final version of the ACA, modified by the Reconciliation Act, moved substantially in the direction favored by the House.

A serious philosophical disagreement between Senate and House Democrats played out in Title IX, and the fight over the Cadillac tax was a symptom. Senate leaders wanted a revenue package financed largely by changes from within the health care sector while House leaders wanted a revenue package financed largely by higher-income taxes on wealthy Americans (plus taxes on employers who don't cover their workers). The income sur-tax on the wealthy included in the November 2009 House health reform bill (5.4 percent on incomes in excess of $500,000 and $1 million for joint returns) would have generated $460.5 billion in revenues by 2019, more than the total revenue generated by the full final version of all Title IX provisions. The final ACA gave both chambers part of what they wanted, though the totality of revenue and savings—including the revenue provisions of Title IX, the Medicare changes in Title III, and the Medicaid changes in Title II—result in about 75 percent of reform financed from within the health sector rather than the 50 percent preferred by House Democrats.

Let's examine the controversial sections in the order of their financial size in the final ACA.

Broadening the health insurance tax base for high-income taxpayers ($210.2 billion, section 9015). FICA—that bite out of everyone's paycheck—stands for the Federal Insurance Contributions Act and has two parts. First, there is the old-age, survivors, and disability insurance tax set at 6.2 percent of wages up to the annual limit ($106,800 in 2010). Second, there is the hospital insurance tax equal to 1.45 percent of wages. The employer pays both, 7.65 percent, and the employee pays a similar amount, withheld from wages. Section 9015 increases the hospital insurance tax by 0.9 percent on an individual taxpayer earning more than $200,000 ($250,000 for married couples filing jointly). This part was included in the December PPACA approved by the Senate and was priced by the JCT at $86.8 billion over ten years.

The reconciliation bill added an important new element to this provision—an Unearned Income Medicare Contribution as an additional hospital insurance tax of 3.8 percent on investment income for taxpayers with adjusted gross incomes in excess of $200,000 ($250,000 for joint returns). The difference between the final JCT estimate for this section of $210.2 billion and the December estimate of $86.8 billion is this provision, which was added in reconciliation, amounting to $123.4 billion over ten years.

Though this provision received scant public attention leading to passage and in the time since passage, it represents a major shift in federal tax policy—for the first time, unearned income will be subject to Medicare taxes, albeit less than for earned income. For progressives, this is an enormous and positive breakthrough in tax policy heretofore considered untouchable; to conservatives the policy is anathema. This provision is a significant factor in the conclusion reached by the Medicare trustees in August 2010 that the ACA will extend the solvency of the Medicare Hospital Insurance Trust Fund from 2017 to 2029.[4] It is impossible to imagine this provision as part of a bipartisan health reform agreement. Had it ever got to that point in negotiations, section 9015 would most certainly have been a deal breaker for Republicans. Because they were not at the table, it was an acceptable, desirable, and doable policy choice for Democrats. And the barn door is now open.

Imposing an annual fee on health insurance providers ($60.1 billion, section 9010).   This is a new fee applying to any entity engaged in the business of providing health insurance with respect to U.S. health risks, beginning after December 31, 2013. The amounts increase yearly: $8 billion in 2014, $11.3 billion in 2015 and 2016, $13.9 billion in 2017, and $14.3 billion in 2018, and are indexed to the rate of premium growth in years after that. The treasury secretary will determine who owes what based on the insurer's share of premiums written in the United States in the prior year. The fee applies only to traditional health insurance and does not apply to employers who self-insure their workforce, even when they use an insurer for administrative services. Government entities are excluded, as are nonprofit insurers when at least 80 percent of their premium revenues come from Medicare, Medicaid, or CHIP.

There are concerns with this fee. Because it does not apply to employer-based self-insured plans, it creates one more incentive for more employers to drop standard coverage and to self-insure. An estimated 59 percent of Americans with employer-based coverage obtained it through self-insured plans in 2010.[5] As more employers do this, the base of remaining traditional coverage shrinks, and the fee hits that shrinking base even harder. During the health reform process in the fall of 2009 and early 2010, congressional and administration staffers considered applying the assessment to self-insured plans as well but were dissuaded from doing so because of strenuous objections from Business Roundtable representatives, who indicated that such a move would lead the Roundtable—the only leading business organization not publicly opposing the reform law—to oppose the entire bill.

To the extent they are able, health insurance companies will pass on the fee to their customers through higher premiums. This places administration and congressional leaders in an uncomfortable position as they pressure insurers to hold down the rate of health insurance premium increases. As the size of the $60 billion fee took shape in the Senate Finance Committee's markup in September 2009, the insurance industry was not in a strong position to block it, having just released a string of critical reports on the expected impact of the reform law on premiums, the final straw for Democrats after a summer of souring relations with the industry. Combined with Title III's reductions in Medicare Advantage payments to private insurers, the insurance industry took the largest hit of any part of the health care sector in paying for the ACA. They will also reap billions in subsidized and unsubsidized premium payments as part of the mandate for most Americans to buy their products. Some cheer this result, and others condemn it. There is no denying it.

Imposing a 40 percent excise tax on high-cost employer-sponsored health coverage—a.k.a. the Cadillac tax ($32 billion, section 9001). This section creates a new 40 percent excise tax on insurers (or the plan administrator in the case of a self-insuring employer) when the aggregate value of employer-sponsored health insurance exceeds set limits. When the tax takes effect in 2018, the threshold limit is $10,200 for individual and $27,500 for family coverage, with adjustments for the age and gender of the workforce. Higher thresholds apply in the case of non-Medicare retirees over age fifty-five as well as for certain health plans where the majority of enrollees are engaged in specified high-risk professions. In 2019, the thresholds will increase by the consumer price index plus 1 percent, and after that by the CPI. Over time, more and more policies will face the threshold if, as expected, premium growth continues to exceed the growth of the CPI. The 40 percent tax applies only to the value of insurance over the threshold, so, for example, an individual policy costing $11,200 in 2018—$1,000 above the threshold—would face a $400 excise tax.

The expectation is that most employers and workers potentially subject to the excise tax will not pay it—and will instead alter their health insurance plans to avoid paying the tax, by reducing benefits, increasing cost sharing, adopting innovative plan designs and more. Further, employers will shift the money they save to higher wages, which, unlike health insurance, will be subject to federal taxes. So the largest portion of the $32 billion in expected new federal revenue will come from higher payroll taxes and not from the excise tax itself. While the 2018 implementation date draws derision from the provision's critics, who claim Congress will blink before allowing the excise tax to take effect, others suggest that employers will not wait until 2018 to begin making changes to avoid the tax and that the beneficial results may be in evidence years before actual implementation.

The label *Cadillac* is used to suggest that only excessively generous health insurance plans will be affected. However, many health insurance plans are expensive not because of excessive benefits or limited cost sharing, but because of older-than-average workforces and because they are located or concentrated in higher-cost regions such as the Northeast, leading some to complain that many "Chevy" plans will also be hit by the tax.[6] To economists hoping to break the back of medical inflation—such as Peter Orszag, former CBO director as well as President Obama's first head of the Office of Management and Budget—this provision is one of the most promising and important long-term reforms in the entire ACA, even in its whittled-down form. It had one other exclusive advantage in that it was the only provision credited by the CBO with both generating revenues and containing costs.

Instead of Cadillac or Chevy, section 9001 could also be called the "incredible shrinking tax." When Senate Finance chair Max Baucus unveiled the provision in the Finance markup in September 2009, it was projected to generate $201.4 billion in federal revenues over ten years; by the time the Senate gave its final approval to the PPACA on December 24—and a narrowed version of the Cadillac tax—its size was estimated by the JCT at $148.9 billion. By March 2010, the final version, amended by the reconciliation sidecar, had shrunk to $32 billion. Chiefly, the initial thresholds were increased from $8,000 ($21,000 for joint returns), exemptions and higher thresholds were added for certain subpopulations, and the start was pushed from 2013 to 2018—leaving some to question whether the tax will ever take effect.

The tax is the remnant of a heavily promoted idea to change the federal tax treatment of health insurance, regarded by health economists of all political stripes as a key engine for the nation's excessive rate of rising health care costs. President Ronald Reagan gave the idea its first prime time exposure as part of his tax reform agenda in 1985 and 1986—and it went nowhere. The idea to restrict the health insurance federal tax exclusion became an early and celebrated way to pay for universal coverage while taming the health inflationary beast, and no political leader embraced the concept as much as Senator Max Baucus, who made it a key part of his November 2008 health reform white paper[7] and continued to promote the idea in public hearings, speeches, and articles. His enthusiasm clashed with opposition from candidate and then president Obama, organized labor, many corporate leaders, the House of Representatives, and others. In July 2009, both the White House and Majority Leader Harry

Reid (D-NV) told Baucus to drop modification of the tax exclusion as a financing source. Senator John Kerry (D-MA) suggested the idea of a Cadillac tax as an alternative revenue source in Finance Committee circles, though not at the ambitious level envisioned by Baucus. Lacking acceptable alternatives at a point when Baucus still hoped to attract Republican votes, he embraced Kerry's revised concept and brought it to the Finance Committee in September.

How Congress and the administration will view the tax when implementation looms in 2017 and 2018 requires knowing the future occupant of the White House, as well as the identity of the majority parties in both branches of Congress at that point. The only thing knowable at this point is that the controversy over section 9001 will not go away.

Imposing an annual fee on manufacturers and importers of branded drugs ($27 billion, section 9008) *and an excise tax on manufacturers and importers of certain medical devices* ($20 billion, section 1405). Section 9008 imposes a new aggregate sector fee on the manufacturers or importers of brand-name prescription drugs, including foreign drug makers. The fee starts in 2011 at $2.5 billion, and then $2.8 billion for 2012 and 2013, $3 billion for 2014–16, $4 billion for 2017, $4.1 billion for 2018, and $2.8 billion for 2019 and years thereafter. Fees will be apportioned by the treasury secretary based on a company's share of the total branded drug sales, which will include drugs sold to or covered by government programs. Section 1405 of the Reconciliation Act imposes a tax on the sale of medical devices by a manufacturer, producer, or importer at 2.3 percent of the sales price, and includes any device defined in section 201(h) of the Food, Drug, and Cosmetic Act intended for humans, except eyeglasses, contact lenses, hearing aids, or anything defined by the HHS secretary as available for the public at retail for individual use.

Both the pharmaceutical and medical-device industries wanted to be constructive participants in the health reform process and wanted the legislation to pass. The pharmaceutical industry, represented by the Pharmaceutical Research and Manufacturers of America (PhRMA), has a long track record of effective lobbying, whether for or against a particular policy, and it brought that experience fully to bear in the 2009–10 process, negotiating the first agreement by any industry with the White House and Senate Finance Committee in June 2009. The original assessment under this section, valued at $22.2 billion over ten years by the JCT, was ratified and reflected in the Senate Finance markup as well as in the PPACA approved by the Senate in December 2009. In their efforts to identify more revenue, congressional and White House leaders decided to expand the assessment to $25 billion in the final March version, to the irritation, though not open opposition, of the drug industry.

The medical-device industry, represented by AdvaMed, brought far less experience to the table and opposed any assessment, fee, tax, or whatever else on its business. But the industry had signed on to the multi-industry letter in May 2009 stating a concerted desire to help achieve $2 trillion in ten-year health system savings, a move that brought AdvaMed representatives to the Senate Finance bargaining table whether they liked it or not—Senate staffers insist they would have been summoned regardless of the $2 trillion commitment. Senate Finance staff analysis pointed to a highly profitable industry whose success is significantly, if indirectly, tied to Medicare, Medicaid, and other government programs—Finance staff estimates that Medicare pays for more than half its business. Finance staffer Jon Selib started the bidding at $60 billion in industry contributions, and the industry reciprocated with a counter offer of zero. Baucus included $38.6 billion in the Senate Finance markup, and Majority Leader Harry Reid dropped it to $19.2 billion in the December PPACA and $20 billion in the final March version, a concession demanded by Senators Evan Bayh (D-IN) and Amy Klobuchar (D-MN) as a condition for their December votes. Also, the House of Representatives included a $20 billion excise tax on medical devices—the only such assessment on a health-related industry included in the November 2009 House legislation; Speaker Nancy Pelosi assured her members of a $20 billion ceiling, and that's where it ended. The House also prevailed in reconciliation regarding the nature of the device industry tax. The Senate had proposed an industry-wide fee resembling the one placed on insurers and drug makers, but the House insisted on a flat and predictable excise tax. The House version put more pressure on smaller device companies and less pressure on the larger players, and the Senate version did the reverse. Unlike the pharmaceutical industry, the medical-device industry continues to publicly oppose the fee and will advocate to repeal it up to and, if necessary, after it takes effect on December 31, 2012.

Excluding unprocessed fuels from the cellulosic biofuel producer credit ($23.6 billion, section 1408).   This section could win the prize for the oddest item in the entire ACA and gives a window into the arcane world of federal tax policy. The provision modifies an existing cellulosic biofuel producer credit to exclude black liquor from eligibility, and the JCT estimates the exclusion will save the federal government about $23.6 billion. What does this have to do with health care? Nothing except that it gets credit for $23.6 billion in revenue to help pay for the ACA.

Black liquor is a byproduct of wood that can be turned into fuel and has been used since the 1930s by pulp and paper companies to power their plants. While Congress never intended it, the IRS ruled in 2009 that the byproduct is eligible for a biofuel producer tax credit that is set to expire at the end of 2012—and the estimated cost to the federal treasury of subsidizing black liquor could reach $23.6 billion.

Congressional Democrats have had black liquor on their radar screen since the IRS ruling and planned to close the loophole to pay for the 2009 extension of unemployment benefits and a tax credit for first-time homebuyers. When it became clear that the black liquor loophole closing would not be needed for that, House leaders included it in their health reform legislation in November 2009. The Senate, with a smaller health reform price tag, left the provision out, keeping it in reserve to pay for other anticipated legislation. In early 2010, as leaders struggled to put a new financing plan together, House, Senate, and White House leaders all agreed that it was time to close the black liquor loophole and that the ACA was the place to do it. Some paper industry representatives claim the tax credit would not be used at all or to the extent claimed by budget estimators. Since the credit has already been repealed, that is one assertion that will never be verified as true or false.[8]

Expanding requirements for reports on payments to corporations ($17.1 billion, section 9006). This section, also known as the 1099 provision, expands the scope of information required to be reported to the IRS by persons engaged in a trade or business who make payments exceeding $600 per year to a single payee, including compensation. The primary purpose of this provision is to help the IRS determine whether those corporate and contractor tax returns are accurate and complete. The expanded scope in the ACA amends section 6041 of the IRS Code to require reporting of all payments exceeding $600 to for-profit corporations made after December 31, 2011, including payments for goods and services. Under prior law, businesses only needed to report services by noncorporate entities, chiefly independent contractors.

This provision began generating strong controversy and opposition from the business community beginning in the summer of 2010 because of the potentially massive paperwork burden it will place on companies of all sizes. The expectation among drafters was that improved reporting would enhance revenue collections by between $2 billion and $3.3 billion per year beginning in 2013, totaling $17.1 billion by 2019. The provision was included in both the House and Senate bills approved in November and December 2009, respectively, as well as in the Senate Finance markup in October. The policy rationale was to address the substantial underpayment of federal taxes by increasing reporting requirements on responsible parties as a way to catch the underpayers. From the early months following passage, this provision emerged as one of the most likely sections to be significantly revised or repealed, and in April 2011 Congress did just that, making section 9006 the first part of the ACA to be repealed and financed by tightening rules on recipients of premium subsidies.

Raising the 7.5 percent floor on the medical-expenses tax deduction to 10 percent ($15.2 billion, section 9013); *limiting health flexible spending arrangements to $2,500* ($13 billion, section 9005); and *conforming the definition of medical expenses for health savings accounts* ($5 billion, section 9003).   These three sections all tighten the rules for individuals and the tax treatment of their medical expenses and alternative insurance policies, including health savings accounts (HSAs) and flexible spending arrangements (FSAs), combining for $33 billion in new revenues through 2019. All three were included in the Senate Finance markup, the December PPACA approved by the Senate, and they were not altered in the legislative outcome in March. The first item was not included in the House-approved legislation in November 2009, while the other two were included.

The first section, 9013, increases the threshold for claiming an itemized deduction for unreimbursed medical expenses for tax purposes from 7.5 to 10 percent of adjusted gross income after December 31, 2012; however, the increased threshold will not apply until 2017 for taxpayers who are turning sixty-five in any of the intervening years. The second section creates a $2,500 cap on the amount of medical expenses available under a flexible spending arrangement that can be used on a pretax basis for unreimbursed medical expenses. The $2,500 limit will increase each year by the consumer price index. An analysis by Hewitt Associates found that 20 percent of U.S. workers contributed to an FSA in 2010, and of those, 18 percent contributed more than the new limit of $2,500, and those who did tended to be individuals earning more than $150,000.[9] A coalition to "Save Flexible Spending Plans"[10] sponsored by the Employers Council on Flexible Compensation[11] was unable to eliminate the provision, though they were successful in incorporating the indexing provision favored by the House.

The third section eliminates nontaxable reimbursements through HSAs, FSAs, and medical savings arrangements for over-the-counter medications unless those drugs are prescribed by a physician—thus conforming the standard for these drugs to the broader IRS deduction for medical expenses.

Eliminating the deduction for expenses allocable to the Medicare Part D subsidy ($4.5 billion, section 9012).   This section alters a feature of the Part D Medicare Drug Program established by Congress and President Bush as part of the 2003 Medicare Drug Improvement and Modernization Act (MMA). Under that law, employers who continue to provide prescription drug coverage to their retirees are eligible for a federal subsidy payment for a portion of each retiree's drug costs, known as the "qualified retiree prescription drug plan subsidy." The subsidy was created as an incentive for employers to continue providing retiree drug coverage because it is cheaper for the government than providing coverage to these retirees through Part D, even with the subsidy. The subsidy amounts to 28 percent of the employer drug costs above the minimum beneficiary threshold ($310 in 2010). Under the MMA, employers were allowed to claim as a tax deduction the amount of money they actually spent on retiree drug costs as well as the value of the subsidy they obtained from the federal government. Section 9012, as of December 31, 2012, disallows the value of the federal subsidy to be claimed as a deductible business expense, providing $4.5 billion to pay for the ACA. As the JCT explains:

> For example, assume a company receives a subsidy of $28 with respect to eligible drug expenses of $100. The $28 is excludable from income under section 139A, and the amount otherwise allowable as a deduction is reduced by the $28. Thus, if the company otherwise meets the requirements of section 162 with respect to its eligible drug expenses, it would be entitled to an ordinary business expense deduction of $72.[12]

And not $100, one might add. Less than a week after President Obama signed the ACA into law, the American Benefits Council, representing about three hundred employers nationwide, urged repeal of this provision as Caterpillar, 3M, and other national corporations revised their financial statements negatively to account for the deduction's new restriction. AT&T projected a $1 billion loss over a period of decades. Companies also suggested they would reexamine the continuation of retiree drug coverage because of the ACA change. But after an initial flurry, the issue has dropped from view.[13]

Codifying the economic substance doctrine and imposing penalties for underpayment ($4.5 billion, section 1409).   Like section 1408 on the cellulosic biofuel producer credit, this section has nothing to do with health care except to provide revenue to pay for it. The section puts into federal law the so-called economic substance doctrine, which is a "common law doctrine that has been applied by courts to deny tax benefits arising from transactions that do not result in a meaningful change to the taxpayer's economic position other than a purported reduction in Federal income tax, even though the purported activity actually occurred."[14] Taxpayers who engage in this activity and do not disclose it to the IRS will face a 40 percent strict liability penalty, while taxpayers who disclose the activity and are found in violation will face a 20 percent strict liability penalty—this is where the estimated $4.5 billion in revenue will be found.

Proposals to codify the economic substance doctrine go back to President Bill Clinton's budget proposal for federal fiscal year 2000, submitted to Congress in February 1999, and codification has been made part of various legislative proposals in subsequent years, never achieving passage until the signing of the ACA in March 2010. This proposal was included in the November 2009 House health reform plan but not in the various Senate versions and was added in the reconciliation package. Critics have complained that the statutory requirements triggering the penalty are untested and ambiguous.[15] The CBO scored them, however, and that is what counted in the health reform process.

Imposing a 10 percent excise tax on indoor tanning services ($2.7 billion, section 9017).   This section imposes a tax on each individual on whom indoor tanning services are performed, equaling 10 percent of the amount paid. The tax applies only to services employing an electronic product designed to induce skin tanning and that uses ultraviolet lamps emitting ultraviolet radiation. The tax is designed to be paid by the individual receiving the service.

The tax was inserted into the final version of the ACA approved by the Senate in December 2009 to replace a proposed 5 percent tax on cosmetic surgery and other similar elective procedures. Derided and praised as the "Bo-tax" because it taxed the wrinkle-smoothing injection Botox and other cosmetic procedures, it would have raised an estimated $5.8 billion, compared with $2.7 billion in estimated revenue from the "tanning tax." In the four weeks between the release of the first version of the ACA in November and the release of the final version, which included Majority Leader Harry Reid's Manager's Amendment, the American Academy of

Dermatology, with support from the American Medical Association and many consumers, raised a storm of objections to the proposed Bo-tax.

The sudden shift in December from cosmetic procedures to tanning caught the Indoor Tanning Association off guard and unable to mount an effective campaign to thwart the tax, which does not apply to similar procedures in physician offices, gyms, or fitness centers. "Repeal the Tan Tax Now," is the association's new motto.[16] But the tax has public support from the same American Academy of Dermatology that opposed the Bo-tax because of the documented link between indoor tanning before the age of thirty-five and a 75 percent increase in melanoma, the deadliest form of skin cancer.

Indeed, the tanning tax could be the most positive revenue source in the entire ACA from a public health and prevention standpoint. Among the estimated 30 million users of tanning beds, about 2.3 million are teenagers.[17] Among all cancers in the United States, the incidence of melanoma is increasing the most rapidly, including an alarming increase among girls and women between the ages of fifteen and thirty-nine, with an estimated annual increase of 2.7 percent among this group between 1992 and 2004.[18] Recent studies have suggested an opiate-like addiction to the treatment by frequent users.[19] Numerous nations have tightened restrictions on indoor tanning, and some—France, Germany, Austria, Britain—have banned access to the treatment by minors. While the U.S. Food and Drug Administration is reviewing the safety of the procedure, the new tax will have some impact in reducing use.

. . .

Another list long ago landed in DC paper-shredders—the list of items *not* included in Title IX, whether for policy or political reasons, and often that categorization is in the eye of the beholder. The health insurance tax exclusion was not touched, albeit broached in the "Cadillac" excise tax; elective cosmetic surgery was not taxed; sugared beverages were not taxed, nor were alcohol, tobacco, or other sources connected with adverse health outcomes (often called "sin taxes," which some staffers made the case to push); nor was online pornography, which got a closer look by Senate Finance staffers than anyone has revealed to date.

The legendary New York Mayor Fiorello LaGuardia said: "Politics is very much like taxes—everybody is against them, or everybody is for them as long as they don't apply to him."[20] The assortment of new taxes, fees, and assessments included in Title IX was assembled to provide narrowly crafted burdens on a range of sources. Some, such as the new information reporting requirement on business, will be eliminated or altered, while most seem likely to stick at least for the foreseeable future.

Since passage, I have participated in debates on the ACA with opponents of the law who invariably seek to shock audiences with statements such as "And they paid for it by doing X" and "They paid for it by doing Y." When it's my turn, I note that there is no way to pay for any significant legislation without disturbing and angering whoever is required to pay. The essential difference in fiscal policy between the ACA and the 2003 Medicare Modernization Act as well as the other signal policy initiatives of the Bush administration (the 2001 and 2003 tax cuts plus wars in Iraq and Afghanistan) is that the Obama administration and the Democratic congressional leaders "paid for it."

14. Title X-Plus—The Manager's Amendment and the Health Care Education and Reconciliation Act

In a "normal" federal legislative process, Title X would never have been advanced as a stand-alone title, and the Reconciliation Act would never have been advanced as a stand-alone bill. Instead, the numerous large and small changes they make—Title X amends provisions in Titles I through IX, and the subsequent Health Care and Education Reconciliation Act (HCERA) amends provisions in Titles I through X—would have been blended into the underlying legislation, and a single, coherent, comprehensive substitute PPACA would have been approved on the floor of the Senate in the case of Title X and by both the Senate and House in the matter of reconciliation. In a normal legislative process, the budget reconciliation process would not have been used at all—though it has been used frequently by both parties over several decades for legislation large and small.

As we have seen, little in the health reform drive from June 2008 until March 2010 resembled a normal legislative process. It was extraordinary whether one views it as extraordinarily good or bad. This strange process reflects deep divisions in American society regarding the future of U.S. health care as well as divisions over the related tax and financing policies to enable it. The unusual process also reflects the changing nature of the U.S. Senate and House of Representatives toward more harshly partisan and divided institutions where behavior has become much more regimented along party lines—Democrat and Republican members who strayed from the party line on health reform found themselves in one of the most uncomfortable positions in their political lives. In a legislative assembly, when individuals like and trust each other, the most difficult challenges can be overcome with seeming ease; and when individuals dislike and mistrust each other, the simplest tasks can be impossible to accomplish. Particularly in the U.S. Senate, this latter dynamic is fully operational (while the House is more stridently partisan, majority rule and the lack of a filibuster means that work gets done). Finally, the difficult process reflects the divisions in the nation over the course and direction of the new Obama presidency in 2009 and 2010, in which health reform was a central, though not sole, top-tier priority.

So the messiness of Title X and the HCERA reflects the messiness all around. For the first few months after President Obama signed both bills, it made difficult even the chore of reading and understanding the underlying ACA law. First, one had to read the underlying text of Titles I–IX—already challenging because of the extent to which the ACA text amends other complex federal statutes; then one had to read Title X in case anything in it changed anything in the previous nine titles; then one had to read the HCERA in case anything in there changed anything in ACA Titles I–X. It was not until late spring 2010 that the Legislative Counsel's Offices in the Senate and House produced a single, consolidated version of the two laws—and for reading purposes only. When in doubt, it's the original text and awkward structure that count.

For this final chapter in Part II, we deviate from the format used in the chapters describing Titles I–IX. This chapter first describes the process leading to the creation of Title X, also called the Manager's Amendment, followed by an overview of the process leading to the creation of the HCERA, also called the reconciliation sidecar. Following these is a selected outline of the key provisions in Title X and the sidecar. Following that is a discussion of several noteworthy provisions not discussed in prior chapters.

THE MANAGER'S AMENDMENT

The Senate Finance Committee finished its markup process on October 16, 2009, following action by the Health, Education, Labor and Pensions Committee (HELP) on the previous July 15. Many titles and large portions of the two bills were complementary, reflecting each committee's singular jurisdiction, and so combining those elements was not onerous. Title I on coverage was shared by both committees, and so combining the HELP and Senate Finance Committee versions involved both significant policy decisions and immense technical and language complexity. Staff of the two committees, along with staffers from Majority Leader Harry Reid's office and Obama administration staff, began meeting in September to accomplish the "merge" as fast as possible. At this point, most political pressure shifted to focus on Reid who, until then, had largely left the committees to their own devices.

In producing a combined bill, Reid had major decisions to make—for example, whether to require the inclusion of a so-called public option in the state exchanges, and whether to include the CLASS Act, just for starters. He and his staff, led by his chief health aide, Kate Leone, also had to round up the votes of sixty members, not to approve a bill, but simply to allow debate to proceed. With sixty Democratic Caucus members (Senator Edward Kennedy, who passed away on August 25, 2009, had been replaced by Democrat Paul Kirk until an election for a permanent successor would be held in January), and only one Republican in play, Senator Olympia Snowe (R-ME), Reid had almost no margin for error. His first mission was not to construct a bill that could pass but to construct a bill that could receive sixty votes to proceed, fully recognizing that more changes would need to be made before a final bill won Senate approval. On November 19, more than two weeks after the House of Representatives approved its version of health reform, Reid unveiled his merged legislative proposal, along with budget scores from the Congressional Budget Office and the Joint Committee on Taxation and the news that he had sixty confirmed votes to proceed. Many of those sixty—all Democratic Caucus members—made it clear their votes to proceed would not be followed by votes to approve the bill without significant changes. On late Saturday evening, November 21, the weekend before Thanksgiving, the Senate voted sixty to thirty-nine to begin debate on the PPACA.

While debate on the Senate floor unfolded, Reid began meeting with all of his fifty-nine Democratic colleagues plus Olympia Snowe to find out what they needed changed before they would commit to a final aye vote for passage. Dick Durbin (IL), Charles Schumer (NY), Patty Murray (WA), Max Baucus (MT), Chris Dodd (CT), and Tom Harkin (IA) were his key lieutenants. With only days to go until Christmas, Reid unveiled his Manager's Amendment, eighty-nine sections of revisions, large and small, noticed and unnoticed, most promoted by one or more Democratic Caucus members (the Snowe chase ended in early December), with many declaring that Reid would not have their vote without the change they wanted. Under the standard legislative process, the amendments would be inserted and melded into the underlying base bill in the appropriate sections, and a single vote would be held to move forward with a substitute bill. In this case, though, Republicans made it clear they would use the rules to require a cloture vote on each individual change—a real threat that would effectively shut down the Senate. As an unorthodox alternative, Reid's team strategized to consolidate all the changes into a separate new Title X, so that all amendments would be subject to only one packaged cloture process and vote. Democratic members and staffers comforted themselves with the knowledge that after the Senate gave the bill approval, the final merger process with the House would produce a coherent single piece of legislation that would wash away the mess. Title X was never intended to have a lifespan of more than a few weeks.

Several days before Christmas, all Democratic Caucus members having been sufficiently satisfied by Reid, all sixty voted to proceed to a vote to adopt the Manager's Amendment, setting the stage for the final Senate vote at 7 a.m. on December 24 to approve the PPACA.

THE RECONCILIATION SIDECAR

In the normal federal legislative process, after both branches have approved major, complex legislation, a bipartisan conference committee with members from both branches is convened to merge the two versions into a single bill for up or down final action in both chambers. When House and Senate leaders and staff returned from the holiday break in early January 2010, there was no discussion of setting up a conference committee. Senate Republican leaders, similar to their stance on the Manager's Amendment, made it clear they would use every procedural device at their disposal to slow down the forming and naming of a conference committee—a delay that could consume literally months. In response, Senate and House Democratic leaders determined to use a process called ping-pong to negotiate in private an agreement on a final bill without a conference and then to have the bill approved consecutively in each branch. The final key Senate action to approve the merged bill would again require sixty votes to overcome a certain filibuster. Between January 5 and 19, key members and staff, directed by the White House, met intensely to negotiate and merge the two immense health reform bills into one unified legislative vehicle.

The January 19, 2010, election of Republican Scott Brown to the Senate seat formerly held by Senator Edward Kennedy and the loss of a sixty-seat Democratic Caucus majority ended ping-pong as an effective legislative strategy. Only one pathway emerged as viable, with two parts. The first part involved the House approving the Senate-enacted PPACA in whole, with no changes, thus eliminating the need for any further Senate vote on the bill, sixty votes or otherwise. The second part involved using a budget reconciliation bill, which would require only fifty-one votes for Senate approval and not be subject to any filibuster, to make changes to the PPACA agreeable to both chambers and the White House.

Senate Republican members had expressed virulent opposition throughout 2008 and early 2009 to the use of reconciliation to pass health reform. Some influential Democrats, especially Budget chair Kent Conrad (D-ND), agreed and cautioned his progressive colleagues that the reconciliation process included strict budget rules that would narrow severely the scope and viability of any health reform legislation. A prime example of the special difficulty is a process, named after the late Senator Robert Byrd (D-WV), lead architect of the reconciliation rules in the 1970s, nicknamed the "Byrd bath," allowing any member to challenge any provision (or portion of any provision) of a reconciliation bill that does not have a direct and substantive, positive or negative impact on the federal budget. In this new post–January 19 context, though, Conrad readily agreed that an appropriately drawn bill that only amended PPACA provisions meeting the Byrd test was legitimate, and he agreed to play the lead role in structuring and shepherding the legislative vehicle to do so.

The House approved the agreed-upon reconciliation legislation on March 21, 2010, immediately after voting to approve the Senate-crafted PPACA. The Senate then began a weeklong process on the bill; closed sessions conducted by the Senate parliamentarian resembled courtroom scenes where Democratic and Republican staffers made their case for any or against the fealty of challenged provisions to the Byrd test. Senate Democratic staffers prepared intensively for the final round, and their hard work showed as all major Republican points of order were ruled for the Democrats, with only two minor provisions struck, and thus requiring one final House vote before the sidecar bill was sent to the president's desk for his signature.

Following are descriptions of major provisions of Title X and then descriptions of major provisions of the Reconciliation Act.

UNDERSTANDING TITLE X

This is an overview of Title X of the ACA, the Manager's Amendment, also titled "Strengthening Quality, Affordable Health Care for All Americans." It has eighty-nine sections and is divided among these eight subtitles (there were no changes to Title VII, biosimilars):

Subtitle A: Provisions Relating to Title I—Private coverage

Subtitle B: Provisions Relating to Title II—Medicaid and CHIP

Subtitle C: Provisions Relating to Title III—Medicare and delivery reform

Subtitle D: Provisions Relating to Title IV—Prevention and wellness

Subtitle E: Provisions Relating to Title V—Health workforce

Subtitle F: Provisions Relating to Title VI—Fraud and abuse and transparency

Subtitle G: Provisions Relating to Title VIII—CLASS

Subtitle H: Provisions Relating to Title IX—Revenue

Following is a brief overview of key sections, with the number of each selected section at the end of each bullet in parentheses. In brackets is the ten-year savings score estimated by the CBO and the JCT (in the case of Title IX). A plus sign (+) means the section will cost the federal treasury billions (B) or millions (M) and a minus sign (−) means the provision will save federal dollars. If there is no bracketed item, the CBO or JCT estimates zero cost or savings. Also included are the names of the key senators associated with each provision.

Subtitle A includes changes to Title I addressing private health insurance coverage. Major amendments include restructuring the ban on lifetime and annual insurance limits, altering rules affecting medical loss ratios, modifying patient protection provisions, and changing the rules on coverage of abortion services. Other new sections include the following provisions:

- Group health plans and health insurance issuers must provide coverage of costs for individuals participating in approved clinical trials (Sherrod Brown, D-OH) (section 10103).

- The federal Office of Personnel Management will facilitate the offering of at least two nonprofit multistate insurance plans to be made available through the insurance exchanges in each state (section 10104).

- Employers offering health coverage to their workers must provide free-choice vouchers to qualified employees if the worker wants to buy a qualified health plan through a state exchange. The voucher's value must equal the contribution the employer would have made to its own plan for the worker. Workers qualify if their required insurance premium contribution would be between 8 and 9.8 percent of their income (Ron Wyden, D-OR) [+$4B] (section 10108).

Subtitle B includes changes to Title II addressing Medicaid and the Children's Health Insurance Program (CHIP). Provisions include 100 percent coverage of incremental Medicaid costs for Nebraska (later removed under the Reconciliation Act), plus additional assistance for Louisiana, and extension of CHIP funding through 2015. New sections include the following provisions:

- A financial incentive is created for states to shift Medicaid beneficiaries out of nursing homes and into home- and community-based services (Maria Cantwell, D-WA, and Herb Kohl, D-WI) (section 10202).

- A Pregnancy Assistance Fund will award competitive grants to states to assist pregnant and parenting teens and women (sections 10212–14).

- The Indian Health Care Improvement Act is reauthorized, including programs to expand the Indian health care workforce, create innovative delivery models, improve behavioral health, enhance health promotion and disease prevention, improve access to services, construct facilities, and create a youth suicide prevention grant program (Byron Dorgan, D-ND) (section 10221).

Subtitle C includes changes to Title III addressing Medicare and delivery-system reform. Major provisions revise the Medicare shared savings program, the payment bundling program, the hospital readmissions program, home health payment reductions, and provider market basket reductions. Other new key sections include the following provisions:

- Medicare coverage and screening will be provided to individuals exposed to environmental health hazards determined under the Comprehensive Environmental Response, Compensation, and Liability Act of 1980 (Max Baucus, D-MT) [+$300M] (section 10323).

- Beginning in 2011, Medicare hospital wage-index and geographic-practice expense floors are established for hospitals and physicians in states where at least 50 percent of the counties are frontier (Kent Conrad and Byron Dorgan, both D-ND) [+$2B] (section 10324).

- The HHS secretary may test value-based purchasing programs for inpatient rehabilitation facilities, inpatient psychiatric hospitals, long-term care hospitals, certain cancer hospitals, and hospice providers (freshmen senators) (section 10326).

- Medicare Part D plans must include medication reviews and a written summary as part of medication therapy management programs (freshmen senators) (section 10328).

- The HHS secretary will develop a Physician Compare website where Medicare beneficiaries can compare measures of physician quality and patient experience (Susan Collins, R-ME, and Joe Lieberman, I-CT) (section 10331).

- The Office of Minority Health is codified within the DHHS. The National Center on Minority Health and Health Disparities at the National Institutes of Health (NIH) is upgraded from a center to an institute. The Offices of Minority Health will monitor health, health care trends, and quality of care among minority patients and evaluate the success of minority-health programs and initiatives (Ben Cardin, D-MD, and Roland Burris, D-IL) (section 10334).

Subtitle D includes changes to Title IV addressing prevention and public health. Amendments include changes to the treatment of co-insurance for preventive services. Following are new additional sections:

- The HHS secretary shall develop a national report card on diabetes, to be updated every two years (Kay Hagan, D-NC) (section 10407).

- An NIH Cures Acceleration Network is created and authorized to award grants and contracts to accelerate the development of medical products and behavioral therapies (Arlen Specter, D-PA) (section 10409).

- The administrator of the HHS Substance Abuse and Mental Health Services Administration will award grants to centers of excellence for the treatment of depressive disorders (Debbie Stabenow, D-MI) (section 10410).

- The HHS secretary may track the epidemiology of congenital heart disease and organize a National Congenital Heart Disease Surveillance System. NIH research on congenital heart disease will be expanded, intensified, and coordinated (Richard Durbin, D-IL) (section 10411).

- A national education campaign for young women and health professionals about breast health and risk factors for breast cancer and enhanced prevention research will be developed by the CDC (Amy Klobuchar, D-MN) (section 10413).

Subtitle E includes changes to Title V addressing health workforce needs:

- A national diabetes prevention program is established at the CDC (freshmen senators) (section 10501).

- The National Health Service Corps is improved by increasing the loan repayment amount, allowing for half-time service and for teaching to account for up to 20 percent of the corps service commitment (Bernie Sanders, I-VT) (section 10501).

- The Community Health Centers and National Health Service Corps Fund is established to expand and sustain the national investment in community health centers under section 330 of the Public Health Service Act and the National Health Service Corps. Mandatory funding for community health centers is increased to $11 billion over five years, from FY 2011 through FY 2015 (Bernie Sanders, I-VT) [+$11B] (section 10503).

Subtitle F includes changes to Title VI of the ACA addressing health care fraud and abuse and related issues:

- Grants to states are authorized to test alternatives to civil tort litigation. These models must emphasize patient safety, the disclosure of health care errors, and the early resolution of disputes. Patients may opt out of these alternatives at any time (Tom Carper, D-DE) (section 10607).

- Liability protections contained in the Federal Tort Claims Act are extended to free clinics (Patrick Leahy, D-VT) [+$100M] (section 10608).

Subtitle H includes changes to Title IX of the ACA, which incorporates revenue items to help pay for the cost of the legislation. Key changes included modifications to the excise tax on high-cost employer-sponsored health coverage, to the limits on flexible spending arrangements, and to the fees on medical-device makers and health insurance providers, elimination of the tax on cosmetic procedures along with the addition of a new tax on indoor tanning services.

Amendments Included in the Health Care and Education Reconciliation Act

These are key provisions of the Reconciliation Act, described below in the following subtitles.

Subtitle A: Provisions Relating to Coverage

Subtitle B: Provisions Relating to Medicare

Subtitle C: Provisions Relating to Medicaid

Subtitle D: Provisions Relating to Fraud, Waste, and Abuse

Subtitle E: Provisions Relating to Revenues

Key Sections of the Amendments

Subtitle A includes changes to the Title I private coverage sections of the ACA. All the sections in Subtitle A add $161.4 billion in costs for 2010–19.

- Financing for premiums and cost sharing for individuals with incomes up to 400 percent of the federal poverty level is enhanced to make subsidized premiums and cost sharing more affordable, especially for those with incomes below 250 percent of the FPL. Starting in 2019, the growth in premium tax credits is constrained if premiums grow faster than the consumer price index, unless spending is more than 10 percent below current CBO projections (section 1001).

- The assessment on individuals who choose to remain uninsured is changed in three ways: (1) income below the filing threshold is exempted, (2) the flat payment is lowered from $495 to $325 in 2015 and from $750 to $695 in 2016, and (3) the percent of income that is an alternative payment amount is raised from 0.5 to 1.0 percent in 2014, 1.0 to 2.0 percent in 2015, and 2.0 to 2.5 percent in 2016 and subsequent years to make the assessment more progressive (section 1002).

- The employer-responsibility policy is changed to subtract the first thirty full-time employees from the payment calculation. The provision changes the payment amount for firms that do not offer coverage to $3,000 per full-time employee. Employers who offer coverage but whose employees receive tax credits will see the aggregate cap on payments increased to $2,000. Also, the assessment for workers in waiting periods is eliminated (section 1003).

- The HHS secretary will be provided with $1 billion to finance the administrative costs of implementing health insurance reform (section 1005).

Subtitle B includes changes to Title III, the Medicare sections of the ACA:

- A $250 rebate is provided for all Medicare Part D enrollees who enter the doughnut hole in 2010. The pharmaceutical makers' 50 percent discount on brand-name drugs beginning in 2011 is expanded to include new federal support to provide 75 percent coverage by 2020 to fill the doughnut hole [+$24.8B] (section 1101).

- Medicare Advantage payments are frozen in 2011. Beginning in 2012, benchmarks are reduced relative to current levels. Benchmarks will vary from 95 percent of Medicare spending in high-cost areas to 115 percent in low-cost areas, with benchmarks increased for high-quality plans. MA plans must spend at least 85 percent of revenue on medical costs or activities that improve quality of care, rather than for profit and overhead [−$17B] (sections 1102–3).

- Cuts for Medicare disproportionate share hospitals will begin in fiscal year 2014 and the ten-year reduction is lowered by $3 billion [+$3B] (section 1104).

- The hospital market basket reduction is changed as follows: −0.3 in FY 2014 and −0.75 in FY 2017, FY 2018, and FY 2019. Providers affected are inpatient hospitals, long-term care hospitals, inpatient rehabilitation facilities, psychiatric hospitals, and outpatient hospitals [−$9.8B] (section 1105).

- An additional payment is provided under the Medicare inpatient prospective-payment system to hospitals in counties in the bottom quartile of counties as ranked by risk-adjusted spending per Medicare enrollee [+$400M] (section 1109).

Subtitle C includes changes to Title II, the Medicaid and public programs sections of the ACA:

- The provision for a permanent 100 percent federal matching rate for Nebraska for Medicaid costs of newly eligible individuals is struck. Federal Medicaid matching payments for the costs of services to newly eligible individuals are set at the following rates: 100 percent in 2014, 2015, and 2016; 95 percent in 2017; 94 percent in 2018; 93 percent in 2019; and 90 percent thereafter. Beginning in 2019, expansion states will receive the same federal Medicaid payments as other states for newly eligible and previously eligible nonpregnant childless adults [+$39B] (section 1201).

- Medicaid payment rates to primary care physicians must be no less than 100 percent of Medicare payment rates in 2013 and 2014. Federal funding will finance 100 percent of the additional costs to States [+$8.3B] (section 1202).

- The reduction in federal Medicaid disproportionate-share hospital payments is lowered from $18.1 billion to $14.1 billion and will begin in fiscal year 2014 [+$4.1B] (section 1203).

Subtitle D includes changes to Title VI, the fraud, waste, and abuse sections of the ACA:

- Funding for the Health Care Fraud and Abuse Control program is increased by $250 million for 2010–19, and the fund is indexed based on consumer price increases [+$300M] (section 1303).

Subtitle E includes changes to Title IX, the revenue sections of the ACA (described in detail in chapter 13). (*Note*: In this Subtitle E outline, a plus sign means that the provision raises federal revenues, not federal costs.)

- A 40 percent excise tax (the "Cadillac" tax) is levied on insurance companies and plan administrators for any health coverage plan when its cost is above a threshold of $10,200 for single coverage and $27,500 for family coverage [+$32B] (section 1401).

- The tax treatment is equalized for earned and unearned income under the Medicare contribution for taxpayers with income above $200,000 ($250,000 for married couples filing jointly). The provision imposes a 3.8 percent tax on income from interest, dividends, annuities, royalties, and rents that are not derived in the ordinary course of trade or business, excluding active S corporation or partnership income [+$210.2B] (section 1402).

- The fee on pharmaceutical manufacturers is changed to the following amounts: $2.5 billion in 2011, $2.8 billion in years 2012–13, $3.0 billion in years 2014–16, $4.0 billion in 2017, $4.1 billion in 2018, and $2.8 billion in 2019 and years thereafter [+$27B] (section 1404).

- The fee on medical-device manufacturers is replaced with an excise tax on the sale of medical devices made by the manufacturer or sold from an importer equal to 2.3 percent of the sales price. The excise tax will not apply to the sale of eyeglasses, contact lenses, hearing aids, or any device generally purchased by the public at retail. The provision is effective for sales after December 31, 2012 [+$20B] (section 1405).

• The fee on health insurance providers is changed as follows: $8.0 billion in 2014, $11.3 billion in years 2015–16, $13.9 billion in 2017, and $14.3 billion in 2018 [+$60.1B] (section 1406).

• • •

The Reconciliation Act, as discussed in the previous chapter on Title IX and revenues, changed both expenses and revenues. Table 9 shows both the major new cost items in the Reconciliation Act as well as the major new revenue provisions.

Including all the cost and revenue provisions in the Reconciliation Act, the cumulative ten-year impact on the federal deficit, as estimated by the CBO, resulted in $14.4 billion in additional savings. The significant new expenses were all high priorities for the Democratic leaders of the House of Representatives, particularly improving the affordability of coverage subsidies. The two items labeled "interactions" refer to the estimated indirect budgetary impact of those provisions; for example, by lowering the cost of the Part C Medicare Advantage program, savings are also realized in the fee-for-service physician expenses in Medicare Part B. In this example, the ten-year savings at nearly $53 billion is substantial, achieved because the final Medicare Advantage provision resembles the House version (where the expected effects were even higher) more than it does the Senate version.

One other important item of note—important from both coverage and budgetary perspectives—involves section 1001 of the Reconciliation Act regarding premium tax credits. The first part improves the affordability of premiums and cost sharing for those receiving coverage subsidies—a concern for House leaders and Senate progressives. The second part addresses only the second decade of the law and, beginning in 2019, "constrains the growth in tax credits if premiums are growing faster than the consumer price index." This change was added to achieve a positive CBO score for the second decade of the law, an important budgetary and political statement. Yet the change, if implemented as written, will result in potentially major increases in premiums and cost sharing that subsidy recipients will be required to pay beginning that year and growing year by year. Addressing this, and thus improving affordability, would have a significant negative impact on the budget outlook for the ACA in its second decade. This provision will be a major challenge for future Congresses as 2019 approaches.

TABLE 9.   Key new expenses (+) and revenues/savings (−)
in the Reconciliation Act

Section	Purview	Impact in 2010–19 (in billions of dollars)
New expenses		
1001–4	Coverage provisions	+160.4
1101	Medicare doughnut hole	+24.8
*	Interaction effects of IPAB	+12.6
1201	Federal funding to states	+8.3
1202	Medicaid payments to primary care physicians	+4.1
New revenues		
Title IX	Revenue provision changes	−155.9
*	Medicare Advantage interactions	−52.9
1102	Medicare Advantage payments	−17.0
1105	Provider market basket updates	−9.8

* Not applicable

The Freshmen's Offensive

Senator Mark Warner (D-VA), the former governor of Virginia and a successful business executive, served on none of the committees involved in health reform, and as a freshman senator first elected in 2008, he had no institutional role enabling him to be a player. He wanted health reform to happen and he wanted to be an active participant, so in September 2009, as Senate Finance was struggling through its markup, he suggested to his freshman Democratic colleagues that they go to the floor as a group to speak in support of reform. When ten colleagues joined him and they all liked the experience, they decided to do it weekly. After a few weeks, Warner suggested that they consider formulating their own package of amendments to the still-unfinished health reform bill, which would not be unveiled until mid-November. A few—Jeanne Shaheen (D-NH), Tom Udall (D-NM), Michael Bennett (D-CO)—got heavily involved, while others got on board for specific amendments.

Their work was not controversial or headline generating, and it was focused on strengthening provisions to control costs and improve the delivery of services. They succeeded in attaching more than a dozen provisions to Harry Reid's Manager's Amendment, including:

- improving the new Center for Medicare and Medicaid Innovation by expanding the scope of the entity's mission, and allowing the Center to focus on targeted geographic regions;
- enlarging the number of disease conditions for which bundled payment can be tied beginning in 2016;
- expanding the reporting on quality measures to include all Medicare providers including psychiatric hospitals, ambulatory surgery centers, and more;
- directing the Independent Payment Advisory Board to examine all health related spending, not just for Medicare, and to make nonbinding recommendations to the private sector on ways to control health spending; and
- restating the mission of the new national quality strategy to develop goals for system efficiency as well as for quality.

Other areas in the freshman package included racial and ethnic health disparities, administrative simplification, data collection, pay for performance testing, medication therapy management in Part D, modernizing computer systems at the Centers for Medicare and Medicaid Services, diabetes coordinated care, and expanded penalties for health care fraud. Once it became clear that the freshman members were serious, their staffers were swarmed with lobbyists and stakeholders hoping to promote ideas and proposals for inclusion in their plan. The members held a press conference on December 8 to announce their package to a full audience. They were flexible in negotiating with their powerful counterparts and staffers and ended up having a real impact on the final version of the ACA adopted on December 24.

Indian Health Improvement and the Problem of Page Length

Here is a real-life legislative dilemma: Senator Harry Reid needed sixty out of sixty members of the Senate Democratic Caucus to vote to approve health reform, or else it would die. Nearly every one of the fifty-nine had a price for his or her vote. Senator Byron Dorgan (D-ND), chair of the Senate Indian Affairs Committee, demanded inclusion in the Manager's Amendment of the entire Indian Health Care Improvement Reauthorization and Extension Act (IHCREA).

It was not an outrageous request. Reauthorization was about nine years overdue, as the prior legislative authorization expired in 2001—and the last legislatively approved reauthorization was in 1992, meaning nearly two decades had passed since the act was last updated. Though the needs were great, neither HELP nor the Senate Finance Committees had put the legislation in their committee markups because neither had jurisdiction. While there was no significant opposition to the legislation—indeed, Republican senators including Minority Whip John Kyl (R-AZ) and Lisa Murkowski (R-AK), supported the reauthorization—no Republicans were willing to support health reform just to win Indian Health reauthorization.

The real problem was, in a word, pages. Without the Manager's Amendment, the PPACA ran to 2,034 pages, a perpetual talking point and visual aid for Republicans to use in lambasting the legislation. Without the IHCREA, the Manager's Amendment—which became Title X—ran another 373 pages, bringing the total bill length to 2,407 pages. The IHCREA itself ran another 274 pages. It was just too much, Democratic leaders feared. It wasn't about cost—the entire reauthorization was subject to appropriation—it was just about page length.

Balanced against the page-length problem were genuine concerns about the health of American Indians and Native Alaskans. Federal responsibility for Indian health is embedded in the U.S. Constitution, treaties, federal law, executive orders, and federal court decisions over many years. The federal government provides health care services to 1.9 million persons through the Indian Health Service (IHS), mostly on or near reservations in thirty-five states through approximately six hundred health care facilities. The larger tribes use authority granted in the 1975 Indian Self Determination Act to run their own health facilities, receiving contract support from the IHS, so-called Section 638 Contract Health Services funding. Total available funding in 2010 was about $6 billion, including payments from Medicare and Medicaid as well as special funding for diabetes.

Despite this support, the health status of American Indians and Native Alaskans is deplorable. As a leader of the National Congress of American Indians noted in testimony before the Senate, life expectancy for those populations is nearly six years less than for any other racial or ethnic group in the United States; they are three times as likely to die from diabetes and six times as likely to contract tuberculosis; infant mortality is 40 percent higher than for nonnatives, and youth aged fifteen through thirty-four commit suicide at three times the national rate.[1]

The Indian Health Care Improvement Reauthorization and Extension

Act of 2009 includes sixty-nine sections geared to reauthorize, modernize, and reform the Indian health care system, and to add Indian health-specific provisions to the Social Security Act.[2] The bill addresses workforce shortages, health services and facilities, the needs of urban Indians, behavioral health programs, Indian youth suicide prevention, and more. The legislation was discussed in numerous public hearings and written testimony and was negotiated with tribes, tribal organizations, and urban Indian organizations over the course of the previous decade. The entire measure is subject to the appropriations process with no dedicated funding included in the act. Despite the lack of dedicated funding, American Indian and Native Alaskan organizations were strongly supportive of the reauthorization to help them improve health programs and systems for their populations.

So how to deal with the page-length problem? Dorgan was told to offer the act as an amendment during floor debate. Knowing the uncertainties of floor debate, especially relating to national health reform, he refused and continued to withhold his support for the full bill without a commitment for inclusion in the Manager's Amendment. The House had included the act in its health reform bill, he argued, and the Senate would not look good ignoring the matter; health reform was polling poorly in North Dakota, and this would be an important deliverable in that state and in others with substantial Indian populations. Could the 247-page bill be shrunk, Dorgan was asked, down to about five pages or so? Finally, Dorgan's chief of staff came up with an idea—incorporation by reference. Here is how the final actual text of the ACA reads:

SEC. 10221. INDIAN HEALTH CARE IMPROVEMENT.

IN GENERAL.—Except as provided in subsection (b), S. 1790 entitled "A bill to amend the Indian Health Care Improvement Act to revise and extend that Act, and for other purposes," as reported by the Committee on Indian Affairs of the Senate in December 2009, is enacted into law.

The remainder of the brief section includes two pages of noncontroversial amendments. "Incorporation by reference" had been used at least a half dozen times in the prior three Congresses relating to Department of Defense appropriations, staff were informed by the Congressional Research Service. So no new legislative process ground was broken with the move. As was intended with so many provisions included in the Senate-approved PPACA, it would all change in the merger process with the House bill so that the final version sent to President Obama for his signature would include the full 247 pages plus whatever was added in merger negotiations. This was just a device to get the measure through the Senate with the least amount of pain, and it worked—Republican complaints about the manner of the inclusion were scarcely heard. After the PPACA's December 24 enactment and prior to the January 19, 2010, election to fill Senator Kennedy's seat, House-Senate negotiations regarding the Indian Health Reauthorization Act had been concluded, and negotiators were pleased with the final result. Then the results from the Massachusetts special election pulled the plug on the merger process. The House approved the Senate PPACA, along with budget-related improvements in a reconciliation bill, the only viable path to a bill signing. Because the Indian Health Improvement Act had no budgetary implications, it was not a candidate for modifications in the reconciliation sidecar. The December 24 incorporation-by-reference version turned out to the final one.

As with nearly all provisions in the ACA, passage of the IHCREA is a historic and positive milestone for American Indians and Native Alaskans. Yet the Indian Health Services is still badly stressed for funding and plagued with management, service, and facilities problems. Most importantly, the persons dying, sick, and at-risk need a lot more support to celebrate the promises incorporated in the ACA.

Conclusion

There was a better national health reform law to be written than the Affordable Care Act. There were better approaches to save money and to restrain the rising costs of health care, better ways to cover uninsured Americans, better methods to improve the quality of medical care and to put the nation on a healthier path, and smarter ways to pay for the whole effort. It is fair to say that the ACA is no American's idea of the best possible reform. And yet—because Americans do not agree at all on what the best possible reform would be—the ACA is close to the best reform that could be achieved in the 111th Congress and close to the best reform achievable at least since 1993–94.

Other comprehensive health reform bills were in play. The most prominent was Oregon senator Ron Wyden's Healthy Americans Act, which at its peak had sixteen cosponsors drawn equally from both parties, several of whom stated publicly they would not vote for it as written. Senator Mike Enzi (R-WY), the ranking Republican on the Health, Education, Labor and Pensions (HELP) Committee, introduced his "Ten Steps to Transform Health Care in America" legislation (S1783) in July 2007; he first filed the bill in July 2007 and never attracted a single cosponsor.[1] Senator Judd Gregg (R-NH) offered his own plan in early June 2009 as an alternative to the HELP legislation then being advanced by committee Democrats; he never filed his proposal as actual legislation.[2] Senator Tom Coburn (R-OK) introduced the Patients' Choice Act (S1099) in the 111th Congress as his own comprehensive plan.[3] Coburn's bill, which he avidly promoted, attracted seven other Republican cosponsors, eight counting himself, one-

287

fifth of the Senate Republican Caucus in 2009 and 2010. Those were the oft-cited alternatives in the Senate health reform debate.

The challenge in passing comprehensive health reform legislation in 2009–10 was not to devise a plan that met any one individual's idea of perfection; many of those plans were available. The challenge was to devise legislation that could win votes from at least 60 senators and 218 representatives—not in all Congresses for all times, just in one, the 111th. It is the same standard that applies to any other federal legislation, no more and no less. The alternatives never came close.

This final chapter offers perspective on the immense and historic health reform laws approved in March 2010. After revisiting a meeting in Minnesota, I present summary conclusions, some looking back on the legislative process and some looking ahead.

MINNESOTA REDUX

In this book's introduction, we visited a pre-health-reform meeting in Minnesota in April 2008. Most participants were 1993–94 veterans from both parties, organized by former senator David Durenberger and policy expert Len Nichols. Based on the discussions, the conveners produced a list of "ten commandments" for congressional health reform. Here I recount the ten along with commentary:

Exercise political will. Presidential leadership is critical.   President Obama repeatedly overruled his advisors who wanted to move incrementally, if at all, to win health reform. He understood that focused and sustained presidential leadership was indispensable to passage, in addition to determined leadership from Speaker Nancy Pelosi, Majority Leader Harry Reid, and other key congressional committee chairmen and leaders.

Communicate to the public. The vision, principles, and goals of health reform must be understood.   Compared with the 1993–94 drive, the 2009–10 effort was more sophisticated and well-resourced to carry a message to the public. The message, though, kept changing, and it was frequently drowned out by opposition messaging.

Choose the right advisors and surrogates. They should be those who have your trust and the trust of the public.   The president does not get to choose who will carry the effort in the House or Senate, though he benefited by having key congressional leaders who had lived through the 1993–94 experience and were determined to engineer a different outcome this time. Similarly, many of the key administration, Senate, and House staff, as well as the staff of key stakeholder organizations, brought years of federal legislative experience to the task, and their institutional memory and savvy proved to be of crucial importance.

Empower the Congress. Delegate to Congress the details of legislation. For better and worse, that is what the Obama administration did. Slow, difficult, and contentious as the process proved to be, had they tried to do it themselves and not delegate, they would have failed as the Clintons did.

Manage partisanship. Focus on messages and policies that bring people together. There were leaders from both parties, especially in Senate and in the Gang of Six, who attempted to achieve a bipartisan outcome. There were outsiders, such as the Bipartisan Policy Center, who also worked hard to make this happen. Could it have been better? Only if one side had capitulated to the other far beyond what either political base would tolerate in 2009 and 2010.

Calibrate the timing. Use all deliberate speed in moving the issue to Congress to begin work. Could the process have moved faster? Yes. Much faster? Not unless Congress had advanced a far less ambitious bill. This book's review of the ten titles should convey why it could not have moved much faster. Legislative health reform always takes far longer than most participants anticipate, and far longer than the public can tolerate.

Manage stakeholders. Keep them in the circle (at the table) but not at the center. Hospitals, physicians, drug companies, and other key constituencies who had opposed reform in 1993–94 were kept at the table, involved, and supportive. The two most challenging constituencies, insurers and business, proved too difficult to convince.

Involve the states. Recognize the steps that states have taken while acknowledging their limitations. The ACA includes numerous provisions respecting the capacity and abilities of states without permitting them to thwart reform. The leading voice for states, the National Governors Association, was ineffective because it was divided by the same partisan dynamics affecting the Congress.

Determine the scope. Decide whether it is better to go after a "big bang" bill linking coverage, cost, and quality or a "baby bang" bill that may be easier to pass.   By early 2009, all key Democratic leaders in the White House, Senate and House agreed that comprehensive legislation addressing access, quality, and costs was the goal.

Negotiate procedural roadblocks. Congressional leaders have to agree on a process before legislative work begins.   Congressional leaders were determined from the start to avoid key errors of the 1993–94 process and held to those choices. House leaders, in particular, merged three committee efforts into one to design their health reform legislation, avoiding a major problem from 1993–94. President Obama decided early not to send his own proposal to Capitol Hill. Senate leaders from both parties began working together in late 2008 to agree on a process. Democrats agreed not to use budget reconciliation to pass the major legislative vehicle, while also deciding to hold the tool in reserve. Even so, it is difficult to agree on a process before it is clear whether there can be agreement on substance. In early 2009, no one knew that the Democrats would have sixty votes in the Senate, and near the end, no one knew that the Democrats would lose that margin.

In the future, the ACA will be judged not on the process, but on its results. Here are summary judgments on both, first looking back on the process and then looking ahead.

CONCLUSIONS: LOOKING BACK

The Affordable Care Act is a landmark in U.S. health reform and a landmark in U.S. social policy legislation.   The law itself is a landmark full of smaller landmarks. The ACA has been compared in scope and significance to the 1935 Social Security Act and the 1965 Medicare and Medicaid Act. It is a legitimate comparison. The ACA is not a once-in-a-generation accomplishment; it is a once-every-other or once-every-third generation achievement. When the Social Security Administration began writing checks in 1940, they were sent to 222,000 beneficiaries, a number that rose to 1.1 million by 1945, and 48.9 million by 2006.[4] When Medicare opened for business in 1966, it brought in 19.1 million elderly enrollees, up to 46.6 million elderly and disabled in 2010.[5] When the ACA is fully implemented, the state exchanges and the expanded Medicaid programs are projected to attract between 32 and 34 million new enrollees, and—as with Social Security and Medicare—that number will only increase over time.

Unlike the ACA, Social Security and Medicare covered eligible Americans in a single government program, indisputably a public program. Reflecting the tenor of the American era in which it was created, the ACA slots half its newly covered enrollees into private insurance plans overseen by state health insurance exchanges, and the other half into state Medicaid programs that often delegate their coverage responsibilities to private carriers.

Beyond—or within—the impact of the overall statute, the ACA is laden with smaller provisions and sections that are rightly regarded as landmarks in their respective policy domains. These include the private-insurance-market reforms, structural changes in Medicaid, Medicare payment innovations, prevention and wellness initiatives, workforce provisions, the Physician Payments Sunshine Act, the Elder Justice Act, the CLASS program, the Indian Health Service Reauthorization Act, the biosimilars title, the fraud and abuse measures, and many more. In many cases, these reforms have been works in progress for a decade or more. It is difficult to cite another federal law that contains so many distinct, far-reaching, and self-contained reform provisions. One purpose of this book is to provide a source to understand and learn about these provisions which have received sparse attention, if any at all, in the torrent of public discussion over the more controversial ACA sections. Were it not for the opportunity provided by the ACA, most of these worthy provisions would have waited years for action, and many would never have moved.

The ACA is also a landmark in social welfare policy. Being uninsured in America is more closely tied to lower household income than to any other variable. The vast majority of those who will obtain affordable health insurance coverage because of the ACA are in the bottom third of the nation's income distribution. Shortly after the ACA achieved final passage in the Senate, Finance chair Max Baucus told a press briefing: "This legislation will have the effect of addressing the maldistribution of income in America, because health care is now a right for all Americans, because health care is now affordable for all Americans."[6] Though he backpedaled from the comment after a conservative backlash, his point is valid—up to a point. Particularly because of the new FICA taxes on high-income earners, the ACA does generate progressive income redistribution; but subsidizing the purchase of insurance is not the same as putting money into lower-income persons' pockets—it is paying insurance companies and medical providers. Given the federal tax code's current regressive subsidization of employer health insurance, it is a form of income redistribution that helps to level the nation's income disparities. One political irony of the

ACA is the extent to which it redistributes income from the wealthier blue states, whose representatives overwhelmingly supported passage, to the lower-income red states, whose representatives overwhelmingly opposed passage.

More than money, politics, or anything else, health reform is about values. The word *values* means many things to different people. My preferred definition is "what I believe is important to me." Discussions about values often start at a high level of abstraction—liberty, equality, security, efficiency, patriotism, faith. It is easy for me to conclude that I value all of these. We test our values and discover how much each really means to us—as individuals, families, communities, nations—only when they come into conflict with each other, when we must choose one over another. Then the question becomes, how much do I value this in relation to that? Then we're talking.

Throughout the health reform debate, members, mostly Republicans, would often say—"Of course we all want everyone to have health insurance," and "We all support universal health care." Some listeners would roll their eyes, though I took them at their word. I believe nearly all 100 members of the U.S. Senate and just about all 435 members of the House of Representatives would like everyone in the nation to have health insurance coverage. Then the question becomes, at what cost? What else of something else that you value are you willing to give up or forgo to advance that value? That is where the real divide occurs. Everyone has a price point above which they will not go to achieve a particular value—for most Democrats on health reform, it was about $1 trillion over ten years, and not much higher.

For Republicans, the acceptable price to achieve the value of universal coverage was substantially lower—we don't know how much lower, just a lot. In 2003, Republicans valued providing prescription drug coverage to Medicare enrollees just barely enough to win passage of their proposed law by a slender margin in the House of Representatives and by a more comfortable margin in the Senate. Still, they offset none of the cost of the new Part D program with one penny of revenue, cuts, or savings—and it's fair to suggest that any attempt on their part to do so would have resulted in a failed attempt at passage. Supporters valued drug coverage enough to create the Part D program, though only enough to add its full cost to the national debt; they did not value it enough to pay for one penny of it.

Democrats in 2009 and 2010 valued achieving comprehensive health reform enough to pay for it, and to pay for it fully, according to the CBO.

They valued achieving near-universal coverage enough to risk the loss of their majorities in the Senate and House to win it. And they valued it knowing that implementation will present them with numerous ongoing and difficult challenges. They put their collective political capital at risk to achieve it knowing that presidents Roosevelt, Truman, Carter, and Clinton had all failed and paid a price for their failure.

Absolutely, there is political calculation to be made and political gain to be achieved if health reform succeeds. It is a mistake, though, to view the lengthy struggle and to see only political calculus. James Morone wrote about the deeper, personal meaning of health reform that emerged over the course of the effort for President Obama:

> He began to win audiences over with stories like the one he told at
> a Democratic fund-raiser in February 2010. An uninsured Obama
> volunteer from St. Louis was dying of breast cancer. As the president
> spoke of her, he left unspoken the fact that his own uninsured mother
> had died of ovarian cancer. The campaign volunteer "insisted she is
> going to be buried in an Obama t-shirt," the president continued.
> "How can I say to her, 'You know what, we're giving up'? How can
> I say to her family, 'This is too hard'? How can Democrats on the Hill
> say, 'This is politically too risky'? How can Republicans on the Hill
> say, 'We're better off just blocking anything from happening'?"[7]

The achievement of national health reform was the achievement of a movement. Movements are, by their nature, messy, undisciplined, and uncoordinated. They are fractious and contentious, often devoting more energy to battling movement allies than to winning over the undecided or overcoming obstacles laid by opponents. This was true of the civil rights movement, the labor movement, the women's movement, the environmental movement, the conservative movement, the right-to-life movement—any drive for social change large enough to move society and too big to be controlled by one group.

Within the health justice movement, there are the true believers who will settle for nothing less than fundamental systemic restructuring, and there are the incrementalists who take what current opportunities permit, make the best of it, and get ready for the next reform opportunity. Sometimes the differences between fundamental and incremental are obscure even to those most closely involved. Was Medicare a radical, systemic change or a giant patch on a dysfunctional system? The answer does not follow a true/false or yes/no dichotomy but fits on a spectrum, and the real answer depends on the nature of the question. So consider the ACA on a spectrum where 0 or 1 represents the least revolutionary of change (say, higher appropriations for an existing program), and 9 or 10 represents fundamental change (say, a Healthy Americans Act or Canadian-style single-payer system), and 5 is the borderline between incremental and radical. Where is the ACA? It is too early to say. For now, it's best to place it right on 5, the holding pattern.

What is more clear is that the passage of the ACA, in addition to representing personal victories for Barack Obama, Nancy Pelosi, Harry Reid, Henry Waxman, Max Baucus, George Miller, Chris Dodd, Charles Rangel, Tom Harkin, Ted Kennedy, and so many other elected leaders, is also the victory of a movement that brought together hundreds of thousands of individuals and organizations to push for reform. These include organizations such as AARP, the American Cancer Society, Families USA, the Catholic Health Association, Health Care for America Now, the Service Employees International Union, Community Catalyst, funders, think tanks, trade associations and industry leaders, and so many committed individuals. At the start of any movement's engagement, many wonder: how much will it take and how long will it take? Nearly always, in my experience and observation, the answer is—a lot more than anyone imagines and a lot longer, too. There's an old saying, "In for a dime, in for a dollar." It fits movement activation and success—more than anyone can imagine.

In the middle and end, health reform in 2009 and 2010 became a clash between two movements—health justice versus tea party, the former longstanding and mature and the latter newly engaged and fast evolving, two movements with diametrically opposite goals, vision, and values. At a deeper and more fundamental level, there is more agreement than either side can see—it can be difficult to discern while the tear gas of legislative, media, and movement conflict fills the air.

Bipartisanship was seriously pursued by a few leaders on both sides and was not possible. "The Democratic reform bill is the first piece of major social legislation to be enacted on a strictly partisan basis," noted John Iglehart in the New England Journal of Medicine.[8] A nagging and unanswerable question is, could the outcome have been different—was there a missed opportunity to achieve bipartisan health reform? Though the question has no definitive answer, I offer an opinion: no.

In January 2010, on CNN's *State of the Union* political talk show, Senator Orrin Hatch (R-UT) noted: "We weren't even involved in this process; we weren't even asked." Hatch's statement is a reasonable one for a House Republican to make, but not for a senator, particular the senior senator from

Utah. Hatch was an active participant in Max Baucus's coffee klatch, which became the Gang of Six only when he publicly dropped out. The Republican senators of the gang—Olympia Snowe of Maine, Charles Grassley of Iowa, and Mike Enzi of Wyoming—met with Democratic senators Baucus, Kent Conrad of North Dakota, and Jeff Bingaman of New Mexico for a full sixty-three hours in negotiations. The Baucus and Grassley staffs operated as a team until the former called off the alliance in early September 2009.[9]

Republican ideas permeate the ACA: The individual mandate was advanced and broadly embraced by Republicans in the Clinton era, including Hatch and Grassley. Private-market subsidies to purchase private insurance was another cornerstone of the 1993 Republican alternative. No public-plan option was a persistent Republican demand. The Elder Justice Act was a priority for Hatch and Grassley. The Physician Payments Sunshine Act was another Grassley passion. Expanded fraud and abuse was a concern for Grassley and Tom Coburn (R-OK). Limiting the tax exclusion for everyone (through the "Cadillac" excise tax), not just the wealthy, was a cornerstone demand of Enzi. The young "invincible" catastrophic coverage option was a Snowe priority. Allowing consumers and businesses to buy health insurance across state lines was a priority for nearly every Republican member. "None of these elements go as far as Republicans would like, but to say their party didn't have a moderating influence would be false," noted Carrie Budoff Brown in *Politico*.[10]

Former Snowe staffer William Pewen observed in a *New York Times* op-ed: "Many Republicans had decided even before Inauguration Day to block reform, including policies that their party had previously supported. In 2003, for example, Republicans enacted legislation that financed end-of-life counseling—yet in town halls last August, they claimed a similar measure would create 'death panels.'"[11]

At the same time, Republican opposition makes sense. For a time, there was a divergence between Republicans such as Senator Jim DeMint (R-SC), who likened health reform to Obama's Waterloo, and Republicans who genuinely engaged, including Grassley, Enzi, Snowe, and others. Ultimately, the imperatives of an acceptable Democratic version of comprehensive reform, with broad Medicaid expansions, the CLASS Act, employer penalties, a heavy federal footprint on state insurance regulatory prerogatives, increased taxes on wealthy Americans—were too tough a bottle of pills for a conscientious Republican to swallow, principled or not. In the end, it was not a hard sell for Republicans to portray this as a Democratic bridge way too far.

Grassley was the enigma. A longtime Baucus pal and ally, a public supporter of an individual mandate until the August town meetings when he became a target of tea party wrath in his home state of Iowa, he was actively and personally courted by Obama who asked him at one point if he would support a bill if he got every concession he was seeking:

"Probably not."

"Why not?" asked an exasperated Obama.

"Because I'd have to have a number of Republicans," said Grassley. "I'm not going to be the third of three Republicans. I've defined a bipartisan bill as broad-based support."[12]

It has been demonstrated in numerous national polls that Democrats and Republicans view the U.S. health care system through diametrically opposing lenses—with Independents in the middle, veering back and forth. The harsh partisan differences in attitudes toward the ACA reflect the sharper partisan divide over health system fundamentals. On basic questions such as, does the United States have the best health care system in the world?—68 percent of Republicans say yes compared with only 32 percent of Democrats.[13] Even the collapsed Republican support for an individual mandate can be understood as the product of an energized and awakened conservative base that rejected out of hand an idea once popular in Republican policy salons. Our political system exists to mediate and moderate divergent views and perspectives. It works best when it can create genuine bipartisan consensus to tackle serious societal challenges. It cannot do that all the time, and that is when elections matter.

Compromises and deals were necessary, not scandalous. "Medical interests alone shelled out more than $876 million in lobbying expenses during the 15 months beginning in January 2009 and ending in March, when Congress passed the sweeping overhaul," according to Roll Call.[14] Unlike the 1993–94 health reform era, when Clinton-plan backers were hugely outspent by reform opponents, the 2009–10 campaign saw more evenly divided spending on both sides. Even the progressive Health Care for America Now coalition enjoyed $51 million in support from the Atlantic Philanthropies and major labor unions. The pharmaceutical industry spent about $150 million to back reform. Although they were matched by U.S. Chamber of Commerce (secretly financed by major insurance companies) and other spending against reform, this time it was a contest between two well-resourced camps.

Along the way, deals were made with hospitals, physicians, home health groups, hospices, the pharmaceutical industry, the Business Roundtable; with standing and ad hoc caucuses in the House of Representatives; and with every single Democratic member of the U.S. Senate. Deals, agreements, compromises, understandings, handshakes, nods, and winks—they are all forms of currency in the process of making policies and laws at every level of government, not just in the United States, but in every legitimate legislative assembly on the globe. Without this currency, business does not get done and comes to a standstill. When matters come to a standstill, that is when we see government shutdowns, deadlocks, coups, impeachments, and other assorted mayhem. While one may agree or disagree with the specifics of a particular deal, one cannot participate in a serious legislative process without them. What was different about health reform then?

One compelling difference was the sheer size, scope, and ambition of the legislation, big in page numbers, sections, dollars, interest groups, members with a stake, and more. One other major difference was the extraordinary media coverage of a complex and controversial legislative battle. Harold Pollack in the *New Republic* called it "the best covered news story, ever."[15] Arguably, the American public that chose to pay close attention had the best tutorial on the legislative process in the nation's history. Anyone could get easy access to legislative proposals, CBO analyses, think tank reports, and a blizzard of daily commentary from journalists, real and pseudo, and anyone else. Every health reform hiccup and burp fed the daily demand for instant news—the more provocative and confrontational, the better. For those uncomfortable with behind-the-scenes agreements, there was plenty to dislike—and pretty much anything in a legislative process can be made to appear sinister and unusually out of order, especially when wealthy stakeholders find it in their interest to make it appear that way.

The most criticized of the "deals" was the agreement between the White House and the Senate Finance Committee with the pharmaceutical industry. Some think the deal went too far, many believe it did not go far enough—and most seem to believe no deal should have been made at all. Reasonable arguments can be advanced to support all three viewpoints. And good arguments can be advanced to support the deal. Had the pharmaceutical industry spent $150 million to oppose health reform instead of supporting it, that would almost certainly have tipped the fragile balance toward a repeat of the Clinton fiasco. Many who decry the deal are much more upset at health reform's passage than at any particular agreement—the PhRMA deal is just one of numerous piñatas on which to vent frustration with the outcome. Those who believe the industry did not pay enough must consider that the agreement was the first of the process, with no benchmark for comparison, and the additional dollars that could have been imposed in the absence of a deal would only have been a mirage had the industry gone to the other side.

The other notorious deal involved Nebraska senator Ben Nelson's agreement with Senate Majority Leader Harry Reid that his state's new Medicaid costs would be covered more generously than any other state's. In mid-December 2009, Reid had zero margin for error—he needed sixty out of sixty members of the Democratic Caucus, including Nelson, or health reform would die. In the Senate package, there was no fiscal capacity at that point to make a similar Medicaid deal for every other state. There was also a presumed Senate-House conference committee ahead where such deals get scuttled. The intense negative public reaction to the "Cornhusker compromise" worked to guarantee its elimination in the final ACA. The question for any leader in Reid's position—are you willing to do what's necessary to move the legislation forward, or are you willing to let it die? In the time and the place, Reid made the right call.

President Obama brought on himself the other major criticism of deal making with his campaign promise that all proceedings and negotiations would be televised on C-SPAN—a commitment breathtaking in its disingenuousness or naïveté. Such a process on complex legislation has never happened for a reason—it is impossible to accomplish real negotiation, compromise, and give-and-take when a negotiator's partisans can hear every word. And though the White House summit in March 2009 and the Blair House summit in February 2010 were attempts to address this procedural promise, no real negotiating took place in either setting, nor could there have been.

In the heat of any legislative or political campaign battle, the daily ticktock, the gossip, the outrages channeled by the partisans—these fade in importance, day by day. People remember the process—often vaguely and inaccurately—though its prominence subsides as the substance and stuff of real-world implementation take precedence.

CONCLUSIONS: LOOKING AHEAD

Like Social Security and Medicare before it, the ACA will be revisited and revised repeatedly for years to come. At the time of their enactments, Social Security and Medicare faced criticism, challenges, and attacks from both sides of the political spectrum. Most Republicans supported Social Security's final passage (eighty-one of ninety-six House Republicans and sixteen of twenty-two Senate Republicans), though strong majorities of them voted against the measure throughout the legislative process, and Republicans regularly threatened the repeal of Social Security and Medicare if given the opportunity. Criticism of Social Security was also strong from the political left because of the large and numerous populations of workers deliberately left out of the new system. These included agricultural workers, domestics, government and hospital workers, employees in firms with fewer than ten workers, and more, such that an estimated two-thirds of African American workers and more than half of all women workers were left outside the law's reach.[16] The National Association for the Advancement of Colored People described the 1935 act as "a sieve with holes just big enough for the majority of Negroes to fall through."[17] Even Frances Perkins, FDR's labor secretary, lamented that "the thing had been chiseled down to a conservative pattern."[18]

Medicare also enjoyed some Republican support at its final passage (seventy Republican votes in the House and thirteen in the Senate) as well as significant opposition in its early years of implementation. The threat of a national physician boycott combined with the challenge and obligation to desegregate all hospitals across the nation, especially in the South, left many wondering if the new law ever could achieve its ambitious aims.[19] The new Medicare program lacked any mechanism to pay for outpatient prescription drugs for enrollees or most nursing home care. It also included an inherently inflationary provider-payment mechanism guaranteeing hospitals and physicians their "usual, customary and reasonable" fees.

In both cases, final legislative enactments in 1935 and 1965, respectively, represented the end of hard-fought campaigns to win passage (the former took two years and the latter took thirteen) and the opening of new chapters as future administrations and Congresses wrestled with changing the programs to meet the evolving needs of the American people. Starting in 1939, Congress enacted four significant laws to fill in the largest holes in the 1935 statute, two of the largest additions occurring during the administrations of Republican presidents: Eisenhower in 1956 signed legislation to provide Social Security income to persons with disabilities, and Nixon in 1972 signed legislation to extend Medicare to persons of any age who were eligible for Social Security Disability Insurance.[20]

Medicare undergoes constant tweaking and altering by Congress. In 1983, the hospital payment system was completely revamped; in 1988, a catastrophic-coverage benefit was added—though repealed in 1989; also in 1989, the physician-payment system was revamped; in 1997, Congress made numerous changes to reduce spending growth to achieve federal deficit reduction; in 2003, the prescription drug benefit was added; and in 2010, the program was altered again through the ACA. Nearly every year, Congress makes numerous smaller changes, some lasting and others not.

As Social Security and Medicare did, the ACA faces immense implementation challenges and political threats. It will take time before Congress can get beyond the animosities engendered in the legislative process so that members can work together on necessary modifications; conversations on smaller alterations began almost immediately after the bill signing. Once Congress starts, it will make modifications often: large and small, substantial and insubstantial, expanding and contracting. The continuing shifts in the partisan composition of the House and Senate will be one influential dynamic, as will the shifting tides of public opinion; also significant will be the fiscal outlook for the health reform program, for both the federal and state governments, and for the national economy. It is just beginning, and unless repeal happens, it will continue without end.

Affordability for new exchange enrollees will be a key test—over the short, medium, and long term—and especially the long term. How much will new enrollees in exchange-sponsored private plans have to pay—in premiums and out-of-pocket costs? How will they respond to the costs they will face? Will they seek medically necessary care in spite of their out-of-pocket costs? How will they regard their new coverage? We know what the law requires. Premiums will be based on family income and will range between 3 and 9.5 percent, and enrollee out-of-pocket costs will range between 6 and 40 percent of family income. Exchange enrollees will choose from four levels of coverage—platinum, gold, silver, and bronze, covering benefit costs at 90, 80, 70, and 60 percent, respectively. Enrollee subsidies are tied to the silver, or 70 percent, "actuarial value" plan. Subsidized enrollees can purchase gold or platinum coverage to reduce their potential out-of-pocket exposure, though they will pay noticeably higher premiums with their own money.

The tradeoff among the four coverage levels is clear—higher premiums in platinum and gold plans bring modest cost sharing, while lower premiums in silver and bronze plans bring much higher out-of-pocket cost exposure. The Massachusetts experience with a similar structure shows that most consumers choose lower-premium options, leaving them vulnerable to high cost sharing in the event of a serious illness. These levels of cost sharing are far beyond those faced today by most workers with private employer-based coverage or those with public coverage through Medicare, Medicaid, or the military's Tri-Care coverage.

Under the ACA structure, it will get much worse for enrollees in the second decade. To achieve savings that would be scored favorably by the Congressional Budget Office, the coverage subsidy provisions were structured so that beginning in 2020, the government share of spending on subsidies will grow only at the level of the consumer price index, while the individual's costs will grow as high as 10 percent per year. So between 2014 and 2019, the individual's premium share is fixed, based on income, at 3 to 9.5 percent of income; that cap is lifted beginning in year 2020. This is, in many respects, the ACA's political equivalent of the Medicare Part D "doughnut hole," something a future Congress will have to address if the coverage is to remain affordable.

Why was it done this way? Earlier versions of the coverage provisions, as estimated by the CBO and by MIT economist Jonathan Gruber (on contract with the U.S. Department of Health and Human Services), showed a politically unacceptable federal price tag for more generous coverage through exchange plans, at total costs as high as $1.6 to 2.3 trillion over the first ten years. The only politically achievable direction was downward, accelerated when President Obama set a $900 billion cap on the cost of the whole legislation in his September 2009 address to Congress. How did the price get down? Three key ways: the start date for the exchange subsidies was pushed back to 2014, the actuarial values were reduced, and the Medicaid expansion was pegged to 133 percent of the federal poverty level instead of 100 percent because it is cheaper to cover these individuals through state Medicaid programs than through private coverage and the exchanges.

The pressures so much in evidence in the legislative process will not go away. As 2014 draws near, increasing concerns will become prominent about the inadequacy of out-of-pocket protections for consumers; as 2020 draws near, stronger concerns will be raised about the future financial exposure of enrollees. At the same time, the fiscal concerns regarding the overall cost of the program will continue to constrain the ability of Congress to respond to these concerns. There are two potential savers: one, a hard-to-predict moderation in medical care inflation, as was experienced in the mid-1990s; and two, other ACA reforms that received low savings scores from the CBO may outperform expectations and provide limited breathing room to address affordability concerns—see the following section for more on this last possibility.

The ACA's fiscal future is as uncertain as its affordability guarantees. Not surprisingly, estimates of the financial impact of the ACA differ widely. Place the CBO estimate in the middle, and rival estimates veer in both directions. The CBO estimated a ten-year federal budget savings of $143 billion between 2010 and 2019 and savings in the second decade "between one quarter percent and one half percent of gross domestic product" or as much as $1 trillion.[21] On the conservative side, Douglas Holtz-Eakin, former CBO head and chief policy advisor to Senator John McCain's presidential campaign, concluded in his analysis: "A more comprehensive and realistic projection suggests that the new reform law will raise the deficit by more than $500 billion during the first ten years, and by nearly $1.5 trillion in the following decade."[22] On the other side of the spectrum, Harvard economist David Cutler and Commonwealth Fund president Karen Davis reached a contrary conclusion, examining the law's likely effect on overall health system spending: "We estimate that, on net, the combination of provisions in the new law will reduce health care spending by $590 billion over 2010–2019 and lower premiums by nearly $2,000 per family. Moreover, the annual growth rate in national health expenditures could be slowed from 6.3 percent to 5.7 percent."[23]

Whom to believe? There are too many uncertainties to say with confidence. In health reform, as in most areas of policy, implementation is everything—and until we know how well the numerous ACA provisions will be implemented, it is impossible to predict what their fiscal impact will be. One certainty is the CBO's track record in estimating the financing of prior major federal health reforms. In 2009, Jon Gabel published a look-back on the CBO's scoring of the three largest federal health reforms since the agency's creation in 1974: the 1983 launch of the Medicare Prospective Payment System for hospitals, the 1997 Balanced Budget Act, and the 2003 creation of the Medicare Part D prescription drug program. In each case, the CBO was wrong, not by a little, but by a lot, and in each case in the same direction—underestimating revenues and savings and overestimating costs.[24] If the CBO is going to be wrong, it is better to be wrong in this direction than the alternative, though errors in this direction do deter Congress from constructing reforms as robust as they might otherwise be. Cutler and Davis point to the CBO's restrictive methodology as a culprit: "Most of the evidence upon which they are based comprises peer-reviewed studies that utilize carefully controlled comparison groups (either randomized trials or the natural equivalent)."[25] If the CBO is again wrong in the historic direction, that could be welcome fiscal news.

If the CBO is wrong, where is the likely error? Optimistic analysts point to the array of payment and financing reform experiments, which Gruber refers to as the "spaghetti approach" to cost control: "Throw everything against the wall, and see what sticks."[26] Former White House Office of Management and Budget director Peter Orszag (also former CBO director) and OMB official Ezekiel Emanuel wrote: "One of the essential aspects of the legislation is that unlike previous efforts, it does not rely on just one policy for effective cost control. Instead, it puts into place virtually every cost-control reform proposed by physicians, economists, and health policy experts and includes the means for these reforms to be assessed quickly and scaled up if they're successful."[27]

Here is a gerund-rich list of reforms culled by the Center for Budget and Policy Priorities that optimists hope will bend the cost curve:[28]

- creating health insurance exchanges
- establishing an excise tax on high-cost insurance plans
- reducing administrative costs
- researching comparative effectiveness
- promoting prevention and wellness
- licensing biologic similars
- strengthening primary care
- establishing quality measures and priorities
- promoting high-value care
- establishing a center for innovation
- enhancing program integrity
- reducing avoidable hospital readmissions
- promoting accountable care organizations
- examining payment bundling
- setting up the Independent Payment Advisory Board

Will they work? Experience suggests some will, some will not, and the ones that work will not perform as well as their biggest cheerleaders brag. Back in 1999, former federal health official Bruce Vladeck described the health sector as obsessed with the "search for the next big thing."[29] The benefits of reasonable innovations get promoted far beyond reasonable expectations, leading to their abandonment when they fail to provide exaggerated returns and spurring the resumption of the search for the next, next big thing. There have never been so many health financing and delivery experiments attempted simultaneously—an immense evaluative challenge. The opportunity for the health delivery system to reinvent itself is here and now. If it fails, blunt cost-control mechanisms are ready and likely to emerge next from the closet.

One other federal financing dynamic will benefit ACA supporters, and that is the increasingly favorable impact of the law on federal deficit reduction. In its March 20, 2010, estimate of the ACA, the CBO estimated a federal budget deficit reduction of $143 billion over ten years, $124 billion of that because of the health-related provisions. In its February 18, 2011, estimate to Congress, the CBO predicted $210 billion in deficit reduction from the health-related provisions. What accounts for the difference? Because of the passage of time, the first estimate looked at federal budget years 2010–19, while the second looked at 2012–21. Because the early years of ACA implementation involve far less of the high-cost savings and revenue activities, the negative impact on the federal deficit of repealing the law will become more financially significant year by year. This nonstop dynamic will be beneficial for the law's defenders and a growing obstacle for opponents.

The ACA has the potential to do enormous good for the health needs of racial and ethnic minorities and more potential to reduce racial and ethnic health disparities than any other law in living memory.   Though it did not get much attention, a June 2010 update on the progress of Massachusetts health reform had some startling news: in 2006, before reform, 89 percent of all white adults and 79 percent of all minority adults had health insurance coverage; in a survey carried out in the fall of 2009, 95 percent of both groups had health insurance coverage.[30] In other words, racial and ethnic disparities as they relate to health insurance coverage had been eliminated, not just reduced. This is an important element of the promise and potential of the ACA—the most dramatic assault on health inequality in America since the 1965 passage of Medicare and Medicaid.

Here are some important numbers: of the forty-seven million uninsured Americans in 2008, 46 percent were white, 15 percent were African American, 31.5 percent were Hispanic, and 7.4 percent were "other"—more than half of all uninsured Americans were members of racial and ethnic minority groups. The proportion of uninsured individuals who are Caucasian is even smaller in many states most hostile to reform—40 percent in Arizona, 44 percent in Florida, 38 percent in Georgia, 39 percent in Mississippi, 25 percent in Texas. Here are a few other numbers: while 17.4 percent of all Americans were uninsured in 2008, the uninsurance rate for whites was 12.7 percent, for African Americans it was 20.6 percent, and for Hispanics it was 32.2 percent. Another key variable is that the minority uninsured population tends to have lower incomes than do the white uninsured. Because the ACA targets its most generous assistance to those with fewer economic resources, the law may trigger bigger drops in uninsurance among minorities than among whites.

Democrats had no incentive to broadcast this during the health reform debate as they faced a backlash from the overwhelmingly white tea party movement. Republicans had no incentive to broadcast this either, opening themselves to charges of opposition based on race and ethnicity. The simple fact is that the ACA's coverage provisions will be significantly helpful to America's racial and ethnic minorities, and they hold the potential, as in Massachusetts, to eliminate or sharply reduce racial and ethnic disparities in health insurance coverage.

Reducing or even eliminating disparities in insurance coverage will not by any means eliminate America's racial and ethnic disparities in health and medical care. Still, health insurance is a vital enabling factor in helping people get the care they need. While the ACA will not eliminate disparities, it will be one of the biggest single steps the nation will ever take to address them. Brian Smedley, a national authority on disparities, provides helpful context:

> But by itself, the legislation will not be enough to address the needs of many people of color . . . the major reasons for the persistence of racial and ethnic health inequalities are socioeconomic inequality and differences in neighborhood living conditions—both of them fueled by residential segregation. These are the issues that policymakers must tackle if we are to improve opportunities for good health for all.[31]

Much more is needed, and the ACA is an important and positive step forward. This is why South Carolina congressman James Clyburn frequently refers to the ACA as the "civil rights act of the twenty-first century."

The country faces the most challenging implementation of a federal law since the civil rights laws of the 1960s. Christopher Jennings, President Clinton's senior health care advisor between 1994 and 2001 and a respected health policy strategist, counts more than 150 policies embedded in the ACA that became effective in 2010, not just affecting coverage but also regarding the workforce, Medicare coverage and quality, fraud and abuse, and more.[32] Most of these are not related to the blockbuster reforms scheduled to take effect in 2014, including the establishment of insurance exchanges in all fifty states, launch of the insurance subsidies, and enforcement of the individual mandate. Not only must the federal government be ready to implement the law, states will also need to adjust. Even states that choose not to establish and operate their own exchanges will be required to open up their Medicaid programs to a large, newly enfranchised population of the uninsured.

This work would be difficult under any circumstances and is especially difficult because of political resistance to the new law—especially from more conservative states that will be disproportionate beneficiaries of the funding flows in the law aimed at states with higher levels of uninsurance. On the day President Obama signed the ACA into law, thirteen states filed legal action in federal court to prevent implementation, a number that continues to grow with an influx of new Republican governors elected in November 2010, all of whom opposed the new law. Identifying challenges, problems, and obstacles to effective implementation is one of the easier assignments for political analysts of the ACA.

Still, there is an element in the timing of ACA implementation that fits in its favor. Arguably, the best time to enact substantive reforms is in the depths of a downturn and to time implementation during a recovery and a renewed period of economic growth. In 1988, Massachusetts enacted an ambitious health reform law under Governor Michael Dukakis during his unsuccessful presidential campaign. Months after signing, the state economy crashed with such a thud that political support for the law also collapsed. Implementation was delayed several times until major reforms were repealed in 1996. Many factors went into the failure, and a key one was bad timing. Had the Clinton reforms been enacted in 1994, implementation would have taken off in 1996 and 1997 when medical care inflation was low and the economy was accelerating toward peak growth, an auspicious environment to implement expansions. As the U.S. economy climbs out of economic doldrums, it may surprisingly be seen as serendipitous timing for the launch of the ACA expansions.

No major health system reform law has ever been implemented without controversy, difficulty, confusion, and consternation. As Daniel Fox and Howard Markel note: "With the temporary exception of Medicare Catastrophic Coverage [enacted in 1988 and repealed in 1989], policy makers who led in enacting major entitlement reform have managed to implement it. Indeed, history teaches that the real work of health reform is just beginning."[33] The ACA can easily be characterized as the most complex and challenging of them all. The end is a new beginning only starting to emerge.

· · ·

Final words. The ACA is a product of naked and enormous self-interest *and* an act of public-interest legislative politics of the highest order; way too expensive *and* not nearly expensive enough; the result of a seriously bipartisan *and* excessively partisan process; covered better than any similar public policy controversy in the history of the modern media *and* not covered well enough at all; done way, way too fast *and* way, way too slowly; and a vitally important piece of social policy legislation that will save or improve the lives of many, many Americans *and* a huge experiment that will harm or burden the lives of many, many Americans (numbers to be determined). On balance, in my view, the advantages and benefits of the law vastly outweigh the disadvantages and harm.

I hope every reader can find ample evidence in this book to justify every assertion above, because each is true. In the polarization that engulfs so much of American politics today, one root cause of this polarization is the either/or mindset that influences so much of the American political class (public officeholders and their staffs and political operatives; political media; partisan voters and participants). Too often in our political dis-agreements, it seems that everyone has to be all right or all wrong, black or white, hot or cold, useful or useless, smart or stupid. Americans do not think in terms of continuums and cling to the mental model that every-thing must be one or the other.

An example of this is Americans' views of foreign health systems—the systems in Australia, Canada, England, France, Germany, Japan, Switzer-land, and elsewhere must either be all good or all bad—there is no per-missible middle ground in the conversation. At times, it seems downright theological. One must either worship at the shrine of the perpetual single payer or bow down before the consumer-driven goddess of the free mar-ket, and no neutrals are allowed.

F. Scott Fitzgerald, back in 1936, wrote: "The test of a first-rate intelli-gence is the ability to hold two opposed ideas in the mind at the same time, and still retain the ability to function."[34] America needs help figuring out how to hold two opposed ideas in its mind at the same time *in order to* retain the ability to function. The polarization and resulting demoniza-tion in our current politics weaken our nation, undermine our ability to address and to fix serious national problems, and lessen our esteem and moral example around the world. On the other hand, our ability to dimin-ish or marginalize this tendency, I believe, would help to strengthen our nation, improve our ability to address and fix serious national problems, and enhance our esteem and moral example around the world. It might even help us to fix health care.

Notes

PREFACE

1. *Charting a Course for Health Care Reform: Moving Toward Universal Coverage, Day 1, Hearing Before the Comm. on Finance,* 110th Cong (March 14, 2007) (statement of Stuart Altman, dean and professor of national health policy, Heller School for Social Policy and Management, Brandeis).

INTRODUCTION

1. A narrative account of the Clinton health reform effort can be found in Haynes Johnson and David Broder, *The System: The American Way of Politics at the Breaking Point* (Boston: Little Brown, 1996). See also Theda Skocpol, *Boomerang: Health Care Reform and the Turn against Government* (New York: Norton, 1997) as well as Jacob Hacker, *The Road to Nowhere* (Princeton, NJ: Princeton University Press, 1999).

2. U.S. Department of Labor, Bureau of Labor Statistics, *Career Guide to Industries, 2010–11 Edition,* last modified December 17, 2009, http://www.bls.gov/oco/cg/cgs041.htm.

PART I. PRELUDES AND PROCESS

1. Katherine Atwood, Graham Colditz, and Ichiro Kawachi, "From Public Health Science to Prevention Policy," *American Journal of Public Health* 87, no. 10 (October 1997): 1603–6.

1. THE KNOWLEDGE BASE—WHY NATIONAL HEALTH REFORM?

1. Howard Rosenthal and Keith Poole, "110th Senate Rank Ordering," *Voteview,* December 2008, accessed January 11, 2011, http://voteview.com/sen110.htm.

2. David Blumenthal and James Morone, *The Heart of Power: Health and Politics in the Oval Office* (Berkeley: University of California Press, 2009), 51.

Unless otherwise noted, all references to presidents in this chapter are taken from this book. Chapter 1 describes FDR's efforts.

3. Ibid., chap. 2.

4. Ibid., chaps. 4 and 5.

5. Ibid., chap. 6.

6. Larry Brown, *Politics and Health Care Organizations: HMOs as Federal Policy* (Washington, DC: Brookings Institution, October 1982).

7. Blumenthal and Morone, *Heart of Power*, chap. 7; Karen Davis, "Universal Coverage in the United States: Lessons from Experience of the 20th Century," *Journal of Urban Health* 78, no. 1 (March 2001): 48.

8. Johnson and Broder, *The System* (see introd., n. 1).

9. Blumenthal and Morone, *Heart of Power*, 112–14.

10. U.S. Census Bureau, "Table HI01: Health Insurance Coverage Status and Type of Coverage by Selected Characteristics: 2009," *Current Population Survey*, last revised September 29, 2010, http://www.census.gov/hhes/www/cpstables/032010/health/h01_001.htm.

11. Fifty-four million is the estimate of the Congressional Budget Office. See the March 20, 2010, CBO letter to House Speaker Nancy Pelosi, http://www.cbo.gov/ftpdocs/113xx/doc11379/AmendReconProp.pdf. The estimate of the Office of the Actuary, Centers for Medicare and Medicaid Services is 56.9 million. See the December 10, 2009, memorandum from Richard S. Foster, CMS chief actuary, http://www.tnr.com/sites/default/files/CMSActuarySenate.pdf.

12. Institute of Medicine, *Coverage Matters: Insurance and Health Care* (Washington, DC: National Academies Press, 2001).

13. Institute of Medicine, "America's Uninsured Crisis: Consequences for Health and Health Care," report brief (Washington, DC: National Academies Press, February 2009).

14. Andrew Wilper et al., "Health Insurance and Mortality in US Adults," *American Journal of Public Health* 99, no. 12 (December 2009): 2289–95.

15. Cathy Schoen et al., "How Many Are Underinsured? Trends among U.S. Adults, 2003 and 2007," *Health Affairs* 27, no. 4 (June 10, 2008): w298–w309, doi:10.1377/hlthaff.27.4.w298.

16. David U. Himmelstein et al., "Medical Bankruptcy in the United States, 2007: Results of a National Study," *American Journal of Medicine* 122, no. 8 (August 2009): 741–46.

17. Daniel M. Fox, *The Convergence of Science and Governance* (Berkeley: University of California Press, 2010), 24–26.

18. Davis, "Universal Coverage," 48.

19. Gerard F. Anderson and Patricia Markovich, *Multinational Comparisons of Health Systems Data, 2009* (New York: Commonwealth Fund, 2009), available at http://www.commonwealthfund.org/~/media/Files/Publications/Chartbook/2010/PDF_Anderson_multinational_comparisons_hlt_sys_data_2009_OECD_chartpack.pdf.

20. For an account of Deming's work in Japan, see David Halberstam, *The*

Reckoning (New York: William Morrow, 1986). For more information about W. Edwards Deming, see his book *Out of the Crisis* (Cambridge, MA: MIT Press, 1982).

21. Donald Berwick, "Continuous Improvement as an Ideal in Health Care," *New England Journal of Medicine* 320, no. 1 (January 1989): 53–56.

22. David Blumenthal, "Quality of Care: What Is It?" *New England Journal of Medicine* 335, no. 12 (September 1996): 891–94.

23. Lucian Leape, "Error in Medicine," *Journal of the American Medical Association* 272, no. 23 (December 21, 1994): 1851–57, doi:10.1001/jama .1994.0352023006.

24. Institute of Medicine, *To Err Is Human: Building a Safer Health System*, eds. Linda T. Kohn, Janet M. Corrigan, and Molla S. Donaldson, Committee on Quality of Health Care in America (Washington, DC: National Academies Press, 1998).

25. See, for example, Arnold Milstein and Helen Darling, "Better US Health Care at Lower Cost," *Issues in Science and Technology*, Winter 2010, available at http://www.issues.org/26.2/milstein.html.

26. Max Baucus, *Call to Action: Health Reform 2009* (Washington, DC: U.S. Senate Committee on Finance, November 12, 2008), http://www.kslaw .com/library/publication/HH111708_BaucusPlan.pdf.

27. Congressional Budget Office, *Economic and Budget Outlook: Fiscal Years 2000–2009* (Washington, DC: January 1999), http://www.cbo.gov/doc .cfm?index=1059&type=0&sequence=1.

28. Congressional Budget Office, *An Analysis of the Administration's Health Proposal* (Washington, DC: February 1994), http://www.cbo.gov/doc .cfm?index=4882&type=0.

29. David Herszenhorn, "Fine-Tuning Led to Health Bill's $940 Billion Price Tag," *New York Times*, March 18, 2010, http://www.nytimes.com/2010/03/19/ us/19score.html.

30. See Congressional Budget Office, *Budget Options, Volume 1: Health Care* (Washington, DC: U.S. Government Printing Office, December 2008); available at http://www.cbo.gov/doc.cfm?index=9925.

31. Harvard School of Public Health and Harris Interactive, "Most Republicans Think the U.S. Health Care System Is the Best in the World. Democrats Disagree," news release, March 20, 2008, http://www.hsph.harvard.edu/news/ press-releases/2008-releases/republicans-democrats-disagree-us-health-care -system.html.

32. Robert Blendon et al., "Health Care in the 2008 Presidential Primaries," *New England Journal of Medicine* 358, no. 4 (January 24, 2008): 414–22.

33. Robert Blendon et al., "Voters and Health Reform in the 2008 Presidential Election," *New England Journal of Medicine* 359, no. 19 (October 30, 2008): 2050–61.

34. Pew Center for the People and the Press, "Distrust, Discontent, Anger and Partisan Rancor: The People and Their Government," Washington, DC, April 18, 2010, http://people-press.org/report/606/trust-in-government.

35. Comments by Brodie made at Minnesota health reform conference, April 26, 2008. Recorded by the author.

2. SOCIAL STRATEGY—MASSACHUSETTS AVENUE

1. Pam Belluck and Katie Zezima, "Massachusetts Legislation on Insurance Becomes Law," *New York Times*, April 13, 2006.

2. Irene Wielawski, *Forging Consensus: The Path to Health Reform in Massachusetts* (Boston: Blue Cross Blue Shield of Massachusetts Foundation, 2007).

3. Sharon Long and Karen Stockley, *Health Reform in Massachusetts: An Update as of Fall 2009* (Boston: Urban Institute and Blue Cross Blue Shield of Massachusetts Foundation, June 2010).

4. Massachusetts Health and Human Services Division of Health Care Finance and Policy, *Primary Care Trends in Massachusetts* (Boston: Commonwealth of Massachusetts, July 2010).

5. Gillian SteelFisher et al., "Physicians' View of the Massachusetts Health Care Reform Law—a Poll," *New England Journal of Medicine* 361, no. 19 (November 5, 2009): e39.

6. Ibby Caputo, "How a Public Option Saved My Life," *Washington Post*, October 13, 2009.

7. John E. McDonough et al., "A Progress Report on State Health Access Reform," *Health Affairs*, 27 no. 2 (March–April 2008), w105–w115, doi:10.1377/hlthaff.27.2.w105.

8. Marian Mulkey and Mark Smith, "The Long and Winding Road: Reflections on California's 'Year of Health Reform,'" *Health Affairs* 28 no. 3 (May–June 2009): w446–w456, doi:10.1377/hlthaff.28.3.w446.

9. "Kucinich Asks Himself a Question," Truthdig, posted on December 3, 2007, http://www.truthdig.com/avbooth/item/20071203_kucinich_asks_himself_a_question/.

10. "News: Rep. Weiner Withdraws Single Payer Amendment from Current Health Care Debate," news release on the website of Anthony Weiner, November 6, 2009, http://www.weiner.house.gov/news_display.aspx?id=1368.

11. Sarah Rubenstein, "Order in the Senate! Single-Payer Advocates Disrupt Hearing," *Wall Street Journal*, May 5, 2009; available at http://blogs.wsj.com/health/2009/05/05/order-in-the-senate-single-payer-advocates-disrupt-hearing/.

12. Senator Ron Wyden, in an interview with the author, April 16, 2010.

13. John Sheils and Randall Haught, "The Cost of Tax Exempt Health Benefits in 2004," *Health Affairs*, Web exclusive, February 25, 2004, http://content.healthaffairs.org/content/early/2004/02/25/hlthaff.w4.106/suppl/DC1., doi:10.1377/hlthaff.w4.106.

14. Congressional Budget Office and Joint Committee on Taxation, Letter to Senators Ron Wyden and Robert Bennett, May 1, 2008, http://cboblog.cbo.gov/?p=91.

15. *Co-sponsorship of S. 334, the Healthy Americans Act,* 110th Cong. (September 24, 2008) (statement by Senator Arlen Specter).

16. Edwin Park, *An Examination of the Wyden-Bennett Health Reform Plan* (Washington, DC: Center for Budget and Policy Priorities, September 24, 2008).

17. Ron Wyden and Robert Bennett, "How We Can Achieve Bipartisan Health Reform," *Washington Post,* August 5, 2009.

18. Wyden interview.

3. POLITICAL WILL I—PRELUDE TO A HEALTH REFORM CAMPAIGN

1. Federal News Service, "The Democratic Debate," *New York Times,* November 15, 2007; available at http://www.nytimes.com/2007/11/15/us/politics/15debate-transcript.html?_r=1. A transcript is also available at http://transcripts.cnn.com/TRANSCRIPTS/0711/15/se.02.html.

2. Richard Deem (senior vice president for advocacy, American Medical Association) in an interview with the author, May 12, 2010.

3. Johnson and Broder, *The System,* 204–10 (see introd., n. 1).

4. Chip Kahn (president, Federation of American Hospitals) in an interview with the author, March 4, 2010.

5. Karen Ignagni (president and CEO, America's Health Insurance Plans) in an interview with the author, May 21, 2010.

6. Ignagni is quoted in "Comments at White House Health Care Forum," RealClearPolitics, March 5, 2009; available at http://www.realclearpolitics.com/articles/2009/03/comments_at_white_house_health.html.

7. Rachel Nuzum, *Policy Points: The Path to a High Performance U.S. Health System* (New York: Commonwealth Fund, March 2009).

8. Richard Kirsch, "What Progressives Did Right to Win Healthcare," *The Nation,* August 9, 2010, http://www.thenation.com/article/153947/what-progressives-did-right-win-healthcare.

9. Jacob Hacker, *Health Care for America: A Proposal for Guaranteed Affordable Health Care for All Americans Building on Medicare and Employment-Based Insurance* (Washington, DC: Economic Policy Institute, January 2007); available at http://www.sharedprosperity.org/bp180/bp180.pdf.

10. Kirsch, "What Progressives Did Right."

11. "Harry and Louise Return, with a New Message," *New York Times,* July 16, 2008.

12. Author's notes, July 31, 2008.

13. Howard Baker, Tom Daschle, and Bob Dole, *Crossing Our Lines: Working Together to Reform the U.S. Health System,* report of the Leaders' Project on the State of American Health Care (Washington, DC: Bipartisan Policy Center, June 2009).

14. Paul Krugman, "Edwards Gets It Right," *New York Times,* February 9, 2007.

15. David Plouffe, *The Audacity to Win: The Inside Story and Lessons of Barack Obama's Historic Victory* (Viking: New York, 2009), 75.

16. Obama campaign statement, May 2008, also submitted to "Affordable Health Care for All Americans," *Journal of the American Medical Association* 300, no. 16 (October 22, 2008): 1927–28, doi:10.1001/jama.2008.515.

17. Kevin Sack, "Health Plan from Obama Spurs Debate," *New York Times*, July 23, 2008.

18. "Obama Flip-Flops on Requiring People to Buy Health Care," Politi-Fact.com, *St. Petersburg Times*, July 20, 2009, http://www.politifact.com/truth -o-meter/statements/2009/jul/20/barack-obama/obama-flip-flops-requiring -people-buy-health-care/.

19. Kenneth Vogel, "HRC: 'Shame on You, Barack Obama,'" *Politico*, February 23, 2008.

20. Tom Daschle, *Getting It Done: How Obama and Congress Finally Broke the Stalemate to Make Way for Health Care Reform* (New York: St. Martin's Press, 2010), 102.

21. Jon LaPook, "My Interview with President Obama," CBS News, July 16, 2009, http://www.cbsnews.com/stories/2009/07/16/health/cbsdoc/main5166421 .shtml.

22. White House and campaign officials in interviews with the author conducted between March and May 2009 in Washington DC.

23. Joint Committee on Taxation, "Tax Expenditures for Health Care," report submitted to the Senate Committee on Finance, JCX-66-08, July 30, 2008.

24. *Health Benefits in the Tax Code: The Right Incentives, Hearing Before the Senate Committee on Finance*, 110th Cong. (July 31, 2008) (statement by Katherine Baicker, professor of health economics, Harvard School of Public Health), http://finance.senate.gov/imo/media/doc/073108kbtest.pdf

25. Kaiser Family Foundation/Harvard School of Public Health, *The Public's Health Care Agenda for the New President and Congress* (n.p.: January 2009), http://www.kff.org/kaiserpolls/upload/7854.pdf.

4. POLITICAL WILL II—A HEALTH REFORM CAMPAIGN

1. Quotations are from *Transcript: Prepare to Launch: Health Reform Summer, Plenary Session 3*, U.S. Senate HELP Committee memo (July 1, 2008), 1–2.

2. Baucus, *Call to Action* (see chap. 1, n. 26).

3. Johnson and Broder, *The System*, 455 (see introd., n. 1).

4. House staff in interviews with the author, conducted April–May 2010.

5. White House, *Fiscal Responsibility Summit (February 23, 2009)*, report of proceedings issued March 20, 2009; available at http://www.whitehouse.gov/ assets/blog/Fiscal_Responsibility_Summit_Report.pdf.

6. White House, "Remarks by the President on Reforming the Health Care System to Reduce Costs," news release, May 11, 2009, http://www.whitehouse

.gov/the_press_office/Remarks-by-the-President-on-Reforming-the-Health
-Care-System-to-Reduce-Costs/.

7. David Kirkpatrick, "White House Affirms Deal on Drug Cost," *New York Times,* August 5, 2010.

8. Drew Armstrong, "Insurers Gave U.S. Chamber $86 Million Used to Oppose Obama's Health Law," *Bloomberg,* November 17, 2010, http://www .bloomberg.com/news/2010-11-17/insurers-gave-u-s-chamber-86-million -used-to-oppose-obama-s-health-law.html.

9. Frank I. Luntz, *The Language of Healthcare 2009,* accessed May 20, 2010, http://wonkroom.thinkprogress.org/wp-content/uploads/2009/05/frank -luntz-the-language-of-healthcare-20091.pdf.

10. Carrie Budoff Brown, "Orrin Hatch Quits Health Care Talks," *Politico,* July 22, 2009, http://www.politico.com/news/stories/0709/25268.html.

11. "Transcript: Sens. Dodd, Grassley on 'FNS,'" *Fox News Sunday,* interview with Senators Dodd and Grassley on *Fox New Sunday with Chris Wallace,* June 14, 2009, http://www.foxnews.com/story/0,2933,526301,00.html.

12. "Grassley Backtracks on Individual Mandate," Live Pulse, *Politico,* September 22, 2009, http://www.politico.com/livepulse/0909/Grassley_backtracks _on_individual_mandate.html.

13. Ben Smith, "Health Reform Foes Plan Obama's 'Waterloo,'" *Politico,* http://www.politico.com/blogs/bensmith/0709/Health_reform_foes_plan_ Obamas_Waterloo.html.

14. David M. Drucker and Emily Pierce, "Reid Loses Patience on Health Bill," *Roll Call,* July 8, 2009.

15. The text of the speech can be found in "Obama's Health Care Speech to Congress," *New York Times,* September 9, 2009, http://www.nytimes.com/ 2009/09/10/us/politics/10obama.text.html.

16. Congressional Budget Office, Letter to Senator Orrin Hatch, October 9, 2009, http://www.cbo.gov/ftpdocs/106xx/doc10641/10-09-Tort_Reform.pdf.

17. Elisabeth Kübler-Ross, *On Death and Dying* (London: Routledge, 1973).

18. Sheryl Gay Stolberg et al., "The Long Road Back," *New York Times,* March 21, 2010.

19. White House, "Putting Americans in Control of Their Health Care," accessed July 10, 2010, http://www.whitehouse.gov/health-care-meeting/proposal.

20. Sheryl Gay Stolberg, "Senate Parliamentarian in Role as Health Bill Referee," *New York Times,* March 13, 2010.

21. Michael Shear, "Obama: This Is What Change Looks Like," *Washington Post,* March 22, 2010.

5. TITLE I—THE THREE-LEGGED STOOL

1. PriceWaterhouseCoopers, *The Impact of Lifetime Benefit Caps,* March 2009, http://www.hemophilia.org/docs/LifetimeLimitsReport.pdf.

2. Congressional Budget Office, Letter to Pelosi (see chap. 1, n. 11).

3. Deborah Stone, "The Struggle for the Soul of Health Insurance," *Jour-*

nal of Health Policy, Politics and Law 18, no. 2 (1993): 287–317; doi:10.1215/03616878-18-2-287.

4. U.S. General Accounting Office, Health, Education, and Human Services Division, "Private Health Insurance: Millions Relying on Individual Market Face Cost and Coverage Trade-Offs," report to the Senate Committee on Labor and Human Resources (Washington, DC: U.S. Government Printing Office, November 1996), 71; available at http://www.gao.gov/archive/1997/he97008.pdf; Geoffrey C. Sandler, "New York Individual Market Rules: The Nuts and Bolts of Rating in the Individual Market," presentation at the National Health Policy Forum, Washington, DC, February 19, 2009, slide 4. Available at: http://www.nhpf.org/library/handouts/Sandler.slides_02-19-09.pdf.

5. Julie Rovner, "Republicans Spurn Once-Favored Health Mandate," NPR, February 15, 2010, http://www.npr.org/templates/story/story.php?storyId=123670612.

6. Stuart M. Butler, "Using Tax Credits to Create an Affordable Health System," Heritage Foundation, July 20, 1990, http://www.heritage.org/research/reports/1990/07/using-tax-credits-to-create-an-affordable-health-system.

7. For an overview of constitutional arguments, see Mark A. Hall, "The Constitutionality of Mandates to Purchase Health Insurance," O'Neill Institute Papers, paper 21 (Washington, DC: Georgetown University, 2009), http://scholarship.law.georgetown.edu/ois_papers/21.

8. For a contrary view, see David Rivkin and Lee Casey, "Mandatory Insurance Is Unconstitutional," Wall Street Journal, September 18, 2009.

9. Massachusetts Department of Revenue, "Individual Mandate: 2008 Preliminary Data Analysis," December 2009, http://www.mass.gov/Ador/docs/dor/News/PressReleases/2009/2008_Health_Care_Report.pdf.

10. Commonwealth of Massachusetts, Division of Health Care Finance and Policy, "Employers Who Had Fifty or More Employees Using MassHealth, Commonwealth Care, or the Health Safety Net in State FY09," June 2010, http://www.mass.gov/Eeohhs2/docs/dhcfp/r/pubs/10/50_plus_employers_final_06-28-10.pdf.

11. Gretchen Livingston, Hispanics, Health Insurance, and Health Care Access (Washington, DC: Pew Hispanic Center, September 25, 2009); available at http://pewhispanic.org/files/reports/113.pdf.

12. Karen Davis, "Expanding Medicare and Employer Plans to Achieve Universal Health Insurance," Journal of the American Medical Association 265, no. 19 (May 15, 1991): 2525–28, doi:10.1001/jama.1991.0346019010.

13. Helen Halpin and Peter Harbage, "The Origins and Demise of the Public Option," Health Affairs 29, no. 6 (June 2010): 1117–25, doi:10.1377/hlthaff.2010.0363.

14. Hacker, Health Care for America (see chap. 3, n. 9).

15. John Shiels and Randy Haught, "The Cost and Coverage Impacts of a Public Plan: Alternative Design Options," Staff Working Paper #4 (Falls Church, VA: The Lewin Group, April 6, 2009); available at http://www.lewin

.com/content/publications/LewinCostandCoverageImpactsofPublicPlan-Alternative%20DesignOptions.pdf.

16. Steffie Woolhandler, Terry Campbell, and David U. Himmelstein, "Costs of Health Care Administration in the United States and Canada," *New England Journal of Medicine* 349, no. 8 (2003): 768–75.

17. H. J. Aaron, "The Cost of Health Care Administration in the United States and Canada—Questionable Answers to a Questionable Question," *New England Journal of Medicine* 349, no. 8 (2003): 801–3.

18. Sarah Kershaw, "Mental Health Experts Applaud Focus on Parity," *New York Times*, March 29, 2010.

19. Bob Curley, "Healthcare Reform Law Gives Big Boost to Addiction Treatment and Prevention," *Join Together*, April 9, 2010, http://www.jointogether.org/news/features/2010/healthcare-reform-law-gives.html.

20. Sara R. Collins, Sheila D. Rustgi, and Michelle M. Doty, "Realizing Health Reform's Potential: Women and the Affordable Care Act of 2010," issue brief, The Commonwealth Fund, July 30, 2010.

6. TITLE II—MEDICAID, CHIP, AND THE GOVERNORS

1. Andrea Sisko et al., "National Health Spending Projections: The Estimated Impact of Reform through 2019," *Health Affairs* 29, no. 10, (September 2010): 5, http://content.healthaffairs.org/cgi/reprint/hlthaff.2010.0788v1, doi:10.1377/hlthaff.2010.0788.

2. CBO estimate of the number of Americans who will enroll in Medicaid because of the ACA was 15–16 million. Its final analysis on March 20, 2010, pegged the number at 16 million. See the March 20, 2010, CBO letter to House Speaker Nancy Pelosi, http://cbo.gov/ftpdocs/113xx/doc11379/AmendRecon Prop.pdf.

3. The definitive work on Medicare's development includes only a handful of references to Medicaid. See Theodore Marmor, *The Politics of Medicare*, 2nd ed. (New York: Aldine De Gruyter, 2000).

4. All data are from the Kaiser Family Foundation's Medicaid/CHIP resources, accessed June 7, 2010, http://www.kff.org/medicaid/index.cfm.

5. Stephen Zuckerman, Aimee F. Williams, and Karen E. Stockley, "Trends in Medicaid Physician Fees, 2003–2008," *Health Affairs* 28, no. 3 (May 2009): w510–w519, doi:10.1377/hlthaff.28.3.w510.

6. Baucus, *Call to Action* (see chap. 1, n. 26), 23.

7. Letter from the National Governors Association to Senators Max Baucus and Charles Grassley, dated July 20, 2009, available at http://www.nga.org/portal/site/nga/menuitem.cb6e7818b34088d18a27811050101oa0/?vgnextoid=9ab46d1d40992210VgnVCM1000005e00100aRCRD.

8. John Holahan and Ireen Headen, *Medicaid Coverage and Spending in Health Reform* (Washington, DC: Kaiser Commission on Medicaid and the Uninsured, May 2010).

7. TITLE III—MEDICAL CARE, MEDICARE, AND THE COST CURVE

1. White House, "Remarks by the President" (see chap. 4, n. 6).

2. Henry Aaron, "Waste, We Know You Are Out There," *New England Journal of Medicine* 359 no. 18 (October 30, 2008), 1865–67, doi:10.1056/NEJM po807204.

3. For only two examples, see Ellen-Marie Whelan and Sonia Sekhar, "Costly and Dangerous Treatments Weigh Down Health Care," Center for American Progress, July 9, 2009, http://www.americanprogress.org/issues/2009/07/costly _and_dangerous.html; and http://seekingalpha.com/article/170346-healthcare -waste-spending-pegged-at-700-billion-thomson-reuters-report.

4. Kaiser Family Foundation, *Medicare at a Glance* (fact sheet) (Washington, DC, January 2010), http://www.kff.org/medicare/upload/1066-12.pdf.

5. Congressional Budget Office, Letter to Pelosi (see chap. 1, n. 11).

6. Centers for Medicare and Medicaid Services, Office of the Actuary, "Estimated Financial Effects of the 'Patient Protection and Affordable Care Act,' as Amended," memorandum from Richard S. Foster, Chief Actuary, April 22, 2010; available at http://www.cms.gov/ActuarialStudies/Downloads/ PPACA_2010-04-22.pdf.

7. Paul N. Van de Water, "Understanding the CMS Actuary's Report on Health Reform" (Washington, DC: Center on Budget and Policy Priorities, May 17, 2010).

8. Jon Gabel, "Congress' Health Care Numbers Don't Add Up," *New York Times,* August 25, 2009.

9. See the Emtala.com website at http://www.emtala.com/.

10. MedPAC, *Report to the Congress: Medicare Payment Policy* (Washington, DC: U.S. Government Printing Office, March 2010), 7.

11. Ibid., 202.

12. Ibid., 203.

13. Visiting Nurse Associations of America, "Healthcare Reform Passage Is a Mixed-Bag for Nonprofit Home Health and Hospice," news release, March 24, 2010, http://vnaa.org/vnaa/g/?h=/html/PR_VNAA_healthcare_reform_3 .24.10.html.

14. Kaiser Family Foundation, *Medicare Advantage* (fact sheet) (Washington, DC: November 2009).

15. MedPAC, *Report to the Congress,* 260.

16. Brian Bandell, "Obama Targets Massive Cuts for Florida's Largest HMO Program," *South Florida Business Journal,* November 17, 2008, http://www .bizjournals.com/southflorida/stories/2008/11/17/story5.html.

17. Baucus, *Call to Action* (see chap. 1, n. 26).

18. MedPAC, *Report to the Congress,* 283–304.

19. Blumenthal and Morone, *Heart of Power* (see chap. 1, n. 2), 198–201.

20. *Medicare's Physician Payment Rates and the Sustainable Growth Rate,* Hearings Before the Subcommittee on Health, Committee on Energy and Commerce, U.S. House of Representatives, 109th Cong. (July 25, 2006) (statement of Donald B. Marron, Acting Director, Congressional Budget Office).

21. Paul Van de Water and James Horney, *Health Reform Will Reduce the Deficit* (Washington, DC: Center for Budget and Policy Priorities, March 25, 2010).

22. Congressional Budget Office, Letter to Senator Mike Crapo, August 24, 2010, http://www.cbo.gov/doc.cfm?index=11820.

23. Baucus, *Call to Action* (see chap. 1, n. 26), 46–48.

24. David Glendinning, "House Passes Health Reform Bill, Debate Moves to Senate," *American Medical News*, November 9, 2009, http://www.ama-assn.org/amednews/2009/11/09/gvl11109.htm.

25. Malcolm Sparrow, "Fraud in the U.S. Health-Care System: Exposing the Vulnerabilities of Automated Payments Systems," *Social Research* 75, no. 4 (Winter 2008), 1151–80.

26. See Debra A. McCurdy, "Medicare 'Trigger' Provision Suspended," January 12, 2009, http://www.healthindustrywashingtonwatch.com/2009/01/articles/legislative-developments/medicare-trigger-provision-suspended/.

27. Tom Daschle, *Critical: What We Can Do about the Health Care Crisis* (New York: St. Martin's Press, 2008), 169.

28. Congressional Budget Office, *Budget Options, Volume 1* (see chap. 1, n. 30), 206.

29. Peter Orszag and Ezekiel Emanuel, "Health Care Reform and Cost Control," *New England Journal of Medicine*, June 16, 2010, http://healthpolicyandreform.nejm.org/?p=3564, doi:10.1056/NEJMp1006571.

30. See "Cornyn Introduces the Health Care Bureaucrats Elimination Act," news release on the website of Senator John Cornyn, July 27, 2010, http://cornyn.senate.gov/public/index.cfm?p=NewsReleases&ContentRecord_id=a79c42ff-ac9b-4e0b-ada7-cd6aa939b3eb&ContentType_id=5b0f9315-c5c5-44f5-854b-3b51718a5c2b&b94acc28-404a-4fc6-b143-a9e15bf92da4&19760459-7424-403a-8038-666e11ddb515&f6c645c7-9e4a-4947-8464-a94cacb4ca65&Group_id=3f81a3bd-e4d7-4d7e-8d6f-25e9b718b7aa.

8. TITLE IV—MONEY, MAMMOGRAMS, AND MENUS

1. Louise Russell, *Is Prevention Better Than Cure?* (Washington, DC: Brookings Institution, 1986).

2. Joshua T. Cohen, Peter J. Neumann, and Milton C. Weinstein, "Does Preventive Care Save Money? Health Economics and the Presidential Candidates," *New England Journal of Medicine* 358, no. 7 (February 14, 2008), 661–63, doi:10.1056/NEJMp0708558.

3. Robert Pear, "New Health Initiatives Put Spotlight on Prevention," *New York Times*, April 4, 2010.

4. Kenneth E. Thorpe, "Prevention Is Not Just Disease Detection," *National Journal*, Expert Blogs: Health Care, May 12, 2010, http://healthcare.nationaljournal.com/2010/05/wisest-use-of-prevention-and-w.php#1583043.

5. Trust for America's Health, *Blueprint for a Healthier America: Modernizing the Federal Health System to Focus on Prevention and Prepared-*

ness (Washington, DC: October 2008), http://healthyamericans.org/report/55/blueprint-for-healthier-america.

6. "Screening for Breast Cancer: U.S. Preventive Services Task Force Recommendation Statement," *Annals of Internal Medicine* 151 (November 17, 2009): 716–26, http://www.annals.org/content/151/10/716.full.

7. Gina Kolata, "Mammogram Debate Took Group by Surprise," *New York Times*, November 20, 2009.

8. Steven A. Burd, "How Safeway Is Cutting Health Care Costs," *Wall Street Journal*, June 12, 2009.

9. "An Update on Health Care Reform," e-newsletter on the website of Senator Benjamin L. Cardin, August, 31, 2009, http://cardin.senate.gov/news/enews/aug31.cfm.

10. Quoted in "Michael Warren, "Doctor's Orders," *National Review Online*, July 22, 2009, reprinted on the website of Senator John Barrasso, http://barrasso.senate.gov/public/index.cfm?FuseAction=PressOffice.Opinion Editorials&ContentRecord_id=a315664d-9d6c-20ff-2e5b-cebdcc88c38d &Region_id=&Issue_id.

11. Author's notes.

12. David S. Hilzenrath, "Misleading Claims about Safeway Wellness Incentives Shape Health Care Bill," *Washington Post*, January 17, 2010.

13. Compare, for example, Jaan Sidirov, "Why Wellness Incentives Belong in the Workplace," *Health Affairs Blog*, January 19, 2010, http://healthaffairs .org/blog/2010/01/19/why-wellness-incentives-belong-in-the-workplace/, and Alan Balch, "Workplace Wellness Programs: The Real Issues," *Health Affairs Blog*, January 28, 2010, http://healthaffairs.org/blog/2010/01/28/workplace -wellness-programs-the-real-issues/.

14. Julie Rovner, "Patient Advocates Fear Bias in Wellness Incentives," *National Public Radio*, October 7, 2009.

9. TITLE V—WHO WILL PROVIDE THE CARE?

1. U.S. Department of Health and Human Services, Health Resources and Services Administration, National Center for Health Workforce Analysis, "The Massachusetts Health Workforce: Highlights from the Health Workforce Profile," accessed June 21, 2010, http://bhpr.hrsa.gov/healthworkforce/reports/statesummaries/massachusetts.htm.

2. MedPAC's website is at http://www.medpac.gov/.

3. Association of Academic Health Centers, *Out of Order, Out of Time: The State of the Nation's Health Workforce* (Washington, DC: 2008): iii–vi.

4. Association of American Medical Colleges, Center for Workforce Studies, "Recent Studies and Reports on Physician Shortages in the U.S." (Washington, DC: November 2009), https://www.aamc.org/download/100598/data/recentworkforcestudiesnov09.pdf.

5. Association of American Medical Colleges, Center for Workforce Studies, "The Complexities of Physician Supply and Demand: Projections through 2025"

(Washington, DC: November 2008), 29, http://services.aamc.org/publications/showfile.cfm?file=version122.pdf.

6. Jesse Smith, "Responding to Physician Shortage," *Physician's News Digest,* April 2006, http://www.physiciansnews.com/cover/406.html.

7. *Primary Care Access Reform: Community Health Centers and the National Health Service Corps, Hearing Before the Senate Committee on Health, Education, Labor and Pensions,* 111th Cong. (April 30, 2009) (statement by Dr. Fitzhugh Mullan, Murdock Head Professor of Medicine and Health Policy, George Washington University), http://help.senate.gov/imo/media/doc/Mullan.pdf.

8. David Goodman and Elliott Fisher, "Physician Workforce Crisis? Wrong Diagnosis, Wrong Prescription," *New England Journal of Medicine* 358, no. 16 (April 17, 2008): 1658–61, doi:10.1056/NEJMp0800319.

9. Eli Y. Adashi, H. Jack Geiger, and Michael D. Fine, "Health Care Reform and Primary Care—The Growing Importance of the Community Health Center," *New England Journal of Medicine* 362, no. 22 (June 3, 2010): 2047–50, doi:10.1056/NEJMp1003729.

10. *Primary Care Access Reform* (Mullan), 8.

10. TITLE VI—THE STEW

1. National Health Care Anti-Fraud Association, "The Problem of Health Care Fraud," accessed June 23, 2010, http://www.nhcaa.org/eweb/DynamicPage.aspx?webcode=anti_fraud_resource_centr&wpscode=TheProblemOfHCFraud.

2. Quoted in John Buntin, "Fraud Fighter," *Governing,* June 2010, 42.

3. Sparrow, "Fraud in U.S. Health-Care System" (see chap. 7, n. 25).

4. U.S. Department of Justice, "Eli Lilly and Company Agrees to Pay $1.415 Billion to Resolve Allegations of Off-Label Promotion of Zyprexa," news release, January 15, 2009.

5. *Combating Fraud, Waste, and Abuse in Medicare and Medicaid, Hearing Before the U.S. Senate Special Committee on Aging,* 111th Cong. (May 6, 2009) (statement by Daniel Levinson, HHS Inspector General), http://oig.hhs.gov/testimony/docs/2009/05062009_testimony_aging.pdf.

6. See "Health Care Fraud and Abuse Control Program Report," the webpage of the U.S. Department of Health and Human Services, Office of Inspector General, http://www.oig.hhs.gov/publications/hcfac.asp.

7. Interview with the author, May 6, 2009.

8. U.S. Department of Justice, "Attorney General Holder and HHS Secretary Sebelius Announce New Interagency Health Care Fraud Prevention and Enforcement Action Team," news release, May 20, 2009, http://www.hhs.gov/news/press/2009pres/05/20090520a.html.

9. Baucus, *Call to Action* (see chap. 1, n. 26), 67.

10. Congressional Budget Office, *Budget Options, Volume 1* (see chap. 1, n. 30), 210.

11. John Iglehart, "The ACA's New Weapon against Health Care Fraud,"

New England Journal of Medicine 363, no. 4 (July 22, 2010): 304–6, doi:10.1056/NEJMp1007088.

12. "Disclosure of Drug Company Payments to Doctors," a page on the website of Senator Chuck Grassley, accessed June 25, 2010, http://grassley.senate.gov/about/Disclosure-of-Drug-Company-Payments-to-Doctors.cfm.

13. Alex Berenson and Reed Abelson, "Weighing the Costs of a CT Scan's Look inside the Heart," *New York Times*, June 29, 2008.

14. Quoted in Theodore R. Marmor, *The Politics of Medicare*, 2nd ed. (New York: Aline de Gruyter, 2000), 3.

15. The website of the Cochrane Collaboration is at http://www.cochrane.org/.

16. For an excellent history of health services research, see chapter 3 of Fox, *Science and Governance* (see chap. 1, n. 17).

17. Fox, chapter 4, and "Consumer Reports Best Buy Drugs," Consumer Reports Health.org, accessed June 24, 2010, http://www.consumerreports.org/health/best-buy-drugs/index.htm.

18. Gina Kolata, "New Therapies Pose Quandary for Medicare," *New York Times*, August 17, 2003.

19. Gail Wilensky, "Developing a Center for Comparative Effectiveness Information," *Health Affairs* 25, no. 6 (November 2006): w572–w585, doi:10.1377/hlthaff.25.w572.

20. Billy Beane, Newt Gingrich, and John Kerry, "How to Take American Health Care from Worst to First," *New York Times*, October 24, 2008.

21. Kavita Patel, "Health Reform's Tortuous Route to the Patient-Centered Outcomes Research Institute," *Health Affairs* 29, no. 10 (October 2010): 1778–82, doi:10.1377/hlthaff.2010.0874.

22. U.S. Department of Health and Human Services, Federal Coordinating Council for Comparative Effectiveness Research, *Report to the President and Congress* (Washington, DC: U.S. Government Printing Office, June 30, 2009).

23. Alicia Mundy, "Drug Makers Fight Stimulus Provision," *Wall Street Journal*, February 11, 2009.

24. Johnson and Broder, *The System*, 271–72 (see introd., n. 1).

25. Betsy McCaughey, "Ruin Your Health with the Obama Stimulus Plan," *Bloomberg*, February 9, 2009, http://www.bloomberg.com/apps/news?pid=newsarchive&refer=columnist_mccaughey&sid=aLzfDxfbwhzs.

26. Earl Blumenauer, "My Near Death Panel Experience," *New York Times*, November 14, 2009.

27. Jason Hancock, "Grassley: Government Shouldn't 'Decide When to Pull the Plug on Grandma,'" *Iowa Independent*, August 12, 2009, http://iowaindependent.com/18456/grassley-government-shouldnt-decide-when-to-pull-the-plug-on-grandma.

28. Harry P. Selker and Alastair J.J. Wood, "Industry Influence on Comparative-Effectiveness Research Funded through Health Care Reform," *New England Journal of Medicine* 361, no. 27 (December 31, 2009): 2595–97, doi:10.1056/NEJMp0910747.

29. Patel, "Health Reform's Tortuous Route," 1781.

30. The website of the National Center on Elder Abuse is http://www.ncea .aoa.gov/ncearoot/Main_Site/index.aspx.

31. MetLife Mature Market Institute, the National Committee for the Prevention of Elder Abuse, and the Center for Gerontology at Virginia Polytechnic Institute and State University, *Broken Trust: Elders, Families and Finances* (Westport, CT: March 2009), available at http://www.metlife.com/assets/cao/ mmi/publications/studies/mmi-study-broken-trust-elders-family-finances.pdf.

32. John Eligon, "Brooke Astor's Son Guilty in Scheme to Defraud Her," *New York Times,* October 8, 2009.

33. Mary Manning, "Alleged Scammers Arrested in 'Neighborhood Assistance' Scheme," *Las Vegas Sun,* April 8, 2009.

34. Hillary Rodham Clinton and Barack Obama, "Making Patient Safety the Centerpiece of Medical Liability Reform," *New England Journal of Medicine* 354, no. 21 (May 25, 2006), 2205–8, doi:10.1056/NEJMp068100.

35. S. 1337: Fair and Reliable Medical Justice Act, 109th Cong., Congressional Research Service Summary, accessed September 9, 2010, http://www .govtrack.us/congress/bill.xpd?bill=s109-1337&tab=summary.

36. Institute of Medicine, *To Err Is Human* (see chap. 1, n. 24).

37. Congressional Budget Office, *Budget Options, Volume 1* (see chap. 1, n. 30), 21–22.

38. Congressional Budget Office, Letter to Senator Orrin G. Hatch (see chap. 4, n. 16).

39. "Obama's Health Care Speech" (see chap. 4, n. 15).

40. U.S. Department of Health and Human Services, "The HHS Patient Safety and Medical Liability Initiative," news release, September 9, 2009, http:// www.hhs.gov/news/press/2010pres/06/patient_safety_and_medical_liability _initiative.html.

11. TITLE VII—BIOSIMILAR BIOLOGICAL PRODUCTS

1. Federal Trade Commission, "Emerging Health Care Issues: Follow-on Biologic Drug Competition" (Washington, DC: U.S. Government Printing Office, June 2009), i, http://www.ftc.gov/os/2009/06/P083901biologicsreport.pdf

2. IMS Health, "IMS Health Reports Global Biotech Sales Grew 12.5 Percent in 2007, Exceeding $75 Billion," news release, June 17, 2008, http:// www.imshealth.com/portal/site/imshealth/menuitem.a46c6d4df3db4b3d88f6 11019418c22a/?vgnextoid=bba69e392879a110VgnVCM100000ed152ca2RCRD &vgnextfmt=default/; Anthony So and Samuel Katz, "Biologics Boondoggle," *New York Times,* March 7, 2010.

3. Gina Kolata, "Costly Cancer Drug Offers Hope, but Also a Dilemma," *New York Times,* July 6, 2008.

4. James Greenwood, "The Biotechnology Industry Organization," *Chain Drug Review,* January 5, 2009.

5. Alfred B. Engelberg, Aaron S. Kesselheim, and Jerry Avorn, "Balanc-

ing Innovation, Access, and Profits—Market Exclusivity for Biologics," *New England Journal of Medicine* 361, no. 20 (November 12, 2009), 1917–19, doi: 10.1056/NEJMp0908496.

6. Federal Trade Commission, "Emerging Health Care Issues," v.

7. Emily Walker, "Obama Pushes for Change on Biologics in Healthcare Bill," *Medpage Today*, January 15, 2010.

8. Julie Donnelly, "Biotech, Pharma Look at What's Next for Biosimilars," *Mass High Tech*, November 10, 2010.

9. Ibid.

10. Alfred Engelberg and Aaron Kesselheim, Authors' Reply, *New England Journal of Medicine* 362, no. 7 (February 18, 2010), 661–62.

11. E. E. Schattschneider, *The Semisovereign People: A Realist's View of Democracy in America* (Belmont, CA: Wadsworth, 1975).

12. TITLE VIII—CLASS ACT

1. U.S. Senate Democratic Policy Committee, *The Patient Protection and Affordable Care Act: Section by Section Analysis*, accessed June 29, 2010, http://dpc.senate.gov/healthreformbill/healthbill96.pdf.

2. 149 Cong. Rec. S12,394-5 (daily ed. Dec. 4, 2009).

3. Congressional Budget Office, Letter to Senator Tom Harkin, November 25, 2009, 5, http://www.cbo.gov/doc.cfm?index=10823.

4. Centers for Medicare and Medicaid Services, Office of the Actuary, "Estimated Financial Effects of the 'Patient Protection and Affordable Care Act of 2009,' as Proposed by the Senate Majority Leader on November 18, 2009," memorandum from Richard S. Foster, Chief Actuary, December 10, 2009; available at http://src.senate.gov/files/OACTMemorandumonFinancialImpact ofPPAA%28HR3590%29%2812-10-09%29.pdf.

5. Ibid., 13–14.

6. From Title VIII: Section 3203 (b)(1)(B) and Section 3208 (c).

7. Daniel G. Fish, "CLASS Act: Health Care Reform Law Includes Custodial Care Coverage," *New York Law Journal*, May 21, 2010.

13. TITLE IX—PAYING FOR THE ACA (OR ABOUT HALF OF IT)

1. The website of the Joint Committee on Taxation is http://www.jct.gov/.

2. Congressional Budget Office, Letter to Nancy Pelosi, Speaker of the U.S. House of Representatives, March 20, 2010, http://cbo.gov/ftpdocs/113xx/doc11379/AmendReconProp.pdf.

3. Joint Committee on Taxation, *Estimated Revenue Effects of the Amendment in the Nature of a Substitute to H.R. 4872, the "Reconciliation Act of 2010," as Amended, in Combination with the Revenue Effects of H.R. 3590, The "Patient Protection and Affordable Care Act ('PPACA')," as Passed by the Senate, and Scheduled for Consideration by the House Committee on Rules on March 20, 2010* (Washington, DC: U.S. Government Printing Office), http://www.jct.gov/publications.html?func=startdown&id=3672.

4. Boards of Trustees of the Federal Hospital Insurance Program and Federal Supplementary Medical Insurance Trust Funds, *2010 Annual Report,* submitted to the Congress on August 5, 2010, http://www.cms.gov/ReportsTrust Funds/downloads/tr2010.pdf.

5. Kaiser Family Foundation and Health Research & Educational Trust, Exhibit 10.1: Percentage of Covered Workers in Partially or Completely Self-Funded Plans, by Firm Size, 1999–2010, in *Employer Health Benefits 2010 Annual Survey* (Menlo Park, CA: Henry J. Kaiser Family Foundation, September 2010), 155, http://ehbs.kff.org/pdf/2010/8085.pdf.

6. Elise Gould and Alexandra Minicozzi, "Who Loses If We Limit the Tax Exclusion for Health Insurance?" *Viewpoints: Tax Notes,* March 9, 2009, http://www.epi.org/publications/entry/who_loses_if_we_limit_the_tax_exclusion _for_health_insurance/.

7. Baucus, *Call to Action* (see chap. 1, n. 26), 80–82.

8. Steven Mufson, "An Elixir for Health Reform? Lawmakers Offer 'Black Liquor,'" *Washington Post,* November 8, 2009.

9. Hewitt Associates, "The Effects of Health Care Reform on Flexible Spending Accounts," accessed September 13, 2010, http://www.hewittassociates.com/ Intl/NA/en-US/KnowledgeCenter/ArticlesReports/ArticleDetail.aspx?cid =8400.

10. The website of Save Flexible Spending Plans is http://www.savemyflex plan.org/.

11. The website of the Employers Council on Flexible Compensation is http://www.ecfc.org/.

12. Joint Committee on Taxation, *Technical Explanation of the Revenue Provisions of the "Reconciliation Act of 2010" as Amended, in Combination with the "Patient Protection and Affordable Care Act,"* (Washington, DC: U.S. Government Printing Office, March 21, 2010), http://www.jct.gov/publications .html?func=startdown&id=3673.

13. Steven Greenhouse, "Companies Push to Repeal Provision of Health Law," *New York Times,* March 29, 2010.

14. Mason L. Crocker, "Codification of the Economic Substance Doctrine," *Lexology,* March 23, 2010, http://www.lexology.com/library/detail.aspx?g= 741576cd-33f8-4b4a-9888-29a643182fc5.

15. Deloitte, *Tax Provisions in the Patient Protection and Affordable Care Act,* March 30, 2010, 18.

16. The Indoor Tanning Association maintains a website at http://www .repealtantax.com/.

17. Blake Ellis, "Tanning Salons Burned by Health Bill," *CNN Money.com,* March 24, 2010, http://money.cnn.com/2010/03/24/news/economy/tanning_tax/.

18. David Fisher and William James, "Indoor Tanning—Science, Behavior, and Policy," *New England Journal of Medicine* 363 no. 10. (September 2, 2010), 901–3, doi:10.1056/NEJMp1005999.

19. C. Mosher and S. Danoff-Burg, "Addiction to Indoor Tanning," *Archives of Dermatology* 146, no. 4 (2010): 412–17.

20. Cited in *ThinkExist.com Quotations*, http://thinkexist.com/quotation/ politics_is_very_much_like_taxes-everybody_is/175328.html accessed

14. TITLE X-PLUS—THE MANAGER'S AMENDMENT AND
THE HEALTH CARE EDUCATION AND RECONCILIATION ACT

1. *Hearing on Reforming the Indian Health Care System, Before the Senate Committee on Indian Affairs*, 111th Cong. (June 11, 2009) (statement of Jefferson Keel, First Vice President, National Congress of American Indians).

2. U.S. Senate Committee on Indian Affairs, "Indian Health Care Improvement Reauthorization and Extension Act of 2009, Section-by-Section Summary," October 13, 2009, http://indian.senate.gov/issues/upload/IndianHealth .CareSectionbySection101309.pdf.

CONCLUSION

1. "Enzi Unveils 10 Steps to Transform Health Care in America," news release on website of Senator Mike Enzi, July 12, 2007, http://www.enzi.senate.gov/ public/index.cfm?FuseAction=NewsRoom.NewsReleases&ContentRecord_id= 931a36ce-802a-23ad-4ba2-3147bdd49a59&Region_id=&Issue_id.

2. Carrie Budoff Brown, "Judd Gregg Gives Health Reform a Go," *Politico*, June 2, 2009.

3. Patients' Choice Act, S. 1099, 111th Cong. (May 20, 2009), Sen. Thomas Coburn, sponsor, http://www.govtrack.us/congress/bill.xpd?bill=s111-1099.

4. Social Security Online: History, "Ratio of Social Security Covered Workers to Beneficiaries, Calendar Years 1940–2009," accessed July 6, 2010, http://www.socialsecurity.gov/history/ratios.html.

5. U.S. Census 2000 on www.Allcountries.org, "Table 164: Medicare Enrollees," accessed July 6, 2010, http://www.allcountries.org/uscensus/164_medicare _enrollees.html.

6. Mike Dennison, "Baucus Criticized for Comments about 'Maldistribution of Wealth,'" *Missoulian*, March 31, 2010.

7. James Morone, "Presidents and Health Reform: From Franklin D. Roosevelt to Barack Obama," *Health Affairs* 29, no. 6 (June 2010): 1096–1100, doi:10.1377/hlthaff.2010.0420.

8. John Iglehart, "Historic Passage—Reform at Last," *New England Journal of Medicine* 362 (April 8, 2010): e48, doi:10.1056/NEJMp1003376.

9. Carrie Budoff Brown, "Both Sides Push Health Debate Myths," *Politico*, February 15, 2010.

10. Ibid.

11. William Pewen, "The Health Care Letdown," *New York Times*, March 15, 2010.

12. Richard Wolfe, *Revival: The Struggle for Survival Inside the Obama White House* (New York: Crown, 2010), 70.

13. Robert Blendon et al., "Voters and Health Reform in the 2008 Presi-

dential Election," *New England Journal of Medicine* 359, no 19 (November 6, 2008): 2050–61, doi:10.1056/NEJMsr0807717.

14. Bennett Roth and Alex Knott, "Medical Interests Spent $876 Million on Reform," *Roll Call*, May 3, 2010.

15. Harold Pollack, "The Best-Covered News Story, Ever," *New Republic*, April 1, 2010, http://www.tnr.com/blog/the-treatment/the-best-covered-news-story-ever.

16. Gwendolyn Mink, *The Wages of Motherhood: Inequality in the Welfare State, 1917–1942* (Ithaca, NY: Cornell University Press, 1995), 127.

17. Ira Katznelson, *When Welfare Was White: The Untold History of Racial Inequality in Twentieth Century America* (New York: W.W. Norton, 2005), 43–48.

18. "Imperfect Healthcare Bill Compared to 1935 Social Security Act," *The Best Possible Life* (blog of the Frances Perkins Center), February 3, 2010, http://bestpossiblelife.wordpress.com/2010/02/03/imperfect-healthcare-bill-compared-to-1935-social-security-act/.

19. Blumenthal and Morone, *Heart of Power* (see chap. 1, n. 2), 195–202.

20. Daniel Fox and Howard Markel, "Is History Relevant to Implementing Health Reform?" *Journal of the American Medical Association* 303, no. 17 (May 5, 2010): 1749–50, doi:10.1001/jama.2010.556.

21. Congressional Budget Office, Letter to Pelosi (see chap. 1, n. 11).

22. Douglas Holtz-Eakin and Michael Ramlet, "Health Care Reform Is Likely to Widen Federal Budget Deficits, Not Reduce Them," *Health Affairs* 29, no. 6 (June 2010), 1136–41.

23. David Cutler, Karen Davis, and Kristof Stremikis, *The Impact of Health Reform on Health System Spending* (New York: Commonwealth Fund, May 2010).

24. Jon R. Gabel, "Congress's Health Care Numbers Don't Add Up," *New York Times*, August 25, 2009.

25. Cutler, Davis, and Stremikis, *Impact of Health Reform*, 8.

26. Karen Tumulty and Kate Pickert, "America, the Doctor Will See You Now," *Time*, April 5, 2010.

27. Peter Orszag and Ezekiel Emanuel, "Health Care Reform and Cost Control," *New England Journal of Medicine*, June 16, 2010, http://healthpolicyandreform.nejm.org/?p=3564, doi:10.1056/NEJMp1006571.

28. James Horney and Paul Van de Water, *House-Passed and Senate Health Bills Reduce Deficit, Slow Health Care Costs, and Include Realistic Medicare Savings* (Washington, DC: Center for Budget and Policy Priorities, December 4, 2009).

29. Bruce Vladeck, "Managed Care's Fifteen Minutes of Fame," *Journal of Health Policy, Politics, and Law* 24, no. 5 (October 1999), 1207–12.

30. Sharon Long and Karen Stockley, *Health Reform in Massachusetts: An Update as of Fall 2009* (Washington, DC: Urban Institute, June 2010), http://bluecrossfoundation.org/~/media/Files/Publications/Policy%20Publications/060810MHRS2009ChartbookFINAL.pdf.

31. Quoted in "Early Diagnoses of the New Law," *New York Times*, March 29, 2010.

32. Christopher Jennings, "Implementation and the Legacy of Health Care Reform," *New England Journal of Medicine*, March 31, 2010, http://health policyandreform.nejm.org/?p=3251, doi:10.1056/NEJMp1003709.

33. Fox and Markel, "Is History Relevant?" 1750.

34. F. Scott Fitzgerald, "The Crack-up," *Esquire Magazine*, February 1936.

Health Reform Timeline

June 16, 2008	U.S. Senate Finance Committee Health Reform Summit
November 12, 2008	Release of Senator Max Baucus's Health Reform White Paper
February 17, 2009	President Obama signs the American Recovery and Reinvestment Act
February 26, 2009	President Obama submits FY 2010 budget plan with $630 billion health care reserve
March 5, 2009	White House Health Reform Summit
May 11, 2009	President Obama and health industry leaders announce $2 trillion savings goal
June 17 to July 15, 2009	Senate HELP Committee markup
July 15 to July 17, 2009	House Education and Labor Committee markup
July 16 to July 17, 2009	House Ways and Means Committee markup
July 16 to July 30, 2009	House Energy & Commerce Committee markup
September 9, 2009	President Obama addresses Joint Session of Congress on health reform
September 22 to October 16, 2009	Senate Finance Committee markup
November 7, 2009	House of Representatives approves the Affordable Health Care for America Act
December 24, 2009	Senate approves the Patient Protection and Affordable Care Act

January 19, 2010	Massachusetts special election for the U.S. Senate
February 22, 2010	President Obama releases recommendations for reconciliation amendments
February 25, 2010	President Obama hosts bipartisan health reform summit at Blair House
March 21, 2010	House of Representatives approves the Patient Protection and Affordable Care Act
March 23, 2010	President Obama signs the Patient Protection and Affordable Care Act
March 26, 2010	Senate and House approve the Health Care and Education Reconciliation Act
March 30, 2010	President Obama signs the Health Care and Education Reconciliation Act

Index

Text: 10/13 Aldus
Display: Aldus
Compositor: BookMatters, Berkeley
Indexer: Gerry Van Raavensway
Printer and binder: Thomson-Shore, Inc.